Grammatical Profiles

COMMUNICATION DISORDERS ACROSS LANGUAGES

Series Editors: Dr Nicole Müller, *University College Cork, Ireland* and Dr Martin Ball, *Bangor University, Wales.*

The discipline of communication disorders has made great strides over the last fifty years and more. We now know much more about the nature and causes of breakdowns in speech and language, both in adults and children. We know more about how to classify these breakdowns, how to describe and analyse pathological speech and language, and how to treat communication disorders. Unfortunately, a large proportion of this work is restricted to a small number of European languages; indeed, much of it is on and in English alone.

Research in communication disorders in languages other than English has seen a marked increase in recent years, as has the investigation of such disorders in speakers of more than one language, and communities where bi- and multilingualism is the norm. This series serves to spotlight new and ongoing research in communication disorders across languages. We aim to do this by including studies of communication disorders (including assessment methods and guidelines for intervention) in particular multilingual communities, studies of the manifestations of specific types of disorder in a range of languages (particularly lesser researched languages), and of communication breakdown in bi- and multilingual speakers. Books in the series are used by practitioners, researchers and students, and they address a range of topics, including speech and language disorders in children, literacy, acquired speech and language disorders in adults, fluency, and voice.

All books in this series are externally peer-reviewed.

Full details of all the books in this series and of all our other publications can be found on http://www.multilingual-matters.com, or by writing to Multilingual Matters, St Nicholas House, 31–34 High Street, Bristol BS1 2AW, UK.

COMMUNICATION DISORDERS ACROSS LANGUAGES: 18

Grammatical Profiles

Further Languages of LARSP

Edited by
Martin J. Ball, Paul Fletcher and David Crystal

MULTILINGUAL MATTERS
Bristol • Blue Ridge Summit

DOI https://doi.org/10.21832/BALL4382
Library of Congress Cataloging in Publication Data
A catalog record for this book is available from the Library of Congress.
Names: Ball, Martin J. (Martin John), editor. | Fletcher, Paul - editor. | Crystal, David - editor.
Title: Grammatical Profiles: Further Languages of LARSP/Edited by Martin J. Ball, Paul Fletcher and David Crystal.
Description: Bristol; Blue Ridge Summit: Multilingual Matters, 2019. | Series: Communication Disorders Across Languages: 18 | Includes bibliographical references and index.
Identifiers: LCCN 2019003479| ISBN 9781788924382 (hbk : alk. paper) | ISBN 9781788924405 (epub) | ISBN 9781788924412 (kindle)
Subjects: LCSH: Language disorders in children—Diagnosis. | Grammar, Comparative and general.
Classification: LCC RJ496.L35 G74 2019 | DDC 618.92/855—dc23 LC record available at https://lccn.loc.gov/2019003479

British Library Cataloguing in Publication Data
A catalogue entry for this book is available from the British Library.

ISBN-13: 978-1-78892-438-2 (hbk)

Multilingual Matters
UK: St Nicholas House, 31–34 High Street, Bristol BS1 2AW, UK
USA: NBN, Blue Ridge Summit, PA, USA.

Website: www.multilingual-matters.com
Twitter: Multi_Ling_Mat
Facebook: https://www.facebook.com/multilingualmatters
Blog: www.channelviewpublications.wordpress.com

The policy of Multilingual Matters/Channel View Publications is to use papers that are natural, renewable and recyclable products, made from wood grown in sustainable forests. In the manufacturing process of our books, and to further support our policy, preference is given to printers that have FSC and PEFC Chain of Custody certification. The FSC and/or PEFC logos will appear on those books where full certification has been granted to the printer concerned.

Typeset by Nova Techset Private Limited, Bengaluru and Chennai, India.
Printed and bound in the UK by the CPI Books Group Ltd.
Printed and bound in the US by NBN.

Contents

Contributors

Shanley Allen is Professor of Psycholinguistics and Language Development at the University of Kaiserslautern (Germany). She has published extensively on the acquisition of morphosyntax and narrative by Inuktitut-speaking children, the acquisition of argument realization, the coordination of speech and gesture in motion events across typologically different languages, and code mixing in bilingual preschool children. She is a series editor of the *Trends in Language Acquisition Research* (TiLAR) book series, is on the editorial board of the *Journal of Child Language*, and is Vice President of the International Association for the Study of Child Language (IASCL).

Maryluz Camargo-Mendoza is an Associate Professor in the Department of Human Communication at the National University of Colombia. She received her PhD in Philosophy and Linguistics from the Universidad Autónoma de Madrid (Spain). Her main areas of interest are Clinical Linguistics and Neuromotor Speech Disorders. She is a member of the editorial board of the journal *Revista de Investigación en Logopedia* and an associate member of the European Huntington's Disease Network.

Özlem Cangökçe-Yaşar has a Bachelor's degree in Linguistics and holds her Master's degrees in Linguistics and Speech & Language Therapy and PhD in Speech & Language Therapy. She is an Assistant Professor of Speech and Language Therapy at Ondokuz Mayis University, Turkey. Her research interests include clinical linguistics and language development in cochlear implanted children. Currently, she is Head of the Speech and Language Therapy Department in the Health Sciences Faculty at Ondokuz Mayıs University, Samsun, Turkey.

Ana Castro is Associate Professor at Escola Superior de Saúde do Instituto Politécnico de Setúbal, Portugal, and a researcher in the group LiFE – Formal and Experimental Linguistics of Centro de Linguística da Universidade NOVA de Lisboa. She earned a PhD in Linguistics from the Universidade NOVA de Lisboa and Université Paris 8 (cojoint programme), and she has been a visitor at MIT, the University of Cambridge and

Laboratório de Psicolinguística e Aquisição da Linguagem (LAPAL) da Pontifícia Universidade Católica do Rio de Janeiro (PUC-Rio). Her research focuses on Language Acquisition and Language Impairment, and currently she is working on the development of assessment and intervention tools for children with language impairment.

Ana Isabel Codesido-García is a full-time Associate Professor of General Linguistics at the University of Santiago de Compostela (Galicia-Spain), where she teaches at graduate and postgraduate academic levels. Her doctoral dissertation (2003) dealt with qualitative assessment and linguistic evaluation of SLI in Spain. As a result of two recent periods as a visiting scholar at the Universidad Nacional (Bogotá, Colombia), she has been involved in a research project with Prof. Maryluz Camargo-Mendoza. Nowadays, her main research fields include Clinical Linguistics, Educational Linguistics and Psycholinguistics, considered from a realistic and ecological perspective. She is also particularly interested in Artificial Intelligence applied to the design of linguistic technologies for people with language difficulties.

Kamil Ud Deen is Professor and Chair in the Department of Linguistics at the University of Hawai'i at Manoa. He obtained his Master's degree from Harvard University, and his doctorate from UCLA. His primary interest is in first language acquisition. He has worked on the acquisition of inflection, both morphological and syntactic, including agreement, tense, mood and aspect. More recently, his interests have focused on the acquisition of reference binding of referential expressions, pronouns and other anaphors. He has worked mostly on Thai and Swahili, but recently his research has extended to languages of the Pacific including Tagalog and Samoan. He has published widely, including a 2005 book, *The Acquisition of Swahili*, and is currently a co-editor of Brief Articles of *Language Acquisition: A Journal of Developmental Linguistics*.

Catherine Dench is a speech-language pathologist who has worked with a variety of populations with communication disorders for more than 30 years. Most recently she has served with Kativik Ilisarniliriniq, the school board of the Inuit in Nunavik, Québec, Canada. She has participated in several research and other projects aimed at developing culturally and linguistically appropriate assessment, intervention and educational materials for Inuit children. She has also taught and facilitated courses for Inuit teachers on evaluating and developing speech and oral/written language skills.

Catarina Dôro graduated in Speech and Language Therapy at Escola Superior de Saúde do Instituto Politécnico de Setúbal, Portugal, in 2017. Currently, her clinical practice includes working with children with language disorders and other pathologies.

Paul Fletcher is Emeritus Professor, Speech and Hearing Sciences, University College Cork, Ireland. He previously held professorial positions at the University of Reading and the University of Hong Kong. He has published widely on language development and language impairment in children speaking English, and more recently on Cantonese- and Mandarin-speaking children. He is a past president of the International Association for the Study of Child Language, and an honorary member of the Irish Association of Speech and Language Therapists. He is co-author (with Ciara O'Toole) of *Language Development and Language Impairment: A problem-based introduction.*

Elena Garayzábal-Heinze moved into academic linguistics via a PhD on language development in special populations after an earlier career in a Special Education School as a speech therapist. She currently is an Associate Professor in the Department of Linguistics at the Universidad Autónoma of Madrid (Spain). Her research interests in clinical Linguistics are mainly focused on the study of the relationships among cognition, language and neurophysiology in rare diseases (Williams syndrome, Smith-Magenis syndrome, Prader Willy syndrome), and also language, speech and communication acquisition both in clinical populations and typically developing children. She has published and presented widely in the area of clinical linguistics and psycholinguistics, and she has supervised several PhD students working with these topics.

Kerry Isakson has a Bachelor's degree in Linguistics and Psychology from Northeastern University, Boston, USA, and is pursuing a Master of Education in Educational Leadership & Policy Studies at Boston University. She is currently manager of the Jumpstart programme at Boston University, including recruiting and mentoring corps members to work with young children in high-need classrooms as well as fostering and maintaining community partnerships.

Svetlana Kapalková is an associate professor of Speech-Language Therapy at the Institute of Psychological and Communication Disorders Study of the Faculty of Education at Comenius University in Bratislava. Her main research fields are child language development in typically developing children, bilingual children and children with communication impairments. Also she is a co-founder of a private centre for children with language disorders: the Institute of child language in Bratislava. As well as authoring many scientific papers, chapters and tools for the assessment of child language, she is also a writer and co-writer of four children's books. She has been a principal investigator and researcher of projects of COST, Open Society Foundation, Jan Hus Educational Foundation, APVV (Slovak Research and Development Agency), VEGA and the Visegard Fund. She is a member of the IASCL, Slovak Association of Speech Therapists, and a member of the editorial board of the international journal *Gramotnost, pregramotnost a vzdělávání* (Literacy, Pre-Literacy and Education).

Thomas Klee is Professor and Head of the Division of Speech and Hearing Sciences at the University of Hong Kong. He trained as a speech-language pathologist and taught at universities in the USA, UK and New Zealand before coming to Hong Kong. His current research was supported by the Marsden Fund of the Royal Society of New Zealand and focuses on improving the way in which children with developmental language disorders are identified and norming the New Zealand MacArthur-Bates Communicative Development Inventory: Words and Sentences.

Kristian Emil Kristoffersen was a professor of linguistics at the University of Oslo from 1998 to 2016, and is now director at Frambu National Resource Centre for Rare Disorders. His research includes studies on acquisition of phonology, grammar and lexicon in typically developing children. He was involved in adapting the MacArthur-Bates Communicative Development Inventories into Norwegian. He has also published several studies on linguistic skills in persons with cri du chat syndrome, within phonetics and phonology, morphology, syntax and lexicon.

Morten Aase Løver has his educational background from the University of Oslo as an MA candidate in linguistics. The subject of his thesis was the acquisition of relative clauses in typically developing children. He is currently employed at the Department of Communication at the University of Oslo.

Carolina Marques graduated in Speech and Language Therapy at Escola Superior de Saúde do Instituto Politécnico de Setúbal, Portugal, in 2017. She works currently as a speech and language therapist and her clinical activity focus mainly in the prevention, evaluation and intervention of language disorders in children.

Vesna Mildner, is tenured professor and Chair of applied phonetics at the Department of Phonetics, Faculty of Humanities and Social Sciences, University of Zagreb. She teaches undergraduate, graduate and doctoral courses and her teaching activities include supervision of doctoral dissertations, BA/MEd theses and award-winning student projects. Her research and teaching focus on speech acquisition, bilingualism, neurolinguistics, speech perception and auditory impairments. Dr Mildner has participated in Croatian and international research projects. Her publications include two books, about 100 book chapters, journal articles and abstracts, as well as book reviews and editorials. She (co)edited several books and proceedings, served as editor-in-chief in journals *Govor* and *Strani jezici* and is currently on the editorial board of several journals. Dr Mildner is regularly asked to peer-review books and articles for Croatian and international publishers. She presented more than 20 invited talks in Croatia and worldwide and has been an active participant and organizer of Croatian and international conferences. Dr Mildner is a member of numerous national and international associations (e.g. International Phonetic Association, International Clinical Phonetics and Linguistics Association).

N. Gabriela Moffatt recently obtained her doctorate in Applied Language and Speech Science at the University of Louisiana at Lafayette, and was a participant in the Southern Regional Education Board's Doctoral Scholars program. She received a BA in Russian at the University of South Carolina in 2008 and a MS in Speech Language Pathology from the University of Louisiana at Lafayette in 2010. She has studied abroad in Russia several times since 2006, with her two most recent trips funded by the Department of State's Critical Language Scholarship initiative. Her research interests include early child language development in culturally and linguistically diverse populations, descriptive assessment, and augmentative and alternative communication. She holds a Certificate of Clinical Competence from the American Speech-Language-Hearing Association (CCC-SLP) and is currently working with medically complex children in Florida.

Nicole Müller is Professor of Speech and Hearing Sciences at University College Cork, Ireland. Before joining UCC in 2017, she held academic positions in the UK, the US, and Sweden. Her research interests are clinical linguistics, cognitive-communication impairments related to neurodegeneration and brain injury, and interaction in the presence of communication impairments. She also has research experience in the Celtic languages, especially Irish. She co-edits the journal *Clinical Linguistics and Phonetics*.

Martina Ozbič was assistant professor at the University of Ljubljana, Slovenia (Department for special pedagogy, BA and MA for speech and language therapy) from 2010 to 2017. Since 2017 she has run her own bilingual private clinical practice in Slovenia. Since 2018 she has been collaborating as a researcher with the *Associazione La Nostra Famiglia* and as a lecturer with the University of Trieste (Italy) in courses for speech and language therapy, and also with the Faculty for applied social sciences in Nova Gorica (FUDŠ), Slovenia. Her current area of research and professional expertise are Slovenian developmental phonology and protracted phonological development (collaboration with UBC Vancouver Canada) and language impairment (COST Action IS1406, *Associazione La Nostra Famiglia*), especially in bilingual children. She has authored and coauthored several papers on phonological development, prevention of specific learning impairment and adaptations of assessment instruments for Slovenian language.

Ana Praprotnik is a speech and language therapist. She received her Master's degree in 2017 on the topic of LARSP (The use of LARSP for the analysis of grammatical competence in 3-year-old children). In 2018 she received her certificate as a neurodevelopmental Bobath speech therapist. She currently works as an SLT with preschool and school-age children with special needs.

Lalitha Raja, is an Assistant Professor in Linguistics, Annamalai University. She was recently a Fellow at the Indian Institute of Advanced Study, Shimla, undertaking post-doctoral research on Optimality Theory in phonological acquisition and in assessment and intervention of phonological disorders. In addition to the post of Assistant Professor, she is in charge of the Centre for Speech and Language Disorder Studies at Annamalai University. She holds a PhD in Linguistics (Psycholinguistics) and her research interests are in Clinical, Psycho and Cognitive Linguistics. She is an Adjunct faculty member for teaching Clinical Linguistics to Speech and Language Pathology students of SRM University, Chennai and Manipal University, Manipal. She is a consultant for four Special Schools in Chennai and Chidambaram. She has presented more than 50 research papers in child language disorders at National and International conferences. Over her research career, she has published one book and more than 40 articles in peer-reviewed journals and proceedings.

Ingeborg Sophie Ribu is a PhD research fellow at the University of Oslo, where she is affiliated with the Research group in Clinical Linguistics and Language Acquisition and the Center for Multilingualism in Society across the Lifespan. Her research interests include lexical and grammatical processing in neurologically healthy and clinical populations, and she has been involved in developing and adapting multiple screening tools for Norwegian. In her PhD project she is developing a screening battery that is sensitive enough to detect language decline in early stages of Alzheimer's disease and Primary Progressive Aphasia.

Tamara Sevšek completed a Master's degree in Speech and Language Therapy and Deaf Education at the University of Ljubljana, Faculty of Education in Slovenia. She is currently employed by a Special Education Primary School as a peripatetic teacher for Extra Professional Support in local Primary Schools and Kindergartens. For a year, she worked for the Association for Down's syndrome in Sožitje, where she was providing support and Speech and Language Therapy for Preschool and School Children with Down's Syndrome. Her main field of interest is researching the development and acquisition of narrative abilities, and providing therapy for children with specific speech and language impairment.

Hanne Gram Simonsen is Professor Emeritus in linguistics at the University of Oslo, now at MultiLing Center for Multilingualism in Society across the Lifespan. Her main fields of research are early language acquisition, in particular acquisition of phonology, morphology and lexicon in a cross-linguistic and multilingual perspective, as well as clinical linguistics including language disorders in children and in adults with aphasia and dementia, and instrumental phonetics. She has been involved in adapting and developing several assessment instruments into Norwegian, including the Mac Arthur-Bates CDI, the Cross-linguistic Lexical Tasks (CLT) and the Comprehensive Aphasia Test (CAT). She is a past President of the International Clinical Linguistics and Phonetics Association (ICPLA) (2014–2018).

Darija Skubic is Assistant Professor of Slovene Language Teaching Methodology at the Faculty of Education, University of Ljubljana, Slovenia. She holds a PhD in teaching the methodology of Slovene language. Her main research areas include developing pre-literacy skills in preschool children and Slovene as a second/foreign language in preschool institutions and primary schools. She published a scientific monograph Pedagogical speech in kindergarten and first grade of primary school (2004) and several scientific articles, e.g. Language support to immigrant children (2018), Vowels in contact: the case of Slovenian-Italian bilingual speakers (with co-author Martina Ozbič, 2018), Preschool teacher's role in development of child's reading literacy (2017), Pre-service preschool teachers' beliefs about foreign language learning and early foreign language teaching in Slovenia (with co-author Mateja Dagarin Fojkar, 2017), Pre-service teachers' beliefs about foreign language learning: a study of three different teacher training study programmes in Slovenia (with co-author Mateja Dagarin Fojkar, 2017), Slovene as the second/foreign language in Slovene pre-school institutions (with co-author Janez Jerman, 2016).

Daniela Slančová is a professor of Slovak language at the Institute of Slovak and Media Studies at the Philosophical Faculty of Prešov University in Prešov, Slovakia. Her main research fields are stylistics and rhetorics, sociolinguistics, child language acquisition and sports linguistics. She has been one of the initiators of research into child language development in Slovakia. Her main publications from the field of language acquisition and child directed speech include: *The speech of authority and love: the nursery school/kindergarten's teachers' child directed speech: a register description* (1999), *Studies on child language* (editor and co-author), 2008; *Ten studies on child language* (editor and co-author), 2018. She has also been a member of the team for adapting CDIs into Slovak (2010). She is the editor in chief of the internet scientific journal *Jazyk a kultúra* (Language and Culture).

Vesna Stojanovik holds an MA in Linguistics and English Language Teaching from the University of Leeds, England and a PhD in Human Communication Sciences from the University of Sheffield, England. She is a Professor of Clinical Linguistics at the School of Psychology and Clinical Language Sciences at the University of Reading, UK. She is also Chair of the British Association of Clinical Linguistics. Vesna's research interests focus on speech, language and communication in children with developmental disorders.

Stephanie F. Stokes is a professor in the Division of Speech and Hearing Sciences at the University of Hong Kong, having previously held professorial posts in England, Australia and New Zealand. She is an academic and speech therapist with expertise in early child language development and language disorders. Stephanie continues to collaborate with several international research teams to improve the effectiveness of early language intervention.

Bror-Magnus S. Strand graduated with an MA in linguistics from the University of Oslo in 2015. He is currently a PhD candidate at UiT – The Arctic University of Norway with a project on dialect acquisition and bidialectalism in Norwegian children. Strand has been involved in projects in lexicography, language infrastructure and psycholinguistics as a researcher or research assistant.

Asifa Sultana is a child language researcher working on Bangla-speaking children's typical and atypical language development. Her research particularly focuses on children's acquisition of morphosyntactic details. She is involved in developing a comprehensive understanding of Bangla-speaking children's typical development which can later be used as a framework to assess the children with a range of language difficulties. The current chapter on the Bangla LARSP model is developed with the same purpose. The chapter presents a micro profile of children's typical development with a particular focus on Bangla verb morphological paradigm. Asifa Sultana is based in Dhaka, Bangladesh, and currently works at the Department of English and Humanities, BRAC University.

Diana Tomić is Assistant Professor of Phonetics, in the Faculty of Humanities and Social Sciences, University of Zagreb. She received her BA in Phonetics and English language and Literature in 2006 and her PhD in Linguistics in 2013 from the University of Zagreb with PhD thesis *Interactions between phonetic and phonological development of the phoneme /r/: a study from age 3 to age 7*. Her research interests are developmental phonology, pronunciation teaching and communication in the sports context. She has published several papers in national and international peer reviewed journals. She teaches phonetic and public speaking courses at the Faculty of Humanities and Social Sciences and Faculty of Kinesiology, University of Zagreb and also serves as a Secretary of Phonetic Journal Govor (Speech) and as a President of the Phonetic Section of the Croatian Philological Association.

Seyhun Topbaş is a Professor of Speech and Language Therapy at İstanbul Medipol University, Turkey. She is one of the pioneers of the Speech & Language Therapy profession in Turkey, and the founder of the first graduate and undergraduate programs in Speech Language Therapy in the country, Dr Topbaş has developed standardized tests and has authored many articles and chapters in international and national journals. She has written and been the editor of three volumes in speech and language disorders as well as an international book published by Multilingual Matters titled *Communication Disorders in Turkish* (co-authored). She is a member of ASHA, CPLOL and a member of IALP, ICPLA, and on the editorial board of the journal *Clinical Linguistics and Phonetics*. Currently, she is Head of the national Association of Speech and Language Therapists in Turkey.

Introduction

The chapters in this collection constitute the third, and for now, at least, the final volume of adaptations of the LARSP assessment system to languages other than English. There are 12 different languages represented in this book and, while most of them belong to various branches of the Indo-European language family, there are also representatives from the Turkic, Dravidian, Bantu and Inuit language families. This linguistic diversity is evidence of the versatility of the linguistic profile approach. Moreover, even within any one-language family there may be considerable differences in how morphology and syntax operate, as witnessed, for example, in the general paucity of inflectional morphology in English as compared to the abundance in Russian. While such differences often result in profile charts that differ considerably from one language to another, they are all recognizably part of the same 'LARSP family'.

The chapters have been arranged in terms of language families and sub-families, and the first eight chapters describe profiles for Indo-European languages. Chapter 1 describes a profile for Norwegian by Ingeborg Sophie Ribu, Hanne Gram Simonsen, Morten Aase Løver, Bror-Magnus Sviland Strand and Kristian Emil Kristoffersen. The addition of Norwegian means that grammatical profiles have now been devised for the majority of the Germanic languages, with N-LARSP joining profiles for English, German, Dutch, Afrikaans, Frisian and Swedish. It is to be hoped that Danish and Icelandic clinical linguists may add those languages to the total sometime in the future.

The next four chapters deal with Slavic languages. Although Bulgarian featured in a previous collection (Vakareliyska, 2016), these chapters represent a major advance in providing grammatical assessment materials for languages in this sub-family. As Slavic languages generally have a larger inflectional morphology than, for example, English, it is interesting to compare how the authors of these chapters deal with incorporating this into their profile charts.

As Moffatt and Müller point out in Chapter 2, there are very few assessment tools for Russian children with language impairment, thus the Russian LARSP will be of particular use to speech-language pathologists both in Russia and elsewhere where Russian speakers have settled. The other profiles in this group are of West Slavic (Slovak by Svetlana

Kapalková and Daniela Slančová), and the two South Slavic languages of Croatian (Vesna Mildner, Vesna Stojanovik and Dijana Tomić) and Slovenian (Darija Skubic, Ana Praprotnik, Tamara Sevšek and Martina Ozbič). Interest was also expressed in devising profiles for Polish, Czech and Serbian, and it is to be hoped that these may be developed in the future.

Romance languages are represented by European Portuguese (Ana Castro, Carolina Marques and Catarina Dôro), and Colombian Spanish (Maryluz Camargo-Mendoza, Ana Isabel Codesido-García and Elena Garayzábal- Heinze). The main Romance languages not yet provided with LARSP-like profiles are now Italian, Catalan and Romanian; again, it is to be hoped that these may one day be developed.

The last Indo-European language covered in this collection is Bangla. Stokes (2012), in the first volume in this set of books on LARSP, described syntactic development in Bengali (Sylheti) children. However, Sultana, Stokes, Klee and Fletcher in this collection examine verb inflection for the purposes of a micro-profile in this area. Combining these two accounts should now provide a comprehensive profile of the language.

The remaining four chapters cover four different language families. Seyhun Topbaş and Özlem Cangökçe Yaşar revisit the TR-LARSP for Turkish that was first described in 2012. In that earlier work, only the first few stages of the TR-LARSP were described; the present chapter presents new acquisition data allowing the full TR-LARSP chart to be presented. R. Lalitha Raja's chapter provides a profile for Tamil, the second Dravidian language with a profile after Varun Uthappa, Shyamala K. Chengappa and Ramesh Kaipa's work on Kannada (2016).

Kamil Ud Deen describes the preliminaries for a profile of Swahili. As this language is widely spoken throughout East Africa, this development is especially welcome. It is to be hoped that some of the Southern Bantu languages might have profiles provided for them in the future, as speech-language pathology is well established in South Africa. Shanley E.M. Allen, Catherine B. Dench and Kerry Isakson contribute the final chapter to this volume. They describe a profile for Inuktitut, this being the first Indigenous language of the Americas to have a LARSP-like profile devised for it. There are notable grammatical differences between Inuktitut and related languages and Indo-European languages; nevertheless, a usable profile is illustrated in this chapter, suggesting that similar assessment tools could be devised for other Indigenous American languages.

Our hope is that the chapters in this collection will not only be of interest, but also of use to those involved in the assessment of the languages covered. We welcome offers of the development of profiles of further languages.

References

Stokes, J. (2012) An investigation of syntax in children of Bengali (Sylheti)-speaking families. In M.J. Ball, D. Crystal and P. Fletcher (eds) *Assessing Grammar. The Languages of LARSP* (pp. 139–148). Bristol: Multilingual Matters.

Uthappa, V., Chengappa, S.K. and Kaipa, R. (2016) K-LARSP: A grammatical profile of Kannada. In P. Fletcher, M.J. Ball and D. Crystal (eds) *Profiling Grammar. More Languages of LARSP* (pp. 118–134). Bristol: Multilingual Matters.

Vakareliyska, C.M. (2016) Language-specific issues for the Bulgarian LARSP profile and adult aphasia examinations. In P. Fletcher, M.J. Ball and D. Crystal (eds) *Profiling Grammar. More Languages of LARSP* (pp. 236–261). Bristol: Multilingual Matters.

1 N-LARSP: A Developmental Language Profile for Norwegian

Ingeborg Sophie Ribu, Hanne Gram Simonsen, Morten Aase Løver, Bror-Magnus Sviland Strand and Kristian Emil Kristoffersen

Introduction

This chapter outlines the Norwegian version of the Language Assessment, Remediation and Screening Procedure (LARSP) profile chart, and the steps undertaken to develop this chart. As a background to the chart the chapter will also give a general overview of Norwegian grammar and what we know about first language acquisition of Norwegian grammar.

The LARSP profiles that exist for other Germanic languages (English, German and Dutch) are structured in quite different ways (Ball *et al.*, 2012) and neither of them can be directly translated into Norwegian and still give a correct and comprehensive overview of the developmental stages of Norwegian child language acquisition.[1] In adapting LARSP to Norwegian, we have tried to strike a balance between the wish to keep the LARSP profiles as similar as possible for reasons of cross-linguistic comparability, and the need for language-specific adjustments. Thus, the Norwegian LARSP chart, as it is outlined below, is inspired by the LARSP charts from other Germanic languages, but adapted in such a way that it accommodates to language-specific features of Norwegian. We have also tried to keep simplicity in mind, so that LARSP can be useful not only for researchers, but also for clinicians. Our aim has been to keep the profile as simple as possible to use in clinical settings, even for clinicians with little linguistic training.

Norwegian – A Grammatical Sketch

Norwegian is a North Germanic language spoken by approximately 5 million people in Norway. Norwegian vocabulary and grammar are

Table 1.1 Inflection of nouns in Norwegian

	Declension 1 (Masc.)	Declension 2 (Fem.)	Declension 3 (Neut.)
Singular indefinite	bil 'car'	jent-e 'girl'	hus 'house'
Singular definite	bil-en	jent-a	hus-et
Plural indefinite	bil-er	jent-er	hus
Plural definite	bil-ene	jent-ene	hus-a

very similar to Swedish and Danish, whereas other Germanic languages are more different. Morphologically, Norwegian is slightly more complex than English. Nouns fall into three declensions based on gender, and are inflected for number and definiteness, cf. the paradigms in Table 1.1.[2]

As for verbs, there is a major division in Norwegian into weak ('regular') and strong ('irregular') verbs, familiar from other Germanic languages. The proportion of strong verbs is similar to that in English, approximately 4%. As in English, there are a number of strong subclasses, some with a relatively high type frequency, others with only a few members.

As for the weak verbs, there are two weak classes in Norwegian, as opposed to only one in English; one larger, with a type frequency of 56% and one smaller, with a type frequency of 40% (Endresen & Simonsen, 2001). Norwegian verb paradigms have seven cells: imperative, infinitive, present, simple past, past participle, present participle and passive,[3] cf. the example paradigms in Table 1.2.

Table 1.2 Inflection of verbs in Norwegian

	Weak verbs: large class	Weak verbs: small class	Strong verbs
Imperative	kast 'throw'	lek 'play'	bit 'bite'
Infinitive	kast-e	lek-e	bit-e
Present	kast-er	lek-er	bit-er
Past	kast-a	lek-te	beit
Past participle	kast-a	lek-t	bitt
Present participle	kast-ende	lek-ende	bit-ende
Passive	kast-es	lek-es	bit-es

Adjectives in Norwegian are inflected for gender (masculine/feminine vs neuter), definiteness (definite vs indefinite), number (singular vs plural), and degree (positive vs comparative vs superlative),[4] with more contrasts applying to adjectives modifying a head noun than to predicative adjectives. An example of adjective inflection in Norwegian is found in Table 1.3.

Table 1.3 Inflection of adjectives in Norwegian

Indefinite			**Definite**
Masc./Fem.	Neuter	Plural	Singular/Plural
fin 'fine'	fin-t	fin-e	fin-e

In the paradigms for personal pronouns, there are distinctions between subject and object case for some pronouns (e.g. *jeg* 'I' vs *meg* 'me'), between masculine, feminine and neuter (only in 3rd person singular: *han* 'he', *hun* 'she' and *det/den* 'it'), and between singular and plural (e.g. *du* 'you.sg' vs *dere* 'you.pl'. Furthermore, among the possessive determiners (with different forms for most persons in the singular and plural) there are distinctions between genders (e.g. *min* 'my.masc' vs *mi* 'my.fem' vs *mitt* 'my.neut'), and between non-reflexive and reflexive forms (*hans* 'his.non-refl' vs *sitt* 'his.refl').

Among nouns, verbs and adjectives, the main mode of inflection is suffixation. Some nouns and verbs, however, have inflection by modification, see e.g. the column for strong verbs in Table 1.2, where the root vowel of the verb *bite* 'bite' varies between *i* and *ei*. A third possibility is that nothing changes from one cell to another in the paradigm, cf. the singular indefinite and plural indefinite of *hus* 'house' in Table 1.1.

Like in other Germanic languages, compounding is a productive morphological process in Norwegian. Compounds in Norwegian are head final, and the head is the part inflected in the compound. Most productive are compounds with nouns as a head, often compounded with another noun *brannmann* (*brann* 'fire' + *mann* 'man') 'firefighter'; *ordbok* (*ord* 'word' + *bok* 'book') 'dictionary'; but other combinations are also very common, e.g. A+N: *tomflaske* (*tom* 'empty' + *bottle* 'flaske') 'empty bottle'; V+N *symaskin* (*sy* 'sew' + *maskin* 'machine') *sewing machine*; N+A *feberfri* (*feber* 'fever' + *fri* 'free') 'without fever'; N+V *korsfeste* (*kors* 'cross' + *feste* 'fasten') 'crucify'; P+V *innby* (*inn* 'in' + *by* 'bid') 'invite'. There are also examples of compounds consisting of more than two words; N+N+N *landslagstrener* (*land* 'country' + *lag* 'team' + *trener* 'coach') 'national team coach'.

As for word order, Norwegian is a verb second (V2) language, which means that the finite verb occurs in the second position in main declarative clauses and WH-questions, cf. (1):

(1)	a.	Jenta	spiller	sjakk.		Main declarative
		Girl.def.sg.	play.pres	chess		
		'The girl plays chess.'				
	b.	Jenta	spiller	ikke	sjakk.	Main declarative,
		girl.def.sg.	play.pres	not	chess	with negation
		'The girl does not play chess.'				

c.	I går	spilte	jenta	sjakk.	Main declarative, preposed adverbial
	yesterday	play.past	girl.def.sg	chess	
	'Yesterday, the girl played chess.'				
d.	Hvem	spiller	sjakk?		WH-question
	who	play.pres	chess		
	'Who plays chess?'				

Northern and Western dialects can also have V3 in WH-questions (Lie, 1992), cf. the two variants in (2) (from Westergaard, 2003):

(2)	a.	Ka	legen	sa?	V3
		what	doctor.def.sg	said	
		'What did the doctor say?'			
	b.	Ka	sa	legen?	V2
		what	said	doctor.def.sg	
		'What did the doctor say?'			

In embedded clauses with sentence adverbials the target word order is generally V3, in particular with the negation adverbial *ikke* 'not', giving the order Subjunction-Neg-V_{fin}, cf (3):

(3)	a.	Jenta	sa	at	hun	ikke	spiller	sjakk.		V3
		Girl.def.sg	said	that	she	not	play.pres	chess		
		'The girl said that she doesn't play chess.'								
	b.	Jenta	spiser	når	maten	ikke	lukter	vondt.		V3
		girl.def.sg	eat.pres	when	food.def.sg	not	smell.pres	bad		
		'The girl eats when the food doesn't smell bad.'								
	c.	Jenta	liker	mannen	som	ikke	er	sint.		V3
		girl.def.sg	like.pres	man.def.sg	who	not	is	mad		
		'The girl likes the man who isn't mad.'								

First Language Acquisition of Norwegian Grammar

To our knowledge, the first published material on acquisition of Norwegian was the psychologist Thomas Parr's diary from 1903 of the early language development of two of his children from 1;6-2;6 years, adapted and published by Helga Eng (1944). It mainly contains data on the children's vocabulary, but Parr also offers some observations of early grammar (the two children seem precocious in both respects).

Vanvik (1971) published the first linguistic study of first language acquisition in a Norwegian context, with a longitudinal diary study of the speech and language development of his own daughter from birth to eight years of age. The primary focus of Vanvik's research was phonetic and phonological development, but he also made a few notes concerning vocabulary and grammar. For example, he noted gender errors around 2½ years, overgeneralizations of verbal inflections between 2 and 7 years, and deviant placement of sentence adverbials between 3 and 4 years.

Simonsen (1983) was a case study (of spontaneous speech) of a boy aged 4;9-4;11, analysing structure and function in his syntactic patterns. Structurally, the child's language was similar to the adult target, with most basic structures established. However, there were larger differences in the use of these structures concerning semantic content to be attributed to his utterances, and the communicative functions they seemed to fill. The full corpus is published as an appendix to the book.

Simonsen (1990) investigated the phonological development of three children aged between 2;0 and 4;1 acquiring Norwegian (as well as one child acquiring Samoan) establishing a longitudinal corpus of spontaneous speech. Even though the focus of this study was phonological, Simonsen included notes on the interaction between phonology and morphology, as well as lists of all the words produced by her participants, thus providing information about early lexical and grammatical skills. The corpora from two of the three Norwegian children are available on CHILDES.

Plunkett and Strömqvist (1992) included some data on Norwegian from the Simonsen (1990) corpus in their study of early acquisition of Scandinavian. In the domain of syntax, they found negation to be well established with the correct word order in main clauses (with the negation marker *ikke* following the finite verb) by the age 2;6. As for morphology, they found that gender assignment for nouns at the early stages seemed uncomplicated, although slightly more complicated for Norwegian than for Danish and Swedish: While gender acquisition in Danish and Swedish is virtually error free around the age of 2 years, Norwegian children make more errors at this stage – mainly in overgeneralization of masculine gender.

Ragnarsdóttir *et al.* (1999) conducted an experimental study of past tense production of Icelandic and Norwegian children at 4, 6 and 8 years (30 children at each stage). For Norwegian they found that the large weak class was clearly acquired first and was approaching ceiling performance already at 4 years; the small weak class was acquired second and the strong class was acquired last; both were still clearly behind the larger weak class at 6 years with an average of 71% correct for the small weak class and 60% correct for the strong class, as opposed to 94% correct for the large weak class.

Anderssen (2005) examined acquisition of prenominal definiteness markers, suffixal definiteness markers and pronouns in three children aged 1;8-3;3 on the basis of a longitudinal spontaneous speech corpus. The two markers of definiteness are illustrated in the examples in (4) (the pattern in (4b) is commonly referred to as 'double definiteness'):

(4) a.	Hus-et			Suffixal marker only
	House.def.neut			
	'The house'			
b.	Det	gaml-e	hus-et	
	the.def.neut	old	house-.def.neut	Prenominal and suffixal marker
	'The old house'			

Anderssen found that the definiteness suffix (4a) was used appropriately in 70% of obligatory contexts (i.e. linguistic contexts requiring the suffix) already at 1;8, and in more than 80% of the obligatory contexts by two years of age. Personal pronouns were also used from 1;8, whereas possessive determiners (e.g. *mitt* 'my' in *huset mitt* 'my house') were acquired somewhat later. Personal pronouns and possessive determiners followed the same developmental trend. As for the prenominal definiteness marker, Anderssen found that it was acquired considerably later.

Concerning early syntactic skills of Norwegian children, Westergaard (2005) investigated the acquisition of verb second word order (V2) in three children longitudinally from the age of 1;8 until around 3 (the same children as the Anderssen corpus above). The main finding of Westergaard's study was that V2 was attested as soon as multi-word utterances appeared in the data, and that non-V2 word order was also produced in the relevant contexts. Furthermore, Westergaard reported mean length of utterance (MLU) values for the three children at around the age of 2, given in Table 1.4.

As for word order in embedded sentences, in particular with adverbials, this seems to be acquired somewhat later. In a study of two boys acquiring North Norwegian, Westergaard and Bentzen (2007) found that in embedded sentences with the negation *ikke*, the target V3 word order (see (3) above)) was not fully mastered until the age of between four and five. Thus, these children seemed to overgeneralize the main clause placement of *ikke* directly after the finite verb, i.e. V2.[5]

In a large population-based study the Norwegian adaptation of the parent report instrument MacArthur-Bates Communicative development inventories (CDI) was used to examine gestural, lexical and grammatical development in 6574 children between 8 and 36 months (Kristoffersen & Simonsen, 2012; Simonsen *et al.*, 2014). It was found that word combinations and possession expressions appeared in the earliest children around 1;6, followed by definiteness at 1;8, plural of nouns, present tense and past

Table 1.4 MLU for three TD children learning Norwegian (from Westergaard, 2005)

CHILD	MLUw
Ina 2;1.29	2.27
Ann 2;1.28	2.27
Ole 1;10.0	2.24

tense at 1;10 (all ages when 25% of the children had started producing these expressions). However, there was extensive variation: the ages when 75% had started using them stretched from 1;10 for word combinations to 2;5 for past tense, and furthermore there was a significant gender difference – with girls clearly ahead of boys.

Adapting LARSP to Norwegian

Procedure

The Norwegian LARSP profile is in many ways influenced by the profiles already developed for other Germanic languages, English and Dutch, as many of the structures described for the other Germanic languages are also found in Norwegian.

The final profile was constructed in three steps. First, a profile was built using data material from three already existing child language corpora. Second, this profile was applied to a new, more controlled set of spontaneous speech data that was specifically collected for this purpose. In the end, data from those two initial steps were combined to form the basis for the final profile chart.

The first step

Data from three of the child language corpora for Norwegian described above (Anderssen, 2005; Simonsen, 1983, 1990) were used to provide language specific information for the N-LARSP chart. Distributed over the two longitudinal corpora (Anderssen, 2005; Simonsen, 1990) there were five children (two boys and three girls) between the ages 1;8 and 4;1 years, corresponding to stages 2 through 6. Morphological information was also extracted from the results from the Norwegian CDI study (Kristoffersen & Simonsen, 2012; Simonsen *et al.*, 2014). The third corpus, Simonsen (1983), was used to form the basis for stage 7. This corpus consists of spontaneous speech data from one child at 4;9-4;11. The number of recorded sessions per child spanned from 6 to 27 sessions in the two longitudinal corpora. All recordings had been transcribed, and these transcriptions served as basis for developing the primary profile chart.

For each child in the Simonsen (1990) and Anderssen (2005) corpora all the utterances from all recordings were analysed on clause, phrase, and word level. If three of the five children used a feature productively at a specific stage, that feature was considered to be acquired and added to the preliminary LARSP chart. Where possible, the features were also compared to norms from the Norwegian CDI study, where a feature is considered to be acquired when it is used by 50% of the children. Following this approach some features were implemented in the profile chart based on spontaneous speech from three to five children, and some were based on parental reports from more than 2000 children. For some features both CDI data and spontaneous speech data were available. For the seventh stage, only data from one child were available.

As these data had been collected for other purposes and at different times, they are not quite comparable with regard to topics covered by the children and the investigators. In the Anderssen corpus (2005) the children talked to their parents and investigators about daily events, differing from one session to the next, and were often engaged in play or artistic activities such as drawing or painting, whereas the children in the Simonsen (1990) corpus talked about daily events, objects and books that were more similar across sessions.

The second step

As a second step, we collected a new set of data containing spontaneous speech, to test out and further develop the LARSP profile that had been proposed in the first step. In order to assure validity and comparability as well as reliability, we chose a multiple case mixed methodology, with both longitudinal and cross-sectional data, as similar designs have been used in norming the LARSP chart in several other languages (see Ball *et al.*, 2012; Fletcher *et al.*, 2016). The methodological design was also meant to replicate an actual clinical assessment situation with a speech therapist and a child under the suspicion of having a language impairment. As already mentioned, our aim is that the N-LARSP profile both can be applied clinically and used in theoretical investigations, e.g. as a basis for cross-linguistic comparison.

Thus, a spontaneous speech material was collected from 16 children between 1;0 and 5;6 years, giving 32 samples, evenly distributed for gender across all seven stages. Each child (except from four of the youngest and four of the oldest) was recorded two times with a six months interval, ensuring they had reached the next stage by the second recording (see Figure 1.1).

The children were recorded at home with a parent present, and spontaneous speech was elicited through play with a set of toys, and for the older children also through story retelling and talking about recent events.

Stage (age)	1 (1;0–1;6)		2 (1;6–2;0)		3 (2;0–2;6)		4 (2;6–3;0)		5 (2;6–3;0)		6 (3;6–4;6)		7 (4;6–5;6)	
sex	F	M	F	M	F	M	F	M	F	M	F	M	F	M
1st session	2	2	2	2	2	2	2	2	2	2	2	2	2	2
2nd session	2	2	2	2	2	2	2	2	2	2	2	2	2	2

Figure 1.1 Recording scheme, N-LARSP (N = 32) F = female, M = male

The recordings were transcribed orthographically[6] by two of the authors (Sloetjes & Wittenburg, 2008) using ELAN (Max Planck Institute for Psycholinguistics, 2008). The transcriptions were divided so that subjects were distributed evenly between the transcribers in regard to stage and sex. It was also divided such that no subject was transcribed by the same transcriber for both sessions. To assess the reliability of the transcriptions, a section of the transcript was swapped and transcribed by the other transcriber. This gave a coefficient of 95%, which we considered satisfactory.

A sample of 100 utterances was extracted from each recording, starting at 11 minutes into the recording. This second data set, then, is based on 100-utterances samples from eight children (four girls, four boys) at each stage, amounting to a total of 56 100-utterances samples. The utterances were coded for the grammatical variables that were proposed in the first step of the procedure. For a variable to make it to the chart, it had to be present in the 100-utterances sample of at least half of the children at each stage.

The third step and the final profile chart

In view of the extensive variation between children – in particular at the younger stages below three years of age – and to get a larger set of children as a basis for the final profile chart, we combined the two data sets and treated them as one, resulting in between eight and 13 children at each stage. By combining the two data sets the number of utterances per child that serve as a basis for further development of the profile chart, varies from child to child and stage to stage. For each of the eight children recruited for this project in particular, only the 100-utterances samples are used as a basis, whereas for the Simonsen and Anderssen corpora, all the utterances from each recording are included. The total number of children included at each stage is shown in Table 1.5.

As above, at least half of the children at each stage have to produce a variable for it to make it into the chart at that particular stage. Some variables approached the threshold for acquisition at multiple stages before reaching the requirement of 50%.

Table 1.5 Number of children at each stage after combining the existing longitudinal corpora with the new recordings

Stage 1	8 children
Stage 2	11 children
Stage 3	13 children
Stage 4	13 children
Stage 5	11 children
Stage 6	9 children
Stage 7	9 children

Form

The N-LARSP chart is modelled after the Dutch GRAMAT (Bol & Kuiken, 1988, 1990) profile in design, as this in our view is a tidier and more user-friendly design than the original LARSP chart, but with a few changes. For instance, the Norwegian profile consists of seven stages, as in the original LARSP profile, and not six, as in GRAMAT (Bol, 2012). The seventh stage is included to also focus on the children's discourse skills. This stage is lacking from the Dutch profile. Although a child's syntax at 4;6 often displays grammatical accuracy and fluency, there are still some grammatical processes to be learned. Those structures that are found are often used with a different function from what is expected, such as temporal sentences with causal meanings, as in (5), or causal structures without causal meaning (Simonsen, 1983), as in (6):

(5)	Hvorfor	fikk	han	ikke	noe	bål	når	man	ikke	hadde
	Why	get.past	he	no	any	fire	when	one	not	have.past

fyrstikker. (Erlend, 5;1)
matches
'Why didn't he get any fire when they didn't have any matches?'

Jeg	hadde	en	tang,	men	den	mistet	jeg	for
I	have.past	one	pliers,	but	that	lose.past	I	because
den	fikk	jeg	av	Astrid	til	jul. (Erlend, 5;1)		
that	get.past	I	from	Astrid	for	Christmas		

'I had a pair of pliers, but I lost them because I got them from Astrid for Christmas'

Furthermore, in the final Norwegian profile a 'rest' level is introduced at the bottom of the chart, corresponding to the summarizing line in the original English LARSP profile. This allows for the therapist to include notes about the child's syntactic and pragmatic knowledge that is not assessed with the profile chart.

MLU was calculated on the basis of 100 transcribed utterances from each child from stage 2 onwards. For the utterances from step 2, this means the same 100 utterances that also served as basis for inclusion in the chart, whereas for the Simonsen (1983, 1990) and Anderssen (2005) corpora 100 consecutive utterances were chosen at a random starting point in each recording.

Section A+B

Sections A and B in N-LARSP incorporate the features described in sections A–D in the original LARSP profile chart. The sections A and B are

Name:	Age:
Date of birth:	Therapist:
Date of recording:	Comments:
A. Unanalyzable utterances	
Incomprehensible:	Incomplete:
Deviant:	Ambiguous:
Minor:	Repetitions:
B. Analyzable utterances	
Total number of utterances	MLU:

Figure 1.2 N-LARSP section A and B

non-language specific, and provide the therapist with space for commenting on the number of analysable and unanalysable utterances as well as MLU.

Unanalysable utterances can be classified either as unintelligible, incomplete, deviant, ambiguous, minor or repetitions. Following Crystal *et al.* (1989), minor sentences are shorter (often one-word) utterances normal in informal speech, such as greetings, yes/no answers, interjections, or stereotypical answers such as nursery rhymes and other memorized utterances (i.e. numbers or the letters of the alphabet), or aphorisms and idioms.

Repetitions refer to the child's immediate repetition of his or her own utterances, or immediate repetitions of the therapist/teacher/investigator's utterances. The category 'deviant' is used to account for utterances that do not fit either normal adult speech or the usage of typically developing children (Crystal *et al.*, 1976, 1989). These responses should be counted and marked under the header 'unanalysable'; they should not be included in the main chart.

Mean length of utterance is calculated on basis of the number of analysable utterances included in the chart. Sections A and B in the N-LARSP chart are shown in Figure 1.2.

Clause, phrase and word levels

Similar to all other LARSP profiles, the Norwegian chart is also divided into clause, phrase and word levels between stages 2 and 6 (1;6-4;6). The clause level refers to how the major utterances are structured, and the phrase level is concerned with the internal structuring of the clauses. The word level gives a representation of the child's morphological knowledge. As the utterances at stage 1 are mainly one-word utterances there is no need to distinguish between clause, phrase and word levels at that stage. At stage 7 the child's language output is so close to adult-like language that the distinction between clause, phrase and word levels is abolished and replaced with room for a detailed description of the child's communicative skills.

Note that in the descriptions below some constructions are mentioned as emerging at earlier stages than they are considered acquired: for a construction to count as acquired at a given stage, it must be present in at least 50% of the children at this stage.

Stage 1 (0;9-1;6)

This first stage is quite similar across languages, and gives an account of single-word utterances.

The children use simple nouns to refer to objects and verbs for action naming. The category 'other' is also provided, and is here used to refer to any other word class than nouns and verbs, such as negations, interrogatives, adjectives, adverbs, pronouns etc.

Examples

V

(7) Se! (Oliver 1;0:7)
'look!'

N

(8) Mann (Emma 1;5:4)
'Man'
Other

(9) Oi (Jakob 1;5.29)
'Oops'

The section for stage 1 in the N-LARSP chart is illustrated in Figure 1.3.

Stage 2 (1;6-2;0)

From this stage on the children are joining words together at both clause and phrase level, and it is therefore sensible to make a distinction between these levels. At this point the children also start to combine and inflect words, and to modify their utterances by means of adverbials and negations. Although much of the children's speech at this point consists of two-word utterances, there is still extensive use of one-word utterances, especially in interrogative and imperative clauses.

We introduced a distinction between NP_{-poss} and NP_{+poss}. This way, possessive expressions are included as a subcategory of NP, but also distinguished from other multi-word NP constructions. An alternative distinction could be NP_{+poss} and NP, but a certain degree of redundancy would follow as NP then could include NP_{+poss}. Possessive expressions were included as we consider their particular onset interesting and relevant to the first stages of multi-word utterances. Naturally, having only

Stage 1. 1;0-1;6	N	V	Other

Figure 1.3 N-LARSP Stage 1

one single NP construction would not accentuate this particular development, because it features a wide array of different constructions. As we can see in stage 2 and 3, the distinction between these two NP constructions is useful, as the two categories do not appear simultaneously.

Examples

Sentence level:
Commands:
V:
(10) Åpne! (Lucas, 1;9.23)
'Open!'
Adv:
(11) Der! (Emilie, 1;11.27)[7]
'There!'

Statements:
AdvX:
(12) Ferdig lese bok nå. (Anne, 2;4.2)
Done read.inf book now
'[I am] Done reading the book now'
NegX:
(13) Ikke nå (Lucas, 2;4.2)
Not now
'Not now'

Phrase level:
(14) NP[$_{-Poss}$]:
En bil (Benedicte, 1;6.0)
'A car'

Word level:
Def.sg.:
(15) Sitte bilen der (Lucas, 1;9.23)
Sit car.def.sg there
'Put the car there'

Figure 1.4 shows the section for stage 2 in the N-LARSP chart.

Towards the end of this second stage, the children start using adverbials and auxiliary verbs extensively, and this pattern will dominate the clause level utterances at the next stage.

	Sentence					Phrase	Word
	Question	Command		Statement			
Stage 2. 1;6-2;0		V	Adv	AdvX	NegX	NP [-Poss]	Def.sg

Figure 1.4 N-LARSP Stage 2

Based on 100 transcribed utterances from the 11 children at stage 2, the MLU for this stage has been calculated to 1.48 words on average.

Stage 3 (2;0-2;6)

When the children reach the third stage, their speech is characterized by an increasing number of multi-word utterances, the sentences and grammar are more complex, and the children start using copula verbs. From this point on compounds, mainly noun-noun but also noun-verb compounds, become productive. The children from the northern part of the country (Anderssen, 2005) produce a substantial amount of adjective–noun compounds, which are not seen at all among the children from the central south-eastern part of Norway. It is therefore appropriate to group all compounds together and treating them like one, instead of treating the different kinds of compounds separately.

The presence of both infinitives and inflected words characterizes the verbs in this and the following stage. This can be seen in the examples below, and has been studied in more detail using the specifically gathered data (see 'The second step' under 'Procedure' above) in Strand (2015). Strand argues that the so-called *Root Infinitives* (or *Optional Infinitives*), where an infinitive verb is the main verb of the clause, are particularly prominent in stage 3 and diminishing in stage 4. Therefore one can argue for a *Root Infinitive stage* in Norwegian comprising both stages 3 and 4 (p. 68). Note, however, that present tense inflection is also present in the data and counted as acquired at stage 3.

In addition to the (indicative) Root Infinitive (see SV, VX and AdvX under Statements below), children also produce a *prescriptive* or *jussive* infinitive (see the examples under Commands below). Children's tendency to use the infinitive in commands was noted as early as in Eng (1944: 6). This structure is also used by parents in all North Germanic languages, particularly in child directed speech (i.a. Johannessen (2013), see also Strand (2015), and the references cited there). Investigating stages 3 and 4, Strand (2015) found that children's prescriptive infinitives complied with the syntactic rules of the adult prescriptive infinitive.

Although the children manage to apply the correct gender marking to nouns in the definite singular form already at stage 2, we see that some of the children still make errors on certain nouns even at stage 3. This is exemplified in (16)a, where Ina uses the masculine *-en*, rather than the neuter *-et* definite marker, compared to the correct neuter form in (16)b:

(16) a. Og hoden (Ina 2;4.28)
And head.def.sg.mask
'And the head'

b. Og hodet
And head.def.sg.neut
'And the head' (correct)

Examples

Sentence level:
Questions:
Q(X):

(17) Hva det? (William, 2;5.22)
What that?
'What is that?'

VS(X):

(18) Er du fire? (Linnea, 2 ;9.15)
Are you four?
'Are you four years old?'

Commands:
VX:

(19) Sette på igjen. (Magnus, 2;3.10)
Put.inf on again
'Put it back on'

VO(X):

(20) Pappa hjelpe meg. (Kari, 2;2.7)
Daddy help.inf. me
'Daddy, help me'

VO:

(21) Hjelp meg! (Ole, 2;5)
Help.imp me!
'Help me!'

Statements:
SV:

(22) Han spise. (Ingrid, 2;4.8)
He eat.inf
'He is eating'

SVO:

(23) Jeg låner den. (Nora, 2;3)
I borrow.pres that
'I'm borrowing it'

SVAdv:

(24) Den virke ikke. (Lucas, 2;4.2)
That work.inf not
'It doesn't work'

SVauxV:

(25) Jeg kan kjøre nå. (Anne, 2;4.2)
I can drive now
'I can drive now'

Phrase level:
NP $_{[+Poss]}$:

(26) Mamma sin (Ingrid, 2;4.28)
Mom hers
'Mom's'

Pers.pron:

(27) Han kræsja med deg. (Emil, 2;3.29)
He crash.past with you
'He collided into you'

Copula:

(28) Her er rumpa (William, 2;5.22)
Here is bum.def
'Here is the bum'

VauxV:

(29) Nå skal kjøre. (William, 2;5.22)
Now shall.pres drive.inf
'Now [I] will drive'

Word level:

Present tense:

(30) Det graver ned elgen. (Lucas, 2;4.2)
It buries down moose.def.sg
'It buries the moose'

Past tense:

(31) Tissa bleie. (Benedicte, 2;1.6)
Pee.past diaper
'[I] peed [in the] diaper'

Compound:

(32) Ho kubestemor. (Ina, 2;6.19)
She cow.grand.mother
'The grandmother-cow'

The section for stage 3 is illustrated in Figure 1.5.

At this stage, MLU was calculated on the basis of 100 utterances from 13 children yielding an average of 2.62 words.

Stage 4 (2;6-3;0)

At the fourth stage we see a further increase in more syntactically complex structures, such as basic that-subjunction and inversion (application of the V2 rule), and more advanced syntax in questions. The latter is exemplified through more complex interrogative clauses and inversion in clauses with topicalized adverbials. We also see the emergence of the

Stage 3.	Q(X)	VS(X)	VX	VO(X)	SV	VO	NP [+Poss]	Pres	Past
2;0-2;6					VX	SVAdv	Pers.pron	Compound	
					SVO	SVauxV	Copula		
							Vaux+V		

Figure 1.5 N-LARSP Stage 3

presentational clause with the expletive pronoun det (it/there), although this last feature is not fully acquired until stage 6.

One peculiar and highly frequent phrasal feature of Norwegian is the repetition of the subject as a pronoun in the right periphery, known as right dislocation. The children are using this feature in an adult-like manner from stage 4 and onwards, as seen in the following example:

(33) De har Porschebil de (Nora, 3;1.13)
They have.pres Porsche.car they
'They have a Porsche (type) car'

Relative clauses start to emerge at stage 3, but are not considered acquired until stage 4. Løver (2015) investigated their development applying a large set of variables, for example the number of different verbs, the structure of the matrix clause and the relative clause, the presence of the subjunction and the placement of sentence adverbials relative to the relative clause verb. Løver found that the development of relative clauses follows a very specific sequence for all children. The initial relative clauses are pragmatically useful and propositionally simple, meaning they only make use of either *be* or *have* in the matrix clause, or no matrix clause at all. There is little use of sentence adverbials, and the grammatical structure of the relative clause is predictable, as the children only use certain structures. Later, they develop on all these points. The constructions get more propositionally complex, and both the structures and the verbs get more diverse. Furthermore, although some children used more relative clauses than others, the sequence of development in itself displayed very little inter-children variation. However, at the point of being produced by 50% of the children at stage 4, the strongest characteristics of the relative clauses are i) that both the matrix clause verb and the relative clause verb to a much larger degree than before are highly lexical, i.e. the children use verbs of concrete observable activities (*cut* or *call)* or states (*lack*), rather than the abovementioned verbs, and ii) the children furthermore never omit the subjunction when it is optional. The first characteristic is a clear sign of development, the latter a non-target form property.

Here at stage 4, one of the children also uses a sentence adverbial within the relative clause, however with main clause word order (see example 41 below). This lends support to the proposal that relative clauses are in fact considered conjoined main clauses by the youngest children (Tavakolian, 1977), and thus have not reached their target form. It was however shown that this is not true for other subordinate structures, which exhibited target-like placement of sentence adverbials in subordinate clauses. This tendency is maintained and – as found in an enlarged set of data – strengthened throughout stage 5, but loses some terrain in stage 6. Not until stage 7 do we see a near target-language form in terms of placement of a sentence adverbial. In fact, Løver (2015) found that most of the variables that he investigated had reached their target form in stage 7.

Examples

Sentence level:
Questions:
QVS:
(34) Hva sier den? (Emil, 2;10.2)
What say.pres that?
'What does that one say?'
VauxSV(O):
(35) Kan du hente noen flere tog? (Magnus, 2;9.22)
Can you fetch.inf some more train.indef.pl.?
'Can you fetch some more trains?'
VauxSV(X):
(36) Skal vi se der? (Emil, 2;10.2)
Shall we look there?
'Shall we have a look there?'
VauxSVX(Y):
(37) Kan du legge babyen oppi der? (Anne, 2;11.17)
Can you put.inf baby.def-sg. up.in there?
'Can you put the baby in there?'

Statements:
Coordination:
(38) Nå må kattepusen gå hjem
Now must cat.pussy.def.sg go.inf home

og sove i senga si. (Emil, 2;10.2)
and sleep-inf in bed.def.sg its
'Now the pussycat has to go home and sleep in its own bed'
Conjunction:
(39) (…) og han er mellom og han er mellom og
(…) and he is middle and he is middle and

hun er stor. (Linnea, 2;9.15)
she is big
'and he is the middle one, and he is the middle one, and she is big'
Relative Clause:
(40) For de menneskene som er døde. (Tomas 2;9)
For the people.def.pl that are dead
'for the people who are dead'
(41) Her er pusekatten er ikke skummel (Ingrid, 2;10.28)
Here is pussy.cat.def is not scary
'Here is the pussycat, it is not scary'

Phrase level:
Inversion:
(42) Nå tar jeg flyet. (Ole, 2;8.5)
Now take I plane.def.sg
'Now I will take the plane'

Word level:
Past participle:

(43) Den er gjemt. (Ina, 2;6.26)
That is hidden
'That one is hidden'

At this forth stage there are no new imperative structures.

Figure 1.6 illustrates the section for stage 4 in the N-LARSP chart.

As mentioned above, this stage is characterized by an increase in syntactic complexity, which also leads to longer utterances. The 13 children forming the basis for this stage have an average MLU of 3.99 words.

Stage 4.	VauxSV(O)	QVS		Coord	Conj.	Inversion	Past participle
2;6-3;0	VauxSVX(Y)	VauxSV(X)		Relative	Right dis		

Figure 1.6 N-LARSP Stage 4

Stage 5 (3;0-3;6)

Only a few new features are considered acquired at stage 5, including VSO-questions and the combination of multiple adverbials. In addition, other subordinate constructions than relative clauses are acquired, mainly sentences beginning with the subjunction at 'that':

(44) Jeg så at den må også være med. (Thea 3;2.5)
I saw that it must also be with
'I saw that it/that one also had to be included'

(45) Den er så trøtt at de (interrupted) (Markus 3;2.13)
It is so tired that they
'it is so tired that they-' (Interrupted sentence)

Note that Thea's sentence in (44) follows the structure for main declarative clauses after the subjunction, with the adverbial *også* following the finite verb, and not the regular pattern for subordinate clauses, with the adverbial preceding the finite verb. Yet, in most cases the children at this stage follow the regular subordination pattern:

(46) Jeg så at den også må være med.
I saw that it also must be with
'I saw that it/that one also had to be included'

Other subordinate constructions, such as subordinate infinitive constructions, are not sufficiently documented in the material, and it is therefore not possible to give a detailed account of the acquisition patterns of these structures. When all types of subordinate clauses are taken together, they are acquired at stage 4. But on closer inspection it is clear that it is the frequent use of relative clauses that account for this early acquisition. It is therefore sensible to look at relatives separately from other kinds of subordinations. As we have seen, relatives are acquired at stage 4, while all other subordinate constructions taken together are acquired at stage 5.

Examples

Sentence level:
Questions:
VSO:

(47)	Har	de	sånn	her	hjul? (Markus, 3;2.20)
	Have	they	such	here	wheels?
	'Do they have these kind of wheels?'				

Commands:
VAdvAdv:

(48)	Se	her	da! (Oscar, 3;0.18)
	Look-imp	here	then!
	'Look here!'		

Statements:
Subordination:

(49)	Begynte	jeg	å	gråte. (Thea, 3;2.5)
	Begin.past	I	to	cry
	'[then] I started to cry'			

No new structures are emerging on the word level at this stage.

The section for stage 5 in the N-LARSP chart is illustrated in Figure 1.7.

The MLU at this stage has been calculated to an average of 4.52 words per utterance on the basis of 100 utterances from 11 children.

Stage 6 (3;6-4;6)

For stage 6 our data support the introduction of the following two constructions: It-clefts and object topicalizations. It-cleft is a sentence pattern in Norwegian used for a range of functions relating to information structure. They are introduced by a formal subject *det* 'it' (hence the name *it*-cleft) and copula, followed by the 'clefted constituent' which is the head of a relative clause.

Object topicalization (OVS) is a non-canonical sentence pattern in Norwegian entailing V2 (which was acquired already at stage 4), i.e. placement of the finite verb in second position. Since also adverbials and wh-phrases can be topicalized, object topicalization is a subtype of a more

Stage 5. 3;0-3;6	VSO	VAdvAdv	Subordination		

Figure 1.7 N-LARSP Stage 5

general pattern. All the same we have chosen to keep object topicalizations as a separate category as this is a high-frequent feature in Norwegian.

Examples

Sentence level:
Statements:
It-cleft:

(50) Det er de som klarer det. (Bjørn, 4;2.17)
It is they who manage it
'They are the ones that can do it'

OVS:

(51) Det liker jeg vel (Sara, 4;2.14)
That like.pres I well
'Of course I like that!'

Even at stage 6, some of the children make a few mistakes in gender assignment, as can be seen in (53) a. vs (53) b.

(52) a. En skjerf! (Bjørn, 4;2.17)
a.masc scarf!
'A scarf!'
b. Et skjerf (correct)
a.neutr. scarf
'A scarf'

At stage 6 these mistakes in gender assignment are exceptional, and the children that do make these mistakes most often seem to incorrectly assign a masculine gender marking to neuter nouns. Three of the children at stage 6 made in total eight gender assignment errors, of which six were neuter nouns inflected as masculine, and two masculine nouns inflected as neuter. By the next stage, stage 7, none of the children made erroneous gender assignments.

Figure 1.8 illustrates the section for stage 6 in the N-LARSP chart.

Recall that passive in Norwegian can be constructed either periphrastically by the use of *være* + *V* 'to be + V' or *bli* + *V* 'become + V', where V is a past participle, or as a morphological passive: *V+s*. At stage 6 four out of nine children start to use passive constructions, but not enough for them to be included in the chart. Only passive constructions with *bli* are found in the material:

(53) Og så var det en hai som ble stoppet ut. (Tomas, 3;10.14)
And then was it a shark that become.past stop.past part. out
'And then there was a shark that had been mounted'

Stage 6. 3;6-4;6			*it*-cleft OVS		

Figure 1.8 N-LARSP Stage 6

At this stage MLU from nine children was calculated to an average of 5.18 words per utterance.

Stage 7 (4;6+)

The last stage of the N-LARSP chart is structured differently than the other stages in the profile chart. At this stage the clinician or researcher is given space to comment on the child's discourse and syntactic comprehension. This final stage is similar to the seventh stage in the original LARSP profile for English.

A central feature at the discourse level is the use of introductory and connecting elements, such as vocatives (*du mamma […]* 'you, mom […]'), subjunctions (*hvis* 'if', *for/fordi* 'because', *for (at/å)* 'so that/in order to' etc.), or conjunctions (*og* 'and', *også* 'also', *men* 'but' etc.). Some examples follow.

(54)	Sånn	jeg	skal	sykle	fordi	at	jeg	skal	kjøre
	Such	I	shall	bike-inf	*because*	that	I	shall	drive-inf

sjakken	til	onkelen	min.	(Per, 4;8:23)
chess.def.sg.	to	uncle.def.sg	mine	

'Thus I will bike because I shall drive the chess to my uncle'

(55)	Vi	får	penger	hvis	vi	tar	flere	liv	av han. (Filip, 5;0:25)
	We get	money	if	we	take	more		life.indef.pl	of him

'We get money if we take more lives from him'

(56)	Hvis	den	lander	på	den	kan kongegrisen
	If	it	land.pres	on	it	can king.pig

angripe	deg. (Filip, 5;0.25)
attack.inf	you

'If it lands on that one, the king-pig can attack you'

(57)	Nå	skal	Pinky	her	for	å	leke	heks. (Sara, 4;7.22)
	Now	shall	Pinky	here	for	to	play	witch

'Now Pinky shall come here to play witch'

In the box for syntactic comprehension the clinician/researcher is expected to comment on how well the child understands the use of complex syntactic features such as passives or ambiguous sentences. Possible discrepancies between a structure used and the function or meaning of the structure should also be noted.

The section for stage 7 in the chart is illustrated in Figure 1.9.

	Discourse			Syntactic comprehension
	Initiators			
	Vocative	Conjunction	Subjunction	
Stage 7. 4;6 +				

Figure 1.9 N-LARSP Stage 7

The average MLU for this last stage is 6.13, calculated on the basis of 100 utterances from nine children.

Rest

At the bottom of the chart we have included space for the clinician or investigator to note down comments about the child's language use, similar to the summarizing line 'comments' in the original LARSP profile by Crystal *et al.* (1989).

Any other complex utterances that do not fit into any previous category can be noted down here, or comments about the children's communicative skills. In short, this section is included to give the therapist room to note down issues that are not addressed in the chart, but that can be seen as relevant for each child's individual syntactic and communicative profile.

Figure 1.10 shows the final section for summarizing comments in the N-LARSP chart.

	Rest	Rest

Figure 1.10 N-LARSP Rest section/summarizing lines

Challenges

The above sections outline how the Norwegian LARSP profile came to be, how it looks and which features that are expected to be observed at each stage by typically developing Norwegian children. However, this cannot be considered the whole truth about Norwegian children's language acquisition, as we have based our design on a relatively small set of utterances from a few children.

A more thorough validation is needed, where larger utterance samples from more children are examined.

Basing a language profile on spontaneous speech has some clear advantages, not least in terms of ecological validity. However, it also entails some challenges. During the development of the N-LARSP we see that some structures are not sufficiently documented when we restrict our material to 100 utterances per child, and that other structures are close to the 50% threshold for acquisition for several stages in a row before being counted as acquired. In certain cases this leads to confusion about the inclusion criteria, as some children who might have produced a feature on level 4 were no longer among the children we examined at level 5. This can be exemplified with the question structure QVSAdv that was first documented by two children at stage 4. At stage 5 the structure is produced by five children, but would have to be produced by at least six children for it to be considered acquired. At level 6 the feature still does not reach the 50% threshold, as the children who produce this feature at the two preceding stages are not subject of investigation at the later stages. The feature is thus documented on several levels, but is not marked as acquired at all in this version of the N-LARSP. It is reasonable to assume that children who produce a given structure at one level will also do this at a later stage, but we have no evidence to support this.

It is also difficult to know how to account for the huge dialectal variation observed in the material, as it is near impossible to make a dialect neutral profile chart for Norwegian. In our initial data we included children from the north of Norway as well as children from the south-eastern part of Norway. As the latter dialect area is the largest in the country it is reasonable to base the chart on the dialect spoken there, and language therapists and researchers making use of the chart should be aware that children from other dialect areas may use other structures than the ones noted in the chart, or that the included structures might not be applicable in all dialect areas.

Conclusion

The purpose of this chapter has been to outline the Norwegian version of the LARSP profile chart, and describe the steps undertaken to develop this chart. The proposed N-LARSP profile is a well-defined developmental profile describing prominent features of both morphology and syntax for typically developing Norwegian children.

Although N-LARSP describes a vast amount of different grammatical milestones throughout the child's development, there should be no doubt that the N-LARSP profile does not give justice to the complete grammatical complexity a child has knowledge of at each given stage. However, this challenge may be mitigated by constructing micro-profiles – a more thorough description of a particular stage; e.g. Garman (1979), or the development of a particular grammatical property; e.g. Fletcher (1979) and Fletcher and Frizelle (2016). As of now, two micro-profiles are available for Norwegian; one that goes in depth on the acquisition of verbal inflection (Strand, 2015), and one that examines the acquisition and use of relative clauses (Løver, 2015). In view of the huge variability seen among the children on and between each stage, it should be an aim to construct other micro-profiles in the future.

In the development of this profile chart for Norwegian, we have kept to the requirement that 50% of the children at each stage should use a certain feature for it to be included at a given stage. Yet we see that some issues (i.e. gender inflection) remain problematic until the later stages. This is indicative of the possibilities that lie within using the LARSP to investigate particular acquisition patterns in detail.

We do not believe that this proposal for an N-LARSP chart should necessarily be an end state of LARSP in Norwegian. Rather, clinical and/or theoretical applications of the chart may require modifications to the selection of syntactic and morphological variables and give new insight into their order of acquisition.

Furthermore, the profile chart should be tested and validated on a larger sample of children, both typically developing children and children with specific language impairment (SLI). It is also of scientific interest to assess bilingual children's syntactic abilities in both or all their languages, if a LARSP profile is available in those languages. This being said, we are convinced that this proposal is an important stepping-stone and a useful tool for Norwegian speech and language therapists.

Notes

(1) Just before finalizing this chapter the LARSP profile for Swedish (SweLARSP) was published (Rosenberg & Mellenius, 2016). As Swedish and Norwegian are very similar languages, it would have seemed natural to model the Norwegian adaptation of LARSP on the Swedish one, but as the latter was not available to us when we started working on the Norwegian profile, we have modeled our LARSP chart mainly on the English and Dutch profile charts.

(2) Some dialects have a two-gender, common–neuter declension system, where the common gender corresponds to masculine.

(3) Norwegian has two passive forms, the morphological passive exemplified here, and an analytic passive with the auxiliary *bli* 'become' and a passive participle (e.g. *bli kastet*). The morphological passive is less frequent and is only used in the present tense. In the child data collected here, only the *bli*-passive was found – although not in enough children to count as acquired.

(4) Since the category of degree will not be in focus in what follows, it is not included here.

(5) It is possible that this is due to dialect variation; however, recent investigations concerning subordinate *at* ('that')-sentences with *ikke* in adults across Norwegian dialects indicate that in these sentences both V2 and V3 are found to an equal amount (Kristine Bentzen, personal communication). Thus variation in adult input may also influence children regarding the placement of *ikke* in subordinate sentences.

(6) In some cases it is also necessary to listen for word tone realizations, in particular for children who do not pronounce /r/. In those cases, word tone may be the only way to distinguish between infinitive and present tense in strong verbs (Simonsen, 1986; Strand, 2015).

(7) From the context it is reasonable to assume that the child used 'there' in the sense of 'put it there'.

References

Anderssen, M. (2005) *The Acquisition of Compositional Definiteness in Norwegian.* Department of Language & Linguistics/Castl, University of Tromsø.

Ball, M., Crystal, D. and Fletcher, P. (2012) *Assessing Grammar: The Languages of LARSP.* Bristol: Multilingual Matters.

Bol, G.W. (2012) Gramat: A Dutch adaptation of LARSP. In M. Ball, D. Crystal and P. Fletcher (eds) *Assessing Grammar: The Languages of LARSP.* Bristol: Multilingual Matters.

Bol, G.W. and Kuiken, F. (1988) *Grammatical Analyse Van Taalontwikkelinsstoornissen.* PhD thesis, University of Amsterdam.

Bol, G.W. and Kuiken, F. (1990) Grammatical analysis of developmental language disorders: A study of the morphosyntax of children with specific language disorders, children with hearing impairment and children with Down's Syndrome. *Clinical Linguistics and Phonetics* 4, 77–86.

Crystal, D., Fletcher, P. and Garman, M. (1976) *The Grammatical Analysis of Language Disability: A Procedure for Assessment and Remediation*. London: Edward Arnold.

Crystal, D., Garman, M. and Fletcher, P. (1989) *Grammatical Analysis of Language Disability* (2nd edn). London: Cole And Whurr.

Endresen, R.T. and Simonsen, H.G. (2001) The Norwegian verb. In R.T. Endresen and H.G. Simonsen (eds) *A Cognitive Approach to The Verb: Morphological and Constructional Perspectives*. Berlin: Mouton De Gruyter.

Eng, H. (1944) *Dr. Parrs Dagbok Over Utviklingen Av Sine Barns Tale*. Hamar, Norway: Pedagogisk Forskningsinstitutt.

Fletcher, P. (1979) Micro-profile of the stage III verb phrase. In D. Crystal (ed.) *Working with LARSP*. London: Edward Arnold.

Fletcher, P., Ball, M. and Crystal, D. (2016) *Profiling Grammar: More Languages of LARSP*. Bristol: Multilingual Matters.

Fletcher, P. and Frizelle, P. (2016) Complex sentences in developmental and impairment: stage V revisited. In P. Fletcher, M. Ball and D. Crystal (eds) *Profiling Grammar: More Languages of LARSP*. Bristol: Multilingual Matters.

Garman, M. (1979) Micro-profile of stage I. In D. Crystal (ed.) *Working with LARSP*. London: Edward Arnold.

Johannessen, J.B. (2013) Two imperative types in all the Scandinavian languages. *The 25th Scandinavian Conference on Linguistics*. Reykjavik, Iceland.

Kristoffersen, K.E. and Simonsen, H.G. (2012) *Tidlig Språkutvikling Hos Norske Barn: MacArthur-Bates Foreldrerapport For Kommunikativ Utvikling*, Oslo, Novus.

Lie, S. (1992) Ka Du Sei? *Maal Og Minne* 1, 62–77.

Løver, M.A. (2015) The Ontogenesis of Relative Clauses in Preschool Children Acquiring Norwegian. MA thesis, University of Oslo.

Max Planck Institute for Psycholinguistics, T.L.A. (2008) *Elan*. Nijmegen, The Netherlands.

Plunkett, K. and Strömqvist, S. (1992) The acquisition of Scandinavian languages. In D.I. Slobin (ed.) *The Crosslinguistic Study of Language Acquisition*. Hillsdale, New Jersey: Lawrence Erlbaum.

Ragnarsdóttir, H., Simonsen, H.G. and Plunkett, K. (1999) The acquisition of past tense morphology in Icelandic and Norwegian children: An experimental study. *Journal of Child Language* 26 (3), 577–618.

Rosenberg, M. and Mellenius, I. (2016) Swe-LARSP: A grammatical profile of Swedish. In P. Fletcher, M. Ball and D. Crystal (eds) *Profiling Grammar: More Languages of LARSP*. Bristol: Multilingual Matters.

Simonsen, H.G. (1983) *En Norsk Femårings Språkbruk: Syntaktiske Mønstre, Struktur Og Funksjon*, Oslo, Novus.

Simonsen, H.G. (1986) Om Toåringers Fonologi – System Og Prosesser. In P.E. Mjaavantn, and L. Smith (eds) *Barnespråk*. Trondheim, Norway: Navfs Senter For Barneforskning.

Simonsen, H.G. (1990) Barns Fonologi: System Og Variasjon Hos Tre Norske Og Et Samoisk Barn. PhD Thesis, University of Oslo.

Simonsen, H.G., Kristoffersen, K.E., Bleses, D., Wehberg, S. and Jørgensen, R.N. (2014) The Norwegian communicative development inventories: Reliability, main developmental trends and gender differences. *First Language* 34, 3–23.

Sloetjes, H. and Wittenburg, P. (2008) Annotation by category – Elan And Iso Ddcr. Sixth International Conference on Language Resources (Lrec 2008).

Strand, B.-M.S. (2015) 'Jeg Lese Denne' – Root Infinitives in Norwegian Child Language and the Functions of Finiteness. MA thesis, University of Oslo.

Tavakolian, S.L. (1977) Structural Principles in The Acquisition of Complex Sentences. PhD thesis, University of Massachusetts, Amherst.

Vanvik, A. (1971) The phonetic-phonemic development of a Norwegian child. *Norsk Tidsskrift for Sprogvidenskap* 24, 269–325.

Westergaard, M. and Bentzen, K. (2007) The (non-)effect of input frequency on the acquisition of word order in Norwegian embedded clauses. In I. Gülzow and N. Gagarina (eds) *Frequency Effects in Language Acquisition: Defining the Limits as An Explanatory Concept*. Berlin/New York: Mouton De Gruyter.

Westergaard, M.R. (2003) Word Order in wh-questions in a North Norwegian dialect: Some evidence from an acquisition study. *Nordic Journal of Linguistics* 26, 81–109.

Westergaard, M.R. (2005) *The Development of Word Order in Norwegian Child Language: The Interaction of Input and Economy Principles in the Acquisition of V2*. Department of Language and Linguistics, University of Tromsø.

Appendices

I. N-LARSP profile chart

<table>
<tr><td colspan="2">Name:</td><td colspan="2">Age:</td></tr>
<tr><td colspan="2">Date of birth:</td><td colspan="2">Therapist:</td></tr>
<tr><td colspan="2">Date of recording:</td><td colspan="2">Comments:</td></tr>
<tr><td colspan="4">A. Unanalysable utterances</td></tr>
<tr><td colspan="2">Incomprehensible:</td><td colspan="2">Incomplete:</td></tr>
<tr><td colspan="2">Deviant:</td><td colspan="2">Ambiguous:</td></tr>
<tr><td colspan="2">Minor:</td><td colspan="2">Repetitions:</td></tr>
<tr><td colspan="4">B. Analysable utterances</td></tr>
<tr><td colspan="2">Total number of utterances</td><td colspan="2">MLU:</td></tr>
</table>

<table>
<tr><td>Stage 1.
1;0-1;6</td><td colspan="3">N</td><td colspan="3">V</td><td colspan="2">Other</td></tr>
<tr><td></td><td colspan="6">Sentence</td><td>Phrase</td><td>Word</td></tr>
<tr><td></td><td colspan="2">Question</td><td colspan="2">Command</td><td colspan="2">Statement</td><td></td><td></td></tr>
<tr><td>Stage 2.
1;6-2;0</td><td colspan="2"></td><td>V</td><td>Adv</td><td>AdvX</td><td>NegX</td><td>NP [-Poss]</td><td>Def.sg</td></tr>
<tr><td>Stage 3.
2;0-2;6</td><td>Q(X)</td><td>VS(X)</td><td>VX</td><td>VO(X)</td><td>SV
VX
SVO</td><td>VO
SVAdv
SVauxV</td><td>NP [+Poss]
Pers.pron
Copula
Vaux+V</td><td>Pres Past
Compound</td></tr>
<tr><td>Stage 4.
2;6-3;0</td><td>VauxSV(O)
VauxSVX(Y)</td><td>QVS
VauxSV(X)</td><td colspan="2"></td><td>Coord
Relative</td><td>Conj.
Right dis</td><td>Inversion</td><td>Past participle</td></tr>
<tr><td>Stage 5.
3;0-3;6</td><td colspan="2">VSO</td><td colspan="2">VAdvAdv</td><td colspan="2">Subordination</td><td></td><td></td></tr>
<tr><td>Stage 6.
3;6-4;6</td><td colspan="2"></td><td colspan="2"></td><td colspan="2">it -cleft
OVS</td><td></td><td></td></tr>
</table>

<table>
<tr><td rowspan="4">Stage 7.
4;6 +</td><td colspan="3">Discourse</td><td>Syntactic comprehension</td></tr>
<tr><td colspan="3">Initiators</td><td rowspan="3"></td></tr>
<tr><td>Vocative</td><td>Conjunction</td><td>Subjunction</td></tr>
<tr><td></td><td></td><td></td></tr>
<tr><td></td><td colspan="3">Rest</td><td>Rest</td></tr>
</table>

II Word list

Adv	adverb
Conj	(any) conjunction
Coord	coordination
Compound	(any) compound
Copula	clause with copula verb (*være*)
Def.sg.	definite singular
It-cleft	cleft sentence (with expletive *det*)
N	noun
Neg	negation (*ikke*)
NP $[_{+poss}]$	possessive noun phrase
NP $[_{-poss}]$	noun phrase (not possessive)
O	object
Pers.pron	personal pronoun
Pres	present tense
Past	past tense
Q	*wh*-word
Relative	(any) relative clause
Right.dis	right dislocated subject
S	subject
Subordination	(any) subordination
V	verb
Vaux	auxiliary verb
X	any clausal element
Y	any clausal element
(…)	optional clausal element

2 Developing a Linguistic Profile for Russian

N. Gabriela Moffatt and Nicole Müller

A cursory inquiry into the existing inventory of assessments available for Russian speakers revealed an unexpected dearth of Russian-specific assessment instruments. Reports from US-based clinicians suggest a tendency to use standard American tests such as (PPVT,[1] EOWPVT, CELF, PLS, etc.), with caveats about how these tests are interpreted. A critical point is that standardized tests often lose validity and reliability once they are appropriated for use with culturally and linguistically diverse children (Caesar & Kohler, 2007). Caruso *et al.* (2015) outline best practice assessment procedures for linguistically diverse individuals, emphasizing that evaluation reports should be 'comprehensive and qualitative in their analysis of the client's/patient's performance and not rely solely on results produced by [standardized, norm-referenced tests],' and 'should provide a clear visual picture of the individual's strengths and weaknesses' (2015: 16).

Russian is the eighth most common L1, with about 171 million first language speakers in 17 countries (Lewis *et al.*, 2016). This number reflects decades of compulsory Russian language education throughout the former Soviet Bloc, as well as ethnic Russians who found themselves outside of Russian borders following the collapse of the Soviet Union in 1991 and continue to thrive there today. The dearth we note is of Russian-specific assessments that exists despite this considerable number of speakers.

That is not to presume that Russian clinicians necessarily welcome ready-made assessment tools. Western observations of speech pathology in the (former) USSR are keen to note a different tradition of assessment that de-emphasizes standardized, norm-referenced tests (Barten & Blank, 1971; Mitchell, 1973) in favour of qualitative, descriptive approaches drawing from multiple reports, informants and observations. Alternatively, factors relating to negative views of disability in Russia (Gaines, 2004), with reports of abuse (Prescott, 2017), corruption and a disinclination to use resources to support more than the basic, life-sustaining needs of children (Templeman, 2004), could also account for the lack of assessment instruments, especially where they concern communication needs that would by implication presuppose cognitive potential in children who present with 'intellectual disability' from birth (Y. Pleshivoy, personal communication, 17 February 2018).

Recent decades, however, have seen an academic and practical interest in the development of Russian receptive and expressive language assessment tools. Sasha Yampolsky (1996) developed a pilot for a Russian version of the Peabody Picture Vocabulary Test as part of a thesis project. The Assessment of the Development of Russian (*Otsenka razvitiya russkogo iazyka* – ORRIA; Babyonyshev *et al.*, unpublished manuscript, 2007) and the Test of Morphological Awareness (Kornilov *et al.*, 2012) are other recent advancements. Elleseff (2014) created the Russian Articulation Screener and the Assessment of Sound and Syllable Imitation in Russian-speaking Infants and Toddlers, which also provides general language development milestones. Eliseeva *et al.* (2016) adapted the MacArthur Communicative Development Inventory (CDI) for infants and toddlers (Fenson *et al.*, 1993).

Excepting the Screener and the Russian version of the MacArthur CDI, these assessments do not appear readily available for clinical use. Additionally, it is unclear whether norm-referenced, standardized assessments for Russian would be embraced by the Russian speech therapy community. Therapists who need to reference test scores already do, namely by translating common English-based tests, with caveats about their use and interpretation with non-English-speaking populations. This practice is supported by a recent claim that a translated version of the Preschool Language Scales, 5th edition (Zimmerman *et al.*, 2011) was a valid and reliable measure of language abilities in a single Russian-speaking bilingual child (Zhukova *et al.*, 2016). Supposing this is true of many other language tests such as the PLS-5, it is likely that norm-referenced, standardized test measures would still only occupy a small role in the entire assessment procedure, with other factors and methods being ascribed equal if not greater significance. What might be useful, though, is an instrument referencing the developmental course for Russian grammatical structure. This type of tool could support clinicians working with Russian-speaking clients by affording them a profile-like reference against which interpretation of findings from naturalistic assessment could be made.

The Language Assessment, Remediation and Screening Procedure (LARSP) is a tool that generates a profile of grammar usage for speakers of English, but it has been successfully adapted for several languages very different from English in syntax and morphology (Ball *et al.*, 2012; Fletcher *et al.*, 2016; see also this volume). LARSP profiles provide a descriptive approach that allows patterns of strengths and weaknesses to emerge from individual clinical samples (Crystal, 1982; Crystal *et al.*, 1989). The profiles are based on the speaker's performance during naturalistic speaking tasks, such as in conversation and narration of wordless storybooks. As such, it aligns with best practices in language assessment for culturally and linguistically diverse populations. A LARSP profile for Russian (RuLARSP) could be seamlessly incorporated into the evaluation procedures of clinicians who already collect conversational language samples as one part of assessment. Eventually, a Russian LARSP could be used in the process of creating an updated developmental reference appropriate for the clinical setting while contributing to the body of literature on Russian language development in children. This chapter describes the development of a Russian version of the LARSP for this purpose, with the hope that it may find utility in the assessment procedures of Russian-speaking clinicians working with Russian-speaking clients.

Descriptive Sketch of Russian Grammar

In this outline of Russian, we will highlight the linguistic properties and terms pertinent to the discussion of Russian developmental grammar. This outline is guided by a variety of reference grammars, but mostly follows the topical progression found in Cubberly's (2002) linguistic introduction to Russian and borrows many of its examples. In this section we address syntax and morphology.

When using example clauses in Russian, constituents will be tagged for categories according to the paradigm in Table 2.1. Prepositions, adverbs, interrogative pronouns, numerals and particles are not tagged but translated. Broad phonemic transcriptions are provided in accordance

Table 2.1 Tagging conventions for nouns, adjectives, verbs and pronouns

Gender	Masculine = masc Feminine = fem Neuter = neut
Number	Singular = s Plural = pl
Case	Nominative = nom Accusative = acc Genitive = gen Dative = dat Instrumental = inst Prepositional = prep
Person	First person singular, First person plural = 1s, 1p Second person singular, Second person plural = 2s, 2p Third person singular, Third person plural = 3s, 3p Infinitive = inf
Tense	Past = past Present or future = nonpast
Aspect	Imperfective = imp Perfective = perf

to the IPA system as illustrated for Russian by Yanushevskaya and Bunčić (2015), who follow the system established by the St. Petersburg school of phonology (see Iosad (2018) for a brief history of and distinctions between the St. Petersburg and Moscow schools of phonology).

We start by providing an illustrative sentence borrowed from Paperno and Sylvester's (1987) book on situational dialogues:

(1) Где мне найти профессора, который ведёт грамматику в американской группе? (p. 57)

Гдé	мнé	найти́	профéссора,	котóрый
gdʲe	mnʲe	najˈtʲi	praˈfʲesara	kaˈtorɨj
where	me.1s.dat	find.perf-inf	professor. masc.s.acc	who.masc.s.nom

ведёт	граммáтику	в	америкáнской	грỳппе?
vʲiˈdʲot	graˈmatʲiku	v	amʲirʲiˈkanskaj	ˈgrupʲi
lead.imp-3s.nonpast	grammar. fem.s.acc	in	American- fem.s.prep	group- fem.s.prep

'Where can I find the professor who teaches grammar to the American group?'

This example contains several key features of Russian grammar, including three of its six cases, use of gender and agreement between nouns and adjectives, impersonal constructions, verb inflection and mutation, and grammatical aspect.

Syntax

Russian's system of inflectional morphology indicates the relationships between sentence constituents, so while constituent order has relative freedom, it does seem to be influenced by a number of factors, including whether there is added emphasis to any element of the sentence, and whether the information being expressed is new or given (Launer, 1974). For example, an interrogative clause in Russian may lead with the object of inquiry at the beginning of the sentence, while the declarative clause in answer to that interrogative clause may have the most important information at the end. For another example, recall that attributive (long form) adjectives generally precede nouns; it is when they follow the nouns that they are considered extremely emphatic (Launer, 1974). In Russian, the neutral element order is SVO (Bailyn, 2001; Cubberly, 2002).

The Subject

In the Subject–Predicate binary, the subject 'refer[s] to a major constituent of sentence or clause structure, traditionally associated with the "doer" of an action' (Crystal, 2008: 461). Cubberly (2002) makes the following generalization: 'For Russian [...] we may state the basic (default) situation to be as follows: nominal subjects are in the Nominative; verb subjects are in the Infinitive; and the subject comes first,' (2002: 186). The verbal subject is achieved similarly to how it is done in English, with the verb phrase containing a verb in infinitive form at the beginning of the clause and often corresponding to the verbal noun in English. See the following examples from Cubberly (2002):

(2)

Переводи́ть	э́тот	текст	без
pʲirʲivaˈdʲitʲ	ˈetat	tʲekst	bʲes
translate.pf-inf	this.masc.s.acc	text.masc.s.acc	without

словаря́	тру́дно. (p. 189)
slavaˈrʲa	ˈtrudna
dictionary.masc.s.gen	difficult

'To translate this text without a dictionary is difficult.'

(3)

Кури́ть	запрещено́. (p. 190)
kuˈrʲitʲ	zaprʲiʃʲːiˈno
smoke.imp-inf	forbidden.neut.s.nom

'Smoking is prohibited.'

Zero subjects also occur in Russian, *because* verbs can inflect for person in the non-past (and therefore technically express personal pronouns inside the verb). In cases where the context is clear, this feature extends to gender and number in past tense forms as well (Cubberly, 2002). Finally, zero subjects occur in examples dealing with natural phenomena such as weather, where English uses 'it' or 'there' (as in, 'it's cold'), and in contexts with generalized subjects. See the following examples from Cubberly (2002):

(4) Холодно. (p. 189)
ˈxoladna
cold.neut.s.nom.short
'It's cold.'

(5)

Здесь	хорошо	работается. (p. 189)
zdʲesʲ	xaraˈʃo	raˈbotajit͡sa
here	well	work.imp-nonpast.refl

'One can work here well.'

The Predicate

The predicate in Russian refers to the verb, any complements bound to it and excluding the object and any adverbial modifiers (Cubberly, 2002). Therefore, the predicate is concerned with 'aspect, tense, mood, voice and number, plus either person (non-past forms) or gender (past forms)' (Cubberly, 2002: 190). This further includes expansions of the verb with stylistic particles and reinforcing verbs, as well as compound verbal predicates and compound nominal predicates, though aspect, tense, number and person have been addressed in earlier sections of this overview, so here we describe mood and predicate phrases.

Grammatical mood

Russian uses various means to express mood, mostly through the use of the particle бы /bɨ/ in a number of different constructions. For example, the conditional mood is formed by combining the conditional clause (если бы /ˈjeslʲi bɨ/ + past tense of the verb) with the main clause (past tense of the verb + бы /bɨ/).

(6) Éсли бы	я	былá	ры́бой,
ˈjeslʲi bɨ	ja	bɨˈla	rɨˈboj
If *part*	I.1s.nom	was.imp-past.fem	fish.fem.s.inst

я	плáвала	бы	в	океáне.
ja	ˈplavala	bɨ	v	akʲiˈanʲi
I.1s.nom	swam.imp-past.fem	*part*	in	ocean.fem.s.loc

'If I were a fish, I would swim in the ocean.'

Conditional meanings can also be expressed using the imperative or by using the preposition без /ˈbʲez/ – 'without', with the particle бы /bɨ/. The subjunctive is rendered using чтобы /ˈʃtobɨ/ plus either a past tense verb or the infinitive of the verb, depending on whether there is a different subject for each verb.

Compound verbal predicates

Compound verbal predicates consist of a main verb in the infinitive form preceded by an inflected modal or phrasal auxiliary verb (Cubberly, 2002). Modal verbs express the speaker's attitude toward the main verb using finite forms of words such as мóчь /ˈmot͡ʃʲ/ – 'be able/can', умéть /uˈmʲetʲ/ – 'be able/can/know how', and хотеть /xaˈtʲetʲ/ – 'want'; using дóлжен /ˈdolʒɨn/ – 'must/ought/should' plus быть /ˈbɨtʲ/ – 'to be' plus short-form adjectives; and through impersonal constructions.

Compound nominal predicates

The compound nominal predicate in Russian includes phrases where the verb joins the subject with a complement, the same as the copula does in English, to express existential, equational, and locational states of 'being' (Cubberly, 2002). That is, the copula achieves these effects:

i. Nadine is **a child**. (equational)
ii. Nadine **is in the room**. (locational)
iii. **There is a child** in the room. (existential)

The Russian verb бы́ть /ˈbɨtʲ/ – 'to be' can achieve these effects, but not as uniformly as English 'is'. In the equational example, бы́ть /ˈbɨtʲ/ does not have a present tense in Modern Russian but does conjugate regularly for future and past tenses. The zero present is followed by the noun in nominative form, while future and past are followed by the noun in instrumental case.

(7)	Наде́жда	–	ребёнок.
	naˈdʲeʒda		rʲiˈbʲonak
	Nadine.fem.s.nom	Ø	child.masc.s.nom
	'Nadine is a child.'		

(8)	Наде́жда	была́	младе́нцем.
	naˈdʲeʒda	bɨˈla	mlaˈdʲent͡sɨm
	Nadine.fem.s.nom	was.imp-past.fem	infant.masc.s.inst
	'Nadine was an infant.'		

(9)	Наде́жда	бу́дет	шко́льницей.
	naˈdʲeʒda	ˈbudʲit	ˈʃkolʲnʲit͡sɨj
	Nadine.fem.s.nom	will-be.imp-nonpast.3s	schoolchild.fem.s.inst
	'Nadine will be a schoolchild.'		

Other forms that perform copular functions include бывáть /bɨˈvatʲ/ – 'to be' (with connotation of regularity) and явля́ться /jaˈvlʲat͡sa/ – 'to be' (formal written style) (Cubberly, 2002).

Zero copula бы́ть /ˈbɨtʲ/ in the present tense holds true for locational uses as well.

(10)	Наде́жда		в	ко́мнате.
	naˈdʲeʒda		f	ˈkomnatʲi
	Nadine.fem.s.nom	Ø	in	room.fem.s.prep
	'Nadine is in the room.'			

(11)	Наде́жда	была́	в	ко́мнате.
	naˈdʲeʒda	bɨˈla	f	ˈkomnatʲi
	Nadine.fem.s.nom	is.imp-past.fem	in	room.fem.s.prep
	'Nadine was in the room.'			

In existential contexts, the present tense of быть is есть – 'to be'. This static form is the original 3rd person singular conjugation for быть and it is used only in present tense (Cubberly, 2002). It is common in constructions for possession and establishing the existence of something in a specific location (Cubberly, 2002), though the form can also be seen in questions, definitions, and contexts where the verb is heavily emphasized (Wade, 2011). Notice how the topic of the sentence below consists of the locational phrase, while the 'new' information appears in the comment. See (12) below for a second example.

(12)	В	кóмнате	есть	ребёнок.
	f	ˈkomnat^{j}i	jes^{j}t^{j}	r^{j}iˈb^{j}onak
	in	room.fem.s.prep	is.imp-nonpast.3s	child.masc.s.nom
	'In the room there is a child.'			

The topic of a sentence may correspond to the grammatical subject of a sentence, but there is no fixed map between these concepts and the clause's structure. Generally, Russian is a topic-first, comment-last language (Cubberly, 2002; Nakhimovsky & Leed, 1987), meaning that the most important information of the clause is usually found at the end of it. Russian features topicalization in sentences, which occurs when 'a constituent is moved to the front of a sentence, so that it functions as topic' (Cubberly, 2002: 488). This occurrence is consistently found within frequently occurring clause structures. For example, the clause, 'У меня есть книга' demonstrates grammatical subject that does not coincide with topic.

(13)	У	меня́	есть	кни́га.
	u	m^{j}iˈn^{j}a	jes^{j}t^{j}	ˈkn^{j}iga
	by	me.1s.gen	is.imp-3s.nonpast	book.fem.s.nom
				Grammatical Subject
	Topic		Comment	
	'I have a book.'			

The complement

The complement is the 'nominal (or post-copula) part' that follows the copula in a compound nominal predicate, and may take the form of a noun phrase, adjectival phrase, passive participles, or non-adjectival attributes (Cubberly, 2002: 210). Noun phrases in the present tense, as mentioned earlier, are kept in the nominative case. In past and future tense, they may be in instrumental case, depending on the permanence of the status or attribute, the same way long- and short-form adjectives connote enduring versus transient qualities. Past passive participles, by virtue of their always representing a limited attribute, are naturally short in these constructions. Non-adjectival attributes include those that use genitive constructions ('rodents of unusual size'), prepositional phrases ('she is from Ipanema'), and conjunctional phrases expressing comparison ('I'm like a bird').

Object

An object is a major constituent in a clause, and Russian uses three objects: direct object, indirect object and double direct object (Cubberly, 2002).

Direct objects in Russian normally take the accusative case, though instances of genitive case usage are possible and can express partitive meaning or the absence or denial of the object, or objects that are hypothetical (Cubberly, 2002).

The indirect object in a clause may be indicated by the dative, instrumental, or genitive case as well as some constructions requiring prepositions and their own associated cases. The use of dative case expresses the traditional sense of indirect object, that it is the recipient of the action expressed by the verb, as in English. An indirect object in instrumental case demonstrates a relational meaning to the direct object, while a small number of reflexive verbs require indirect objects to be governed by the genitive case, but are considered rare (Cubberly, 2002).

The double direct object functions as 'a further definition of the first', so it has a relational meaning to the direct object and therefore is governed by the instrumental case (Cubberly, 2002: 222). In the following sentence, 'Nadine' is the double direct object.

(14)	Мы	назва́ли	до́чку	Наде́ждой.
	mɨ	na'zvalʲi	'dot͡ʃʲku	na'dʲeʒdaj
	we.1p.nom	name.perf-past.pl	daughter.fem.s.acc	Nadine.fem.s.inst
	S	V	O_d	O_{dd}

'We named our daughter Nadine.'

Morphology

Russian accounts for case, grammatical gender, number and tense through a system of inflectional markers. There may be several possible endings for a given word, depending on which configuration of these elements is being expressed. Though Russian has a robust number of inflections, it is true that some of them appear and sound the same as others, requiring additional information from other words in a sentence or context to accurately discern the function of an inflected word that would be otherwise ambiguous.

Case

There are the six main cases in the Russian grammatical system: nominative, accusative, genitive, dative, prepositional/locative, and instrumental. Nominative case expresses the subject of a sentence, as well as the form found in the dictionary. Accusative case expresses the direct object in a sentence, as well as duration, motion and destination. Genitive case expresses possession, negation, separation, absence, and partitive nuances of some words. Dative case expresses the indirect object or recipient in a sentence and can indicate movement and general direction. Prepositional/Locative case is used only with prepositions and nearly always concerns locational meanings. Instrumental case expresses how an action is carried out in a sentence, which can be an abstract concept. In prepositional phrases, instrumental case can indicate the use of an object, as well as some locational concepts.

Gender

There are three grammatical genders in Russian: masculine, feminine and neuter. In nominative case, masculine nouns end in a hard consonant, though some do not (such as words for male relatives, like па́па /papa/ – 'papa', and nouns ending in -тель /t^{j}il^{j}/, like преподава́тель / pr^{j}ipada'vat^{j}il^{j}/ – 'instructor'). These are declined following the same patterns as feminine nouns, but they agree with masculine adjectives and verbal inflection. Most nouns ending in -а, -я and -ь in the nominative case are feminine, like ма́ма /'mama/ – 'mama', тётя /'t^{j}ot^{j}a/ – 'aunt', and цель /t͡sel^{j}/ – 'goal', while most nominative case nouns that end in -о and -е and all nouns ending in -ё are neuter.

Number

Russian has singular and plural forms. Singular words fit into semantic classes of abstract (e.g. 'sadness'), collective (but singular, e.g. 'mankind'), uncountable mass (e.g. 'milk'), or names.

Pronouns

Like other languages, Russian uses two different registers of address to indicate respect or familiarity. This is accomplished by its T and V forms of 'you'. The T form, used in the informal register between familiar persons (friends, family), is the 2nd person singular, ты. The V form (used with superiors, strangers) appears the same as 2nd person plural, вы. The formal register is also indicated in verb conjugation by the use of the 2p verb form in singular contexts.

(15)	1s	я	/ja/
	2s	ты	/tɨ/
	3s	о́н/она́/оно́	/on/ /a'na/ /a'no/
	1p	мы	/mɨ/
	2p	вы	/vɨ/
	3p	они́	/a'n^{j}i/

Pronominal declension of personal and non-personal pronouns requires gender and number agreement with respect to verbs and modifiers.

The inflectional system also applies to pronouns. See Table 2.2 for a summary of first and second person pronouns by case and Table 2.3 for a summary of third person personal pronouns by gender, number and case. Some of these forms are ambiguous without context, as they are identical to other case forms, especially feminine pronouns. This is true of case endings for adjectives, too. The addition of 'н' is added to pronouns when preceded by a preposition.

Adjectives

Qualitative adjectives have two forms: long and short. The short form can be used in the predicative position only, whereas the long form may

Table 2.2 First and second person pronouns by case

Case	Pronouns			
	1s	2s	1p	2p
Nominative	я /ja/	ты/tɨ/	мы /mɨ/	вы /vɨ/
Acc./Gen.	меня́ /mʲiˈnʲa/	тебя́ /tʲiˈbʲa/	нас /nas/	вас /vas/
Prepositional	мне /mnʲe/	тебе́ /tʲiˈbʲe/	нас /nas/	вас /vas/
Dative	мне /mnʲe/	тебе́ /tʲiˈbʲe/	нам /nam/	вам /vam/
Instrumental	мно́й /mnoj/	тобо́й /taˈboj/	на́ми /ˈnamʲi/	ва́ми /ˈvamʲi/

Table 2.3 Third person personal pronouns in Russian by case, gender and number

Case	Masc. S.	Fem. S.	Neuter S.	Plural
Nominative	он /on/	она́ /aˈna/	оно́ /aˈno/	они́ /aˈnʲi/
Acc./Gen.	(н)его́ /jiˈvo/	(н)её /jiˈjo/	(н)его́ /jiˈvo/	(н)их /ix/
Prepositional	нём /nʲom/	ней /nʲej/	нём /nʲom/	них /nʲix/
Dative	(н)ему́ /jiˈmu/	(н)ей /jej/	(н)ему́ /jiˈmu/	(н)им /im/
Instrumental	(н)им /im/	(н)ей /jej/	(н)им /im/	(н)и́ми /ˈimʲi/

Note. The н- is added to personal pronouns when they follow prepositions.

be in either the predicative or attributive position, but is most often in the regular attributive position. The message intent determines which form is used. Short-form adjectives are used for temporary or situation-specific qualities, whereas long adjectives refer to constant or general qualities.

(16)	Она́	– краси́вая	де́вушка.
	aˈna	kraˈsʲivaja	ˈdʲevuʃka
	she.3s.fem.nom	beautiful-fem.s.nom	girl.fem.s.nom
	‘She is a beautiful girl.’		

In example (16), the message is about an ongoing nature of the attribute, not specific to one instance but an enduring quality. The long-form adjectival ending here is marked for feminine singular nominative, as indicated by the -ая /aja/ ending attached to the word stem красив-. In example (17) below, there is specific context, or instance, in which ‘she’ was noted to be beautiful, so the short-form adjective is used, as indicated by the -а ending added to the красив- /kraˈsʲiv/ stem.

(17)	На	вечери́нке	она́	была́	так	краси́ва.
	na	vʲit͡ʃʲiˈrʲinkʲi	aˈna	bɨˈla	tak	kraˈsʲiva
	at	party.fem.s.prep	she.3s.fem.nom	was.imp-fem.past	so	beautiful-fem.s.nom
	‘At the party she was so beautiful.’					

The long form consists of a stem and appropriate ending that agrees in number, case and gender with the word it is modifying. However, short-form adjectives exist only in nominative form with endings indicating gender and number only, e.g. -Ø for masculine, -а for feminine, -о for neuter and -ы or -и for plural. A vowel is inserted where the masculine zero ending would result in a consonant cluster at the coda, so the long-form adjective близкий /ˈblʲiskʲij/ ('near') would be shortened thus: бли́з**ок** /ˈblʲizak/ (masc.), близк**а́** /ˈblʲiska/ (fem.), бли́зк**о** /ˈblʲiska/ (neut.) and бли́зк**и** /ˈblʲiskʲi/ (pl.). Notice how feminine and neuter endings are indistinguishable in the transcription, as unstressed /o/ reduces to /a/.

Aspect

Crystal (2008) defines aspect as the grammatical category that describes 'the way the grammar marks the duration or type of temporal activity denoted by the verb' (2008: 38). In Russian, aspect is often explained in terms of the contrast between imperfective and perfective verbs. The imperfective is used where aspect is irrelevant (a simple statement of fact) or when the emphasis is on a process, repetition, duration or habit. The perfective emphasizes completion and implies a resulting state. It also emphasizes the point of onset of the action itself. Verbs occur in pairs where a logical aspectual distinction can be made, often denoted using prefixes, though internal modification of a verb can also achieve aspectual pairing, as in the verbs забыва́ть /zabɨˈvatʲ/ (imperfective) and забы́ть /zaˈbɨtʲ/ (perfective), meaning 'to forget.' Some perfective–imperfective verb pairs are minimal pairs distinguished only by word stress, as in the example, среза́ть /srʲiˈzatʲ/ (imperfective) and сре́зать /ˈsrʲezatʲ/ (perfective) 'to cut down.' Aspectual pairs sometimes derive from different roots. For example, иска́ть /iˈskatʲ/ – 'to search' is the process and its aspectual complement is найти́ /najˈtʲi/ – 'to find', because it entails completion or result. Some verbs inherently imply one aspect or the other and therefore cannot be in a pair (such as рабо́тать /raˈbotatʲ/ – 'to work', which is a process and therefore only imperfective).

Tense

Only imperfective verbs have a present tense, while the present tense form of perfective verbs semantically signifies the perfective future (intent to complete). Verb conjugation typically follows one of two patterns, depending on the ending of the stem in the infinitive form. See Table 2.4 for the conjugation patterns for regular verbs.

The past tense form is -л- /l/ plus one of the four gender/number markers (masc. -Ø; fem. -а; neut. -о; pl. -и /i/ or -ы /ɨ/), which replace the non-finite ending. Sometimes the result would be a phonotactically unacceptable consonant cluster, in which case no special ending is added. See Table 2.5 for examples of past tense. Observe how, again, feminine and neuter endings are indistinguishable when the final vowel is unstressed.

Table 2.4 Regular present tense verb conjugation patterns

Form	Conjugation type			
	I		II	
Infinitive	чита́ть 'to read'	/t͡ʃʲiˈtatʲ/	говори́ть 'to speak'	/gavaˈrʲitʲ/
1s. – 'I'	чита́**ю**	/t͡ʃʲiˈtaju/	говор**ю́**	/gavaˈrʲu/
2s. – 'you'	чита́**ешь**	/t͡ʃʲiˈtajiʃʲ/	говор**и́шь**	/gavaˈrʲiʃʲ/
3s. – 'she/he/it'	чита́**ет**	/t͡ʃʲiˈtajit/	говор**и́т**	/gavaˈrʲit/
1p. – 'we'	чита́**ем**	/t͡ʃʲiˈtajim/	говор**и́м**	/gavaˈrʲim/
2p. – 'You all'	чита́**ете**	/t͡ʃʲiˈtajitʲi/	говор**и́те**	/gavaˈrʲitʲi/
3p – 'they'	чита́**ют**	/t͡ʃʲiˈtajut/	говор**я́т**	/gavaˈrʲat/

Note. 2nd person plural appears the same for V-form 2nd person singular.

Table 2.5 Examples of past tense verb formation

Infinitive	Masc. S.	Fem. S.	Neut. S.	Plural
нести /nʲiˈsʲtʲi/ – 'to carry'	нёс-Ø /ˈnʲos/	несла́ /nʲiˈsla/	несло́ /nʲiˈslo/	несли́ /nʲiˈslʲi/
читать /t͡ʃʲiˈtatʲ/ – 'to read'	чита́л /t͡ʃʲiˈtal/	чита́ла /t͡ʃʲˈtala/	чита́ло /t͡ʃʲˈtala/	читали́ /t͡ʃʲˈtalʲi/
говорить / gavaˈrʲitʲ/ – 'to speak'	говори́л /gavaˈrʲil/	говори́ла /gavaˈrʲila/	говори́ло /gavaˈrʲila/	говори́ли /gavaˈrʲilʲi/

*Irregular verb.

Both imperfective and perfective verbs can be used in the past tense. Negation of imperfective verbs in past tense indicates that the action did not take place (was not initiated), while negation of the perfective verb indicates that the action was started but not completed (Wade, 2011). Similarly, the imperfective future focuses on the process, while perfective future focuses on the completion.

Word formation

Russian derivational morphology consists of three main types of word-building: affixation (prefixes and suffixes), compounding, and abbreviations (Cubberly, 2002). We limit our focus to affixation, as that bears greater relevance to early Russian than other means. Affixation is the joining of a bound morpheme to a lexical root or stem. Russian primarily uses prefixes and suffixes to derive new words. Prefixes occur at the beginning of a word, and therefore can only cause semantic changes (as opposed to changing a word's part of speech), as they do not impact the syntactic functions of inflectional endings by nature of their positioning (Townsend, 1975). Prefixes historically derive from prepositions, many of which are still in use in Modern Russian (their basic meanings are provided in parentheses, but their exact nuance can shift depending on context): в /v/ (in), из /iz/ (out of), на /na/ (on), с /s/ (with, from), у /u/ (by, from), к /k/ (to, towards), от /ot/ (from), до /do/ (until), за /za/ (behind), to list a few. In verbs, prefixes are used to derive the perfective form from the imperfective form.

In this grammatical sketch of Russian, we touched on several aspects of the language that may be of special interest in the discussion of early acquisition. Specifically, we discussed categories that are represented in the inflectional system, though we also introduced features that are of interest to other researchers in the Russian developmental literature, such as topicalization.

Grammatical Acquisition in Russian

A preliminary Russian profile chart

Following from this analysis of Russian grammar, and from examination of classic and recent studies of Russian first language acquisition (especially Gvozdev's diary study, as brought together in his 1949 publication and further descriptions of that work in Slobin (1966) and El'konin (1973); Gagarina (2003, 2008), Gagarina and Voeikova (2009,) Babyonyshev (1993), and the descriptive works of Ceytlin (2000, 2009)), the first author (Moffatt, 2018) drew up a preliminary chart of structures at the two- and three-element levels for clauses and phrases (labelled stages II and III in the English LARSP chart). Once structures were tentatively placed into developmental stages based on this earlier work, there were still gaps in the profile, especially where it concerned phrase structures. In contrast, there were excessive numbers of prepositions and conjunctions represented in the profile, creating a visual and practical imbalance. Too many individual items within these categories could impact the profile's clinical utility by obscuring patterns for the sake of detail, while diminishing the space available for other developmentally informative structures.

In order to produce a more user-friendly profile chart, further child language data in the CHILDES database was accessed, and the resultant analyses are discussed in the next section.

The CHILDES data

As a next step in the construction of the RuLARSP profile chart, the first author analysed the currently available longitudinal child language data in the CHILDES database (MacWhinney, 2000). The Russian child language datasets in the CHILDES database originated from studies by Protassova (1997) and Bar-Shalom and Snyder (1997), whose work and naturalistic data contributions have provided a basis for many ideas concerning Russian acquisition in the developmental literature (see also Bar-Shalom, 2002; Gleason *et al.*, 2010; Janssen, 2014; Kallestinova, 2007;

McCoy, 2003). The children in these collections are Varya and Tanya. Varya's recordings span the age range 1;6 to 2;10, and Tanya's from 2;5 to 2;11. Varya is regarded in the developmental literature as a precocious early talker (Polinsky, 2006), while Tanya (a pseudonym) demonstrates language skills consistent with Russian heritage speakers, such as relatively rigid word order, low and late use of oblique cases, and the use of English words (O. Glotova, personal communication, 2018). A detailed analysis of the language samples in the CHILDES database is presented in Moffatt (2018), and we do not have space here to present these. However, to illustrate the process, the stages of acquisition for two different patterns are shown: two-element prepositional phrases, and personal pronouns.

Two-element phrases containing preposition + noun and preposition + pronoun appeared in both children's speech. Tables 2.6 and 2.7 depict the frequency these phrase types in the first 400 utterances for each sample in both corpora.

The use of personal pronouns by both children is reported in Tables 2.8 and 2.9. In the timeframe from age 1;8 to 2;0, Varya increased her use of first and third person pronouns, though she had been using them consistently before then. Tanya saw a gradual increase in her use of first and third person pronouns from 2;9 to 2;11.

Varya exhibited incremental increases in 1st person pronoun use until age 1;10, when she nearly doubled their frequency, despite the large difference in sample sized from 1;8 to 1;10, suggesting the increase was even more dramatic. Her productive use of that pronoun category appeared to have started at around 1;7 and stabilized later. Tanya appeared to use 1st person pronouns sporadically until around 2;10, when she also significantly increased her use of them. The first person pronoun category encompasses all case forms: я – *ja* 'I', меня – *menja* 'me', and мне – *mnje*

Table 2.6 Two-element prepositional phrases: Varya

				Varya			
Age	1;6	1;7	1;8b	1;10	2;0	2;4	2;10
Utterances	400	400	400	400	400	400	400
PREP N	13	5	16	21	37	30	24
PREP PR	2	0	5	8	18	14	22

Table 2.7 Two-element prepositional phrases: Tanya

				Tanya			
Age	2;5	2;6	2;7	2;8	2;9	2;10	2;11
Utterances	233	304	195	302	123	400	400
PREP N	13	24	32	45	26	53	30
PREP PR	1	0	1	2	3	15	18

Table 2.8 Personal pronouns: Varya

	Varya						
Age	1;6	1;7	1;8b	1;10	2;0	2;4	2;10
Utterances	405	400	400	400	400	400	400
PRONP1S	1	2	5	39	66	61	38
PRONP2S	1	2	3	5	21	14	24
PRONP3S	17	9	6	40	22	33	13
PRONP1P	0	0	1	2	6	1	6
PRONP2P	0	0	0	0	0	0	1
PRONP3P	1	1	5	2	5	12	9

Table 2.9 Personal pronouns: Tanya

	Tanya						
Age	2;5	2;6	2;7	2;8	2;9	2;10	2;11
Utterances	233	304	195	302	123	400	400
PRONP1S	0	2	2	2	9	19	14
PRONP2S	0	0	0	0	0	1	1
PRONP3S	0	5	12	5	5	11	31
PRONP1P	0	0	1	1	1	2	9
PRONP2P	0	0	0	0	0	0	0
PRONP3P	1	0	0	4	3	2	10

'me', as do all the other pronoun categories listed in these tables. The order in which pronouns appeared to stabilize seemed to be as follows:

Personal Pronouns: 3S → 1S → 2S → 3P → 1P → 2P (Varya)
Personal Pronouns: 3S → 1S → 3P → 1P → 2S → 2P (Tanya)

Both children demonstrated later learning of 2nd person singular pronouns compared to their other learned pronouns (there were actually zero instances in Tanya's corpus, possibly due to limited exposure as a heritage learner), with 3rd person singular appearing to have stabilized first. The 2nd person plural pronoun appeared only late for Varya. Varya was consistent in her use of 1st person plural pronouns, but their rate was comparatively low in her corpus. Tanya increased her use of these pronouns by 2;11.

These analyses fed into the choice of structures at the clause, phrase, and word levels of the profile chart for Russian (see Figure 2.1). The developmental stages on the chart lack specific age ranges, to avoid the pitfalls of making assumptions about chronological age where we simply do not have enough data. Further work is needed to properly populate the Stage V tier and beyond.

Name	Age	Sample Date	MLUw	Notes:
Unanalyzed Unintelligible	Symbolic Noise	Deviant	No. Utterances	
Problematic Incomplete	Ambiguous	Stereotype	Interaction Type	

	MAJOR		**MINOR** Responses		Vocatives	Other			
Stage I	Conn	Quest	Comm	Statements	Phrases	Words: V	Words: N	Words: Pr	Prep:
			'V'	V N A	Adjective NN Aux Neg Ø	ROOT Inf.	ROOT Nom.pl	Pron: 3S	в(о)
Stage II	*a* *u*	'Q' Q	'V'$_{INF}$ VI	AA SV VA SA VC SC VO Other	Prep N Neg X DN VV надо/нельзя PPPAST Other	3S -ла	Acc -у Gen -ы Prep -е Dat -е	1S Acc/Gen Dat	у/на для/из
Stage III	*c*	QX	VI.X Давай	X+S:NP X+A:AP SVO AVO SVA VOO SVC VCA Other	X+V:VP X+O/C:NP Prep Pr Num Aux V Neg V надо/нельзя V Other	1S -л 1P -ли	Gen -а Ins -ом Dat -у	3P 1P 4+	к(о) с(о)
Stage IV	*c* *s* Other	QXY Other	Пусть Other	XY+S:NP XY+A:AP SVOA SVOO SVAA SVOC AAVO Other	XY+V:VP XY+O/C:NP Adjective N Adjective Adjective N Other	3P F.A. -ло 2S	Inst -ой Prep -ах Inst -ами Gen -ов	2S Inst 2P Prep	под по
Stage V		Emphatic Order		XYZ+S:NP XYZ+A:AP	XYZ+V:VP XYZ+O/C:NP Num N N/Pr c N/Pr N Prep N Num (Adjective) N Neg X Neg Y	2P	Gen Ø Dat -ам		

Figure 2.1 The RuLARSP chart

A departure from the original LARSP is the expanded focus on pronouns. Crystal *et al.* (1989) address only two kinds of pronouns: those that act as the head of a noun phrase and those that do not. In the early stages, this approach has been considered as well, but it was found that it would either obscure too much information or, if used in conjunction with other codes for pronouns, add too much burden to the process of profiling itself. Our stance from the beginning has been to find the most economical set of codes that yielded the most useful information. To this end, the total number of initial pronoun codes was ultimately increased because they demonstrated to be developmentally informative in the small sample size. It was also decided to incorporate the nonpersonal pronouns as a group subsumed under the '4+' item in the column, rather than focus on individual pronoun types within the category. Interrogatives are not included in that group, as they are indicated elsewhere in the chart under the 'Questions' heading. Finally, a way to consider the application of case to pronouns as a category itself was examined, because the pronouns have their own declension patterns and it would be unwieldy to tease out, for example, when a child had acquired the dative feminine demonstrative pronoun. The profile includes them in a dedicated column (Word: Pr) within the Word section.

A tentative order of preposition acquisition was derived from the CHILDES data, and this is shown in the Prep column in the rightmost position in the chart. The Word section of the chart has three columns: the leftmost for verbal morphology (Words: V), to the right of that a column for nominal morphology (Words: N), and finally the pronoun morphology already referred to.

Another difference between RuLARSP and the original profile chart for English is the omission of tally boxes for ellipticals. Russian uses a high degree of elision, and it did not seem practical to count all occurrences of elliptical phenomena. They are counted in isolated constructions (NEG Ø, НАДО/НЕЛЬЗЯ), but otherwise any further consideration of ellipticals would result in a busy set of boxes before one gets to read the main part of the chart itself. For this same reason, we did not code for nominative case at all. Nominative is the default of any noun or pronoun, and counting it simply would have overwhelmed the process of coding and counting for users of the profile. The word 'Nom' was included in the 'Words: N' column to show the developmental pattern, but this may have been an unnecessary and potentially confusing inclusion in an already burgeoning category box. Rather, it might be beneficial to alter the code to 'Nom.pl' to allow for a place to count nominative-only plurals.

A box for MLUw has tentatively been placed in the top portion of the chart. Having used the profile on multiple samples, we can see the utility of this measure in the implementation of the profile. The use of metrics such as MLU is not widely practiced in Russia (the Russian MacArthur CDI being an exception), and literature on Russian language development refers to it very little. But it is practiced elsewhere where the chart in its current form may find use (i.e. in the West). We found the metric more helpful than chronological age when comparing children's profiles. Beneath the MLUw box, there are now boxes to display other practical information about the sample, such as the total number of utterances the child produced and the type of interaction during which the sample was collected. Narratives, for example, might result in more frequent use of 3rd person pronouns and past tense forms.

Following the analysis of the CHILDES data, the first author applied the profile of Figure 2.1 to new child data that she had collected. For the purpose of profiling, boxes were added to the top of the chart, following the model of the revised LARSP (Crystal *et al.*, 1989). The profile now includes spaces to count unanalysable and problematic structures. This includes unintelligible utterances, symbolic noise, deviant structures, as well as incomplete, ambiguous and stereotyped structures. The overall shape of the profile is wider than it is long, creating empty space in the top right corner. This space may be used later when the profile is expanded for use with children who operate at stage V and beyond.

New data

We present here just four of the 11 participants described in Moffatt (2018), choosing those which best illustrate a progression in terms of grammatical acquisition. Each sub-section that follows, therefore, is about one participant in the cohort. The information presented here about each child is taken from a basic information and language development survey that was completed by a parent. In the survey, parents were asked for basic health history, family composition and for parental impressions about their child's receptive and expressive language use. In the following sections, summaries of the information that these families provided are included, followed by a completed profile of the language sample. The age of the children at the time of sampling is shown in the years; months format and the first initial of their name is used as an identifier.

Z 1;7

Z was a 19-month-old boy living with his parents and grandparents in a southwestern province in the Russian Federation. The family reported that the only language spoken in the home was Russian and that every member of the household was monolingual. Z was reported to be in good health at birth with no history of ear infections. His parents estimated that he could say 20 to 40 words and felt that he could understand what people said to him. His parents reported that he began talking at 1 year of age, and they believe his language is like that of his peers. The total recording time was 41 minutes and consisted of different periods of unstructured play between mother and child. Z's MLUw was calculated to be 1.11. Figure 2.2 depicts Z's profile for this sample. His utterances consisted of single elements, mostly nouns. He did produce verb roots and one clear imperative, 'дай!' – *daj* 'give'. He produced frequent unintelligible utterances and used a significant amount of onomatopoeia to interact with his mother. At the time of language sampling, Z appeared to be operating primarily at the stage I level, because of his use of a handful of single-element statements, vocatives, and root forms of words. He did use the imperative form, though this may have been rote learnt.

Z's age of 1;7 would be appropriate for a child operating at stage I if we compare across languages. However, one would expect a move into more stage II structures shortly with this child.

T 2;0

T was an only child who lived with his monolingual Russian-speaking family in a southwestern province in the Russian Federation. He was born at 41 weeks and had no reported birth complications. His parents reported that he used between 20 and 40 words and could form simple sentences, though he might answer questions with single words. They reported that T did not have trouble expressing himself, but other people would have difficulty understanding him. They reported he had recently improved his intelligibility and that could answer simple WH-questions. The recording lasted for 32 minutes and consisted of shared pre-literacy activities. Figure 2.3 depicts the profile for this sample. T produced numerous single-element statements and few comprising two elements. He also produced questions and used the imperative form. However, the command he used was the same word expressed multiple times, suggesting it may have been rote learnt. T used adjectives, though not in phrases yet. He also produced a DN structure a couple times, as well as used negation to express the absence of an object. He did not use any personal pronouns, but did use two other demonstrative pronouns. In this sample, T was still producing many root words for nouns and verbs, but had also begun using case inflection on nouns using accusative and genitive. In the sample, T seemed to be operating primarily at stage I, though with early development of stage II structures, and with mixed skills at the word level.

In this respect, T, at age 2;0, would be considered slightly delayed if the age ranges of stages I and II of the English LARSP (Crystal *et al.*, 1989) were applied. However, his acquisition of some case endings suggests his morphology is perhaps somewhat in advance of his syntax, an observation that would be consistent with the Gagarina's (2003) notion that 'morphological richness ... compensates for the syntactic poverty (and vs)' (2003: 135).

M 2;7

M was living with her family in a north-eastern province of Ukraine with her mother, father, older sister and grandmother. The parents reported that they were bilingual Russian-Ukrainian but stated that they only used Russian in the home. M was born at term with no reported complications at birth or any reported history of ear infections. Her parents

Name "Z"	Age 1;7	Sample Date	MLUw 1.11	Notes:
Unanalyzed Unintelligible 41	Symbolic Noise 24	Deviant	No. Utterances	
Problematic Incomplete	Ambiguous	Stereotype	Interaction Type	Repetitions 17

	MAJOR		**MINOR** Responses 2	Vocatives 3	Other
Stage I	Conn	Quest	Comm	Statements	Phrases
			'V'	V N 5 A	Adjective NN Aux Neg Ø
Stage II	a u	'Q' Q	'V'INF VI 1	AA SV VA SA VC SC VO Other	Prep N Neg X DN VV надо/нельзя PPPAST Other
Stage III	c	QX	VLX Давай	X+S:NP X+A:AP SVO AVO SVA VOO SVC VCA Other	X+V:VP X+O/C:NP Prep Pr Num Aux V Neg V надо/нельзя V Other
Stage IV	c s Other	QXY Other	Пусть Other	XY+S:NP XY+A:AP SVOA SVOO SVAA SVOC AAVO Other	XY+V:VP XY+O/C:NP Adjective N N/Pr c N/Pr Adjective Adjective N Other
Stage V		Emphatic Order		XYZ+S:NP XYZ+A:AP	XYZ+V:VP XYZ+O/C:NP D Adjective N N Prep N Neg X Neg Y Other

Words: V	Words: N	Words: Pr	Prep:
ROOT 3	ROOT 6		в(о)
Inf	Dim.	3S	у/на
3S	Nom.pl	1S	для/из
-ла	Acc -у	Acc/Gen	к(о)
1S	-ин	Dat	с(о)
-ся	Gen -ы	3P	под
-л	Prep -е	1P	по
1P	Dat -е	4+	
-ли	Gen -а	2S	
3P	Ins -ом	Inst	
F.A.	Dat -у	2P	
-ло	Inst -ой	Prep	
2S	Prep -ах		
2P	Inst -ами		
	Gen -ов		
	Gen Ø		
	Dat -ам		

Figure 2.2 RuLARSP profile: Z 1;7

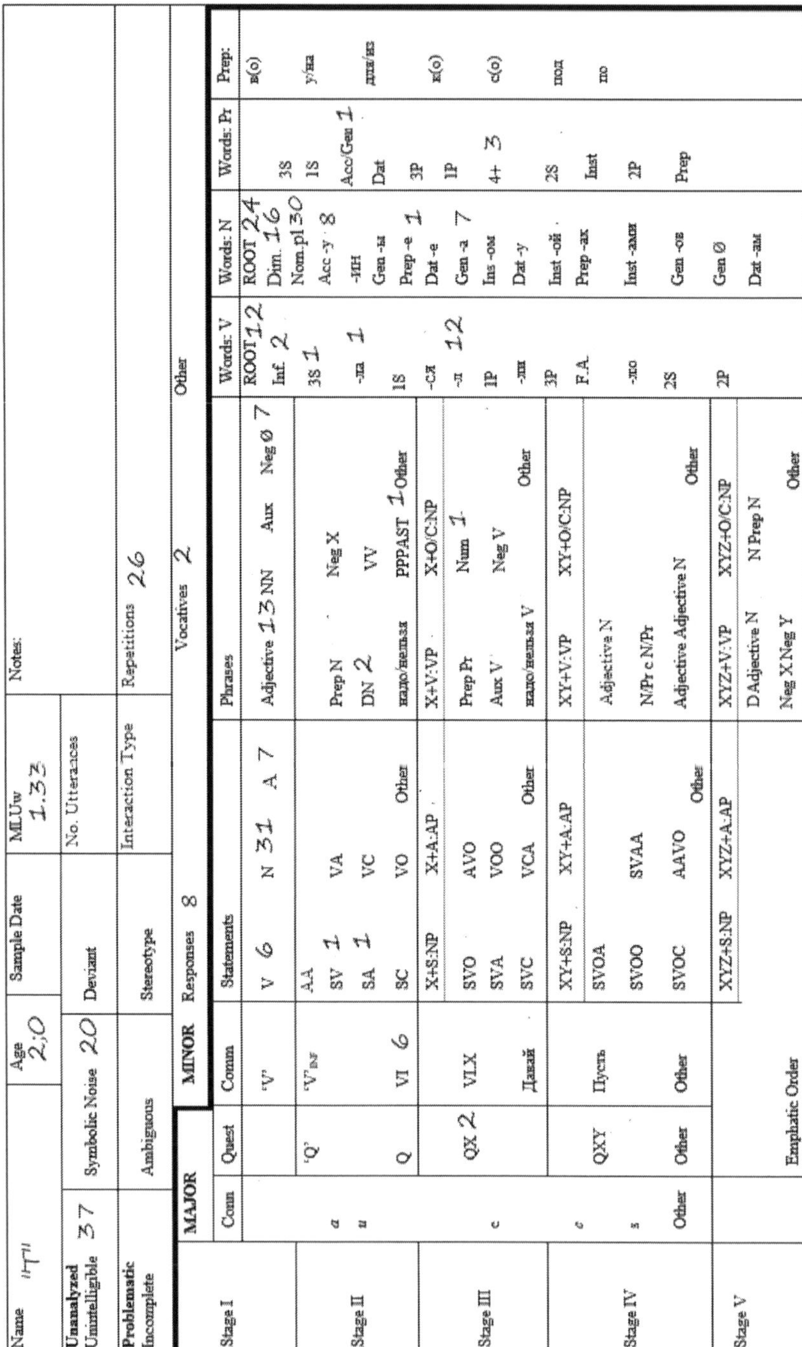

Figure 2.3 RuLARSP profile: T 2;0

estimated that she had an active vocabulary of greater than 100 words and could form sentences. The total recording time was 50 minutes and consisted of shared pre-literacy activities. M's MLUw was calculated to be 3.35. Figure 2.4 depicts the profile for this sample. M's sample featured an extensive spread into two- and three-element clauses and stage IV phrases, as well as expansions at every tier. She used a variety of case endings, verb inflections, and pronouns. However, some of these higher frequencies are due to the fact that M said 'я не знаю' /ja nʲi ˈznaju/ – 'I don't know' 58 times in her sample. This brings to light an important consideration for the RuLARSP. In the English version, the sentence 'I don't know' is considered a stereotype, because it cannot be ascertained that the child is using it productively. The decision was made to code these instances, because they demonstrate so many grammatical categories. It may be the case that 'I don't know' in Russian must also be labelled as a stereotype, to avoid inflating or overestimating the child's skills. If this had been done, the profile would have fewer instances of certain structures (such as SV at the clause level, neg V at the phrase level, 1s pronoun, etc.) but the overall spread would still suggest someone moving into stage IV.

M, at age 2;7, and at the beginning of stage IV, would be similar in age to the suggested age range of Crystal *et al.*'s (1989) English LARSP stage IV; though, of course, it must be borne in mind that the ages are averages, and some children will progress somewhat more quickly and others more slowly through the stages.

P 4;0

P was an only child living with her mother, father and grandmother in a north-eastern region in Ukraine. Her parents reported that they only spoke Russian in the home, but they themselves were bilingual and P was attending a Ukrainian preschool. No health issues at birth or history of ear infections were reported for P. P began talking at around 1;0 and her family had had concerns about her language development. At the time of data collection, the parents said P was capable of forming sentences, but others would only sometimes be able to understand her. They reported feeling that she had come a long way and wondered if she would need speech therapy. The recordings totalled 24 minutes over two sessions and consisted of shared preliteracy activities and unstructured conversation between mother and child. P's MLUw was 3.17. Figure 2.5 depicts the profile for P for this language sample.

At the clause level, P produced clause types at stage II, III and IV, although her overall number of clauses was relatively low. She demonstrated phrase patterns at these levels too, producing a variety of phrases, some of which were not originally on the profile. At the word level, P demonstrated that she could use the different cases in singular contexts, but produced relatively fewer examples of plural nouns with case. She produced a variety of prepositions, as well. She did not produce the full range of pronouns in this sample.

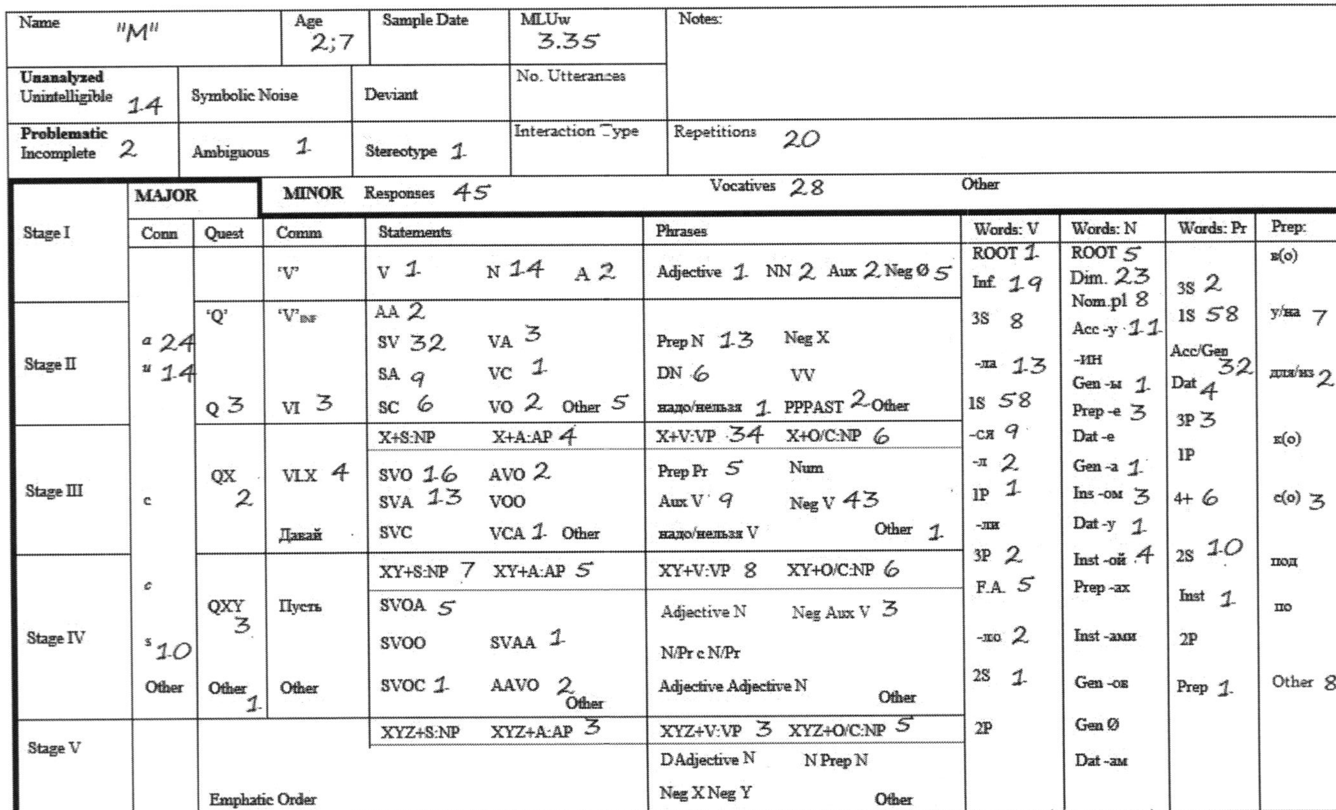

Name "M" | Age 2;7 | Sample Date | MLUw 3.35 | Notes:
Unanalyzed Unintelligible 14 | Symbolic Noise | Deviant | No. Utterances
Problematic Incomplete 2 | Ambiguous 1 | Stereotype 1 | Interaction Type | Repetitions 20
MINOR Responses 45 | Vocatives 28 | Other
MAJOR

	Conn	Quest	Comm	Statements	Phrases	Words: V	Words: N	Words: Pr	Prep:
Stage I			'V'	V 1 N 14 A 2	Adjective 1 NN 2 Aux 2 Neg Ø 5	ROOT 1 Inf. 19 3S 8	ROOT 5 Dim. 23 Nom.pl 8	3S 2	в(о)
Stage II	а 24 и 14	'Q' Q 3	'V'INF VI 3	AA 2 SV 32 VA 3 SA 9 VC 1 SC 6 VO 2 Other 5	Prep N 13 Neg X DN 6 VV надо/нельзя 1 PPPAST 2 Other	-ла 13 1S 58	Acc -у 11 -ин Gen -ы 1 Prep -е 3	1S 58 Acc/Gen 32 Dat 4 3P 3	у/на 7 для/из 2
Stage III	с	QX 2	VLX 4 Давай	X+S:NP X+A:AP 4 SVO 16 AVO 2 SVA 13 VOO SVC VCA 1 Other	X+V:VP 34 X+O/C:NP 6 Prep Pr 5 Num Aux V 9 Neg V 43 надо/нельзя V Other 1	-ся 9 -л 2 1P 1 -ли	Dat -е Gen -а 1 Ins -ом 3 Dat -у 1	1P 4+ 6	к(о) с(о) 3
Stage IV	с s 10 Other	QXY 3 Other 1	Пусть Other	XY+S:NP 7 XY+A:AP 5 SVOA 5 SVOO SVAA 1 SVOC 1 AAVO 2 Other	XY+V:VP 8 XY+O/C:NP 6 Adjective N Neg Aux V 3 N/Pr с N/Pr Adjective Adjective N Other	3P 2 F.A. 5 -ко 2 2S 1	Inst -ой 4 Prep -ах Inst -ами Gen -ов	2S 10 Inst 1 2P Prep 1	под по Other 8
Stage V		Emphatic Order		XYZ+S:NP XYZ+A:AP 3	XYZ+V:VP 3 XYZ+O/C:NP 5 D Adjective N N Prep N Neg X Neg Y Other	2P	Gen Ø Dat -ам		

Figure 2.4 RuLARSP profile: M 2;7

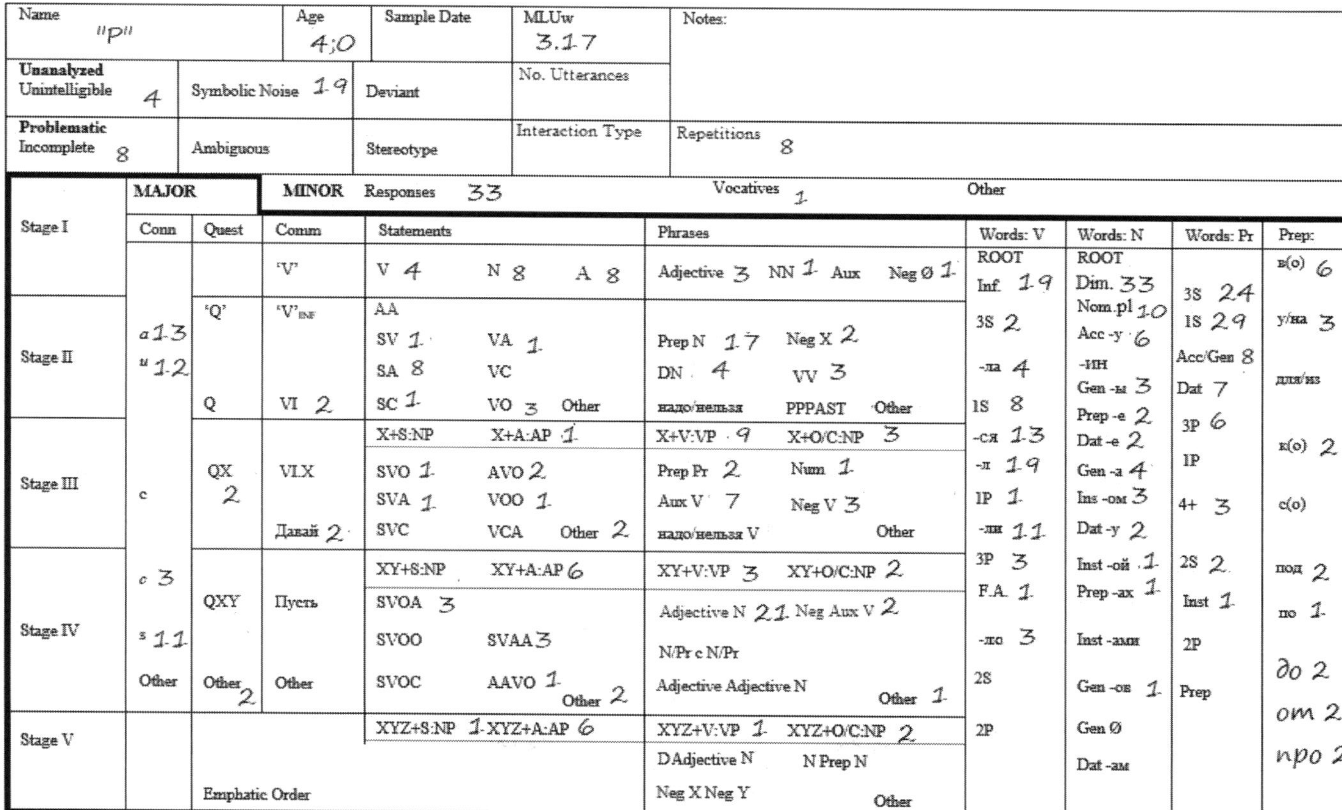

Figure 2.5 RuLARSP profile: P 4;0

P, therefore, is a good example of a child who has a virtually complete first four stages. At age 4;0, this would be somewhat older than one would expect for an English child (though the English child would have had a much simpler inflectional morphology to acquire). The addition in future of studies of older children will show whether the recursion stage in Russian is shorter than in English to balance the morphology.

Conclusion

This study was limited by the relatively small number of participants whose language samples were profiled using the new tool, which restricts the overall making of generalizations about developmental stages of Russian acquisition. Most of the participants were monolingual, but some of them lived in bilingual communities, though their families maintained Russian-language dominance in the home. While the CHILDES corpora were longitudinal, the new child data were cross-sectional. This made it difficult to make generalizations about a single child's level of skill. It would be beneficial to see how the profile tracks development in six-month intervals.

The age range of the CHILDES dataset was also a limiting factor. The two children were under three years old, and this set the upper limit on stages that could be arranged in the profile. The first four stages of the profile may therefore be used to examine the language of early Russian learners but does not deal with complex grammar and discourse markers that may appear in older children and adults. Nor does it address errors. Furthermore, because the profile is based on a limited set of child data, it is not intended to be used in isolation or to justify the application of diagnostic labels. Rather, it is meant to supplement other forms of assessments and contribute to an overall descriptive portrait of a child's language skills. Studies focusing on older children and adults are needed to establish the latter stages of the profile, especially the development of recursion. Russian children acquire forms relatively early but take several years to complete their systems. Therefore, the chart should be expanded to accommodate maturation of systems and identify incomplete acquisition.

In conclusion, we hope to have expanded the knowledge base about early child Russian in these first steps to creating a profiling tool that is clinically useful for describing the grammatical strengths and weaknesses in a given Russian language sample.

Note

(1) PPVT – Peabody Picture Vocabulary Test-4 (Dunn & Dunn, 2004); EOWPVT – Expressive One-Word Picture Vocabulary Test-4 (Martin & Brownell, 2011); CELF – Clinical Evaluation of Language Fundamentals-4 (Semel *et al.*, 2006); PLS – Preschool Language Scales-4 (Zimmerman *et al.*, 2002).

References

Babyonyshev, M. (1993) The acquisition of Russian case. In C. Philips (ed.) *Papers on Case and Agreement II (MIT Working Papers in Linguistics 19)* (pp. 1–44). Cambridge, MA: MIT.

Babyonyshev, M., Hart, L., Reich, J., Kuznetsova, J., Rissman, R. and Grigorenko, E.L. (2007) *Otsenka razvitiya russkogo yazy'ka* [Assessment of the Development of Russian]. Unpublished assessment.

Bailyn, J. (2001) On scrambling: A reply to Bošković and Takahashi. *Linguistic Inquiry* 32, 635–658.

Ball, M.J., Crystal, D. and Fletcher, P. (eds) (2012) *Assessing Grammar: The Languages of LARSP*. Bristol: Multilingual Matters.

Bar-Shalom, E. (2002) Tense and aspect in early child Russian. *Language Acquisition* 10 (4), 321–337. DOI: 10.1207/S15327817LA1004_2

Bar-Shalom, E. and Snyder, W. (1997) Optional infinitives in Russian and their implications for the pro-drop debate. In M. Lindseth and S. Franks (eds) *Formal Approaches to Slavic Linguistics: The Indiana Meeting 1996*. Ann Arbor: Michigan Slavic Publications.

Barten, S. and Blank, M. (1971) Soviet research on speech and language: An American perspective. *Early Childhood Development and Care* 1 (1), 3–14.

Caesar, L. and Kohler, P. (2007) The state of school-based bilingual assessment: Actual practice versus recommended guidelines. *Language, Speech, and Hearing Services in Schools* 38 (3), 190–200.

Caruso, C., Concepcion-Escano, Y. and Elleseff, T. (2015) *Technical Manual: A Guide for the Appropriate Assessment of culturally & Linguistically Diverse and Internationally-adopted Individuals*. New Jersey: New Jersey Speech-Language-Hearing Association. Retrieved from https://www.njsha.org/resources/committee-resources/pdfs/CLDguide.pdf

Ceytlin, S.N. (2000) *Jazyk i rebenok: Lingvistika detckoj rechi*. Moscow: Vlados.

Ceytlin, S.N. (2009) *Ocherki po slovoobrazovaniju b formoobrazovaniju v detskoj rechi*. Moscow: Znak.

Crystal, D. (1982) *Profiling Linguistic Disability*. London: Edward Arnold Ltd.

Crystal, D. (2008) *A Dictionary of Linguistics and Phonetics* (6th edn). Oxford: Blackwell.

Crystal, D., Fletcher, P. and Garman, M. (1989) *The Grammatical Analysis of Language Disability* (2nd edn). London: Cole and Whurr, Ltd.

Cubberly, P. (2002) *Russian: A Linguistic Introduction*. Cambridge: Cambridge University Press.

Dunn, L. and Dunn, D. (2004) *Peabody Picture Vocabulary Test-4*. London: Pearson.

El'konin, D.B. (1973) General course of development in the child of grammatical structure of the Russian language (According to A. N. Gvozdev). In C.A. Ferguson and D.I. Slobin (eds) *Studies of Child Language Development* (pp. 565–583). New York: Holt, Rinehart and Winston.

Eliseeva, M.B., Vershinina, E.A. and Ryskina, V.L. (2016) Makarturovskii oprosnik: Russkaia versiia. Otsenka rechevogo i kommunikativnogo razvitiia detei rannego vozrasta. Ivanovo: Listos.

Elleseff, T. (2014) *Russian Articulation Screener*. Somerset, NJ.: Smart Speech Therapy.

Fenson, L., Dale, P.S., Reznick, J.S., Thal, D., Bates, E., Hartung, J.P., Pethick, S. and Reilly, J.S. (1993) *The MacArthur Communicative Development Inventories: User's Guide and Technical Manual*. Baltimore: Paul H. Brokes Publishing Co.

Fletcher, P., Ball, M.J. and Crystal, D. (eds) (2016) *Profiling Grammar: More Languages of LARSP*. Bristol: Multilingual Matters.

Gagarina, N. (2003) The early verb development and demarcation of stages in three Russian-speaking children. In D. Bittner, W.U. Dressler and M. Kilani-Schoch (eds) *Development of Verb Inflection in First Language Acquisition*. New York: Mouton de Gr.

Gagarina, N. (2008) *Stanovlenie grammatičeskich kategorij russkogo glagola v detskoj reči*. St. Petersburg: Nauka.
Gagarina, N. and Voeikova, M. (2009) Acquisition of case and number in Russian. In U. Stephany and M. Voeikova (eds) *Development of Nominal Inflection in First Language Acquisition: A Cross-linguistic Perspective* (pp. 179–215). Berlin: Mouton de Gruyter.
Gaines, D. (2004) Geographical perspectives on disability: A socio-spatial analysis of the mentally disabled population in Russia. *Middle States Geographer* 37, 80–89.
Gleason, J.B., Phillips, B.C. and Ely, R. (2010) Alligators all around: The acquisition of animal terms in English and Russian. In *Crosslinguistic Approaches to Psychology of Language: Research in the tradition of Dan Slobin*. Taylor & Francis: New York, NY.
Gvozdev, A.N. (1949) *Formirovanije u rebenka grammaticheskogo stroja russkogo jazyka*. [The formation of the child's grammatical structure of Russian.] Moscow: Akademija Pedogogicheskih Nauk RSFSR.
Iosad, P. (2018) Phonology in the Soviet Union. In B.E. Dresher and H. van der Hulst (eds) *The Oxford History of Phonology*. Oxford: Oxford University Press. Manuscript in preparation.
Janssen, B. (2014) Frequency effects on the acquisition of Polish and Russian gender morphology. In *Dutch Contributions to the Fifteenth International Congress of Slavists, Minsk: Linguistics* (SSGL 40): Amsterdam, NY.
Kallestinova, E. (2007) Three stages of root infinitive production in early child Russian. *First Language* 27 (2), 99–131.
Kornilov S.A., Rakhlin N.V. and Grigorenko E.L. (2012) Morphology and developmental language disorders: New tools for Russian. *Psychology in Russia: State of the Art* 5, 371–387.
Launer, M.K. (1974) *Elementary Russian Syntax*. Cambridge, MA: Slavica Publishers.
Lewis, M.P., Simons, G.F. and Fennig, C.D. (eds) (2016) *Ethnologue: Languages of the World, Nineteenth edition*. Dallas, Texas: SIL International. Retrieved from: www.ethnologue.com/statistics/size (accessed 06 June 2016).
MacWhinney, B. (2000) *The CHILDES Project: Tools for Analyzing Talk* (3rd edn). Mahwah, NJ: Lawrence Erlbaum Associates.
Martin, N.A. and Brownell, R. (2011) *Expressive One-Word Picture Vocabulary Test* (4th edn). Novato, CA: Academic Therapy Publications.
McCoy, S. (2003) Connecting information structure and discourse structure through "Kontrast": The case of colloquial Russian particles -TO, ŽE, and VED. *Journal of Logic, Language, and Information* 12 (3), 319–335.
Mitchell, J.C.E. (1973) Aspects of speech therapy in the U.S.S.R. including the role and training of the Russian logopedist. *International Journal of Language & Communication Disorders* 8, 74–78.
Moffatt, N. (2018) The Development of a LARSP-like profile for Russian. Unpublished PhD dissertation. University of Louisiana at Lafayette. USA.
Nakhimovsky, A. and Leed, R. (1987) *Advanced Russian*. Bloomington, IN: Slavica Publishers.
Paperno, L. and Sylvester, R. (1987) *Getting Around Town in Russian: Situational Dialogs*. Bloomington, IN: Slavica Publishers.
Polinsky, M. (2006) Acquisition of Russian: Uninterrupted and incomplete scenarios. *Glossos* 8, 1–64.http://www.seelrc.org/glossos/issues/8/
Prescott, E. (2017) Russia's disabled 'orphans': Suggestions for institutional change. *International Immersion Program Papers*, 58. Chicago: University of Chicago Law School.
Protassova, E. (1997) Transition from Babbling to Word Structure. *Papers and Studies in Contrastive Linguistics* 33, 153–158.

Semel, E.M., Wiig, E.H. and Secord, W. (2006) *CELF4: Clinical Evaluation of Language Fundamentals*. San Antonio, TX: The Psychological Corporation.

Slobin, D.I. (1966) The acquisition of Russian as a native language. In F. Smith and G.A. Miller (eds) *The Genesis of Language*. Cambridge: The Massachusetts Institute of Technology.

Templeman, S. (2004) Social work in the new Russia at the start of the millennium. *International Social Work* 47 (1), 95–107.

Townsend, C. (1975) *Russian Word Formation*. Cambridge, MA: Slavica Publishers.

Wade, T. (2011) *A Comprehensive Russian Grammar* (3rd edn). Chichester: Wiley-Blackwell.

Yampolsky, S. (1996) *A Pilot Russian Version of the Peabody Picture Vocabulary Test – revised*. Boston, MA: MGH Institute of Health Professions.

Yanushevskaya, I. and Bunčić, D. (2015) Russian. *Journal of the International Phonetic Association* 45 (2), 221–228.

Zhukova, M.A., Kornilov, S.A., Simmons, E. and Grigorenko, E.L. (2016) Diagnosing speech development with the help of 'preschool language scales': A case analysis. *Voprosy Psikhologii* 2016 (5), 154–164.

Zimmerman, I.L., Steiner, V.G. and Pond, R. E. (2002) *PLS-4: Preschool Language Scale-4*. Psychological Corporation.

Zimmerman, I.L., Steiner, V.G. and Pond, E. (2011) *Preschool Language Scales* (5th edn) Edition (PLS-5). San Antonio, TX: Pearson.

3 Language Assessment, Remediation and Screening Procedure for Slovak-speaking Children

Svetlana Kapalková and Daniela Slančová

Introduction

The adaptation of LARSP to Slovak (LARSPsk) was based on LARSP in English (abbreviated in this chapter as LARSPe) (Boehm *et al.*, 2005; Crystal, 1979, 1992; Crystal *et al.*, 1989), the typology of the Slovak language, Slovak syntactic tradition and research findings on language acquisition in Slovak-speaking children. Unlike LARSPe, which is based on the procedures of phrasal syntax, we used as a theoretical basis a syntax based on the relationships between sentence elements. As reported by Ivanová (2011: 13), '... syntax, which is traditionally developed in the European context, is appropriate to describe languages with a free word order. Such syntax studies the sequence of relationships between pairs of sentence elements, where the verb is usually the primary element of the entire sentence.' This approach is combined with certain procedures of semantic syntax and its basic postulate, according to which verb is referred to as the core of the sentence (Ivanová, 2011: 13).

The Grammatical Description of Slovak

Slovak is a West-Slavic language. It is basically an inflecting language (mostly in declension) with some introflecting (as a secondary feature of declension), analytic (in conjugation) and agglutinative (in gradation) features. It marks itself off as a relatively simple language and a relatively regular one (Novák, 1977). Slovak nominal morphology is characteristic of a relatively regular declension according to three grammatical genders (masculine, feminine, neuter). It has six cases. Locative is always prepositional, while the remaining cases, apart from nominative, are either with or without preposition. There are two numbers – singular and plural.

Verbal morphology has a regular conjugation in three persons of both singular and plural. There are three tenses – present, preterite and future. The forms of antepreterite are rare. The present has a synthetic form (in the 1st person singular *vidím* = I see); the preterite is analytical (in the 1st person singular masculine *videl som*, feminine *videla som*, neuter *videlo som* = I saw); the future is analytical for imperfects (*budem vidieť* = I will be seeing), and synthetic for perfectives (*uvidím* = I will see). The endings of the 1st (*-m*) and 2nd (*-š*) persons singular and plural (*-me*, *-te*) in the present tense are the same for all verbs. Slovak has a typical Slavic imperfective/perfective aspectual distinction in verbs, expressed in three moods (indicative, imperative, conditional) and two voices (active and passive). The passive and conditional are expressed analytically. There are more reflexive passive forms than analytical ones. Other verbals include adjectival participles, transgressive, and infinitive. The transgressive is rather rare in spoken language. Gradation of adjectives is both synthetic and analytical; gradation of adverbs is of a synthetic character and is in most instances regular. In the morphological system of modern literary Slovak, its inflectional character is not reinforced; the agglutinative features are slightly supported (Dolník, 2000).

Syntactically, Slovak is characterized by asymmetric predication with a potential subject. Word order is relatively free, determined by meaning, functional perspective, pragmatics, stylistics, or the rhythm of the utterance. Subject–verb–object is the basic word order in simple sentences without context. There is fixed word order within attributive nominal phrases and other phrases (clitic sequences). Predicative verbs agree in person and number with their subjects. Adjectives agree in gender and case with the noun they modify. There is a high degree of redundancy: the same gender and number information may be repeated several times in the sentence.

Generally, there are fewer infinitive constructions and nominal forms, although there also exists a strong tendency toward nominalization, especially in writing (cf. Kesselová & Slančová, 2010).

Research Findings on the Grammatical Development of Slovak-speaking Children

Research into child language does not have a long tradition in Slovak psycholinguistics. More intensive research into the language development of Slovak-speaking children, especially in the early stages, was first conducted in the late 1990s. Two research aspects – longitudinal (Fečková Kapalková, 2002; Slančová, 2008, 2018; Slančová & Kičura Sokolová, 2018) and quantitative (Kapalková *et al.*, 2010) – are relevant for the adaptation of LARSPsk.

Within the longitudinal research, the sample consisted of six children coming from all over Slovakia. Children were recorded on video for one hour per month from their birth to 5 to 6 years of age in standard situations (feeding, bathing, playing) based on mutual interaction between children and their communication partners. Children came from complete families, with their mothers being university graduates in humanities, linguistics or logopedy. This selection was based on the assumption of optimal speech development induced by the children's parents, especially by their mothers.[1] The families were monolingual. At the time of the first recording, all children were first-born, except for one second-born child.

Quantitative research is a follow-up to studies dealing with the adaptation of the McArthur-Bates Communicative Development Inventories (CDI) to Slovak. Similarly to CDI, the Slovak adaptation – the Test of Communicative Behavior (Test komunikačného správania, TEKOS) consists of two parts: TEKOS I: Words and Gestures (8–16 months) and TEKOS II: Words and Sentences (17–30 months). The Slovak version was standardized on a sample of 1715 Slovak-speaking children (Kapalková *et al.*, 2010; Dale & Penfold, 2011: 67–68) which in addition to providing developmental percentile norms also represents a data source for further research into the language development of Slovak-speaking children. Findings from both types of research were used for the adaptation of LASRPsk.

Longitudinal research data were collected from three children: one boy (age 0;05-3;04) and two girls (age 0;8-3;6; 1;6-4;1) were used. The sample used for the adaptation of LARSPsk was chosen from the six longitudinally observed children mentioned above. Data from TEKOS II were also used to study both nominal and verbal grammatical categories. Findings reported by Kesselová *et al.* (2013), Kesselová (2014a, 2014b), Slančová and Sokolová (2012), Sokolová (2013) and Kičura Sokolová (2013, 2014) are relevant for the adaptation of LARSPsk. When devising LARSPsk, we follow the assumption that LARSP is not a detailed linguistic description of syntactic development, but represents a simplified picture for the purposes of clinical practice.

Adaptation of LARSPe for Slovak-speaking Children

Stages of normal grammatical development in Slovak-speaking children

To identify particular stages of grammatical development, the number of words or clauses produced by a child in an utterance was used as a primary criterion. The number of words in a child's utterance is considered a criterion until the number of words in a child's single-clause utterance equals or exceeds four or more words. If a child's utterance consists of two or more clauses, then, the main criterion is the number of clauses in a child's utterance. The number of words in a child's utterance was selected as a criterion for the following reasons:

(a) The number of words in an utterance indicates grammatical development. This was confirmed by both the adaptation of MLU to Slovak, which compared MLU in morphemes based on the complex morphemic analysis (cMLUm), MLU in morphemes based on the specific morphemic analysis derived from the developmental data of Slovak-speaking children (sMLUm), MLU in syllables (MLUs) and MLU in words (MLUw) during the longitudinal development of three children. It was also confirmed by TEKOS II: Words and Sentences – three longest sentences subtest (Kapalková *et al.*, 2010, 2011; Slančová *et al.*, 2011). There were strong correlations between data on language development in Slovak-speaking children: cMLUm : sMLUm = 0.996; sMLUm : MLUs = 0.997; MLUs : MLUw = 0.980; cMLUm : MLUs = 0.998; cMLUm : MLUw = 0.976; sMLUm : MLUw = 0.989 (Slančová *et al.*, 2011).

(b) A sentence element can be expressed by more than one word (e.g. prepositional case, ALOC: *na stole*[2] 'on table'), by a multi-word grammatical form (e.g. the analytical future tense: P(Vf) *bude syčať* '(it) will fizz'), by a complex verbal predicate (VVP) or by a complex verbo-nominal predicate (VNP). An utterance may also include a non-grammatical connection between synsemantic (auxiliary) and autosemantic (full) words, e.g. conjunction + autosemantic word; particle + autosemantic word.

(c) Due to the fact that the production of every word[3] in early stages is an indicator of development, this phenomenon also needs to be taken into account in the adaptation of LARSP to Slovak.

In single-clause utterances produced by Slovak children, four stages of development are distinguished according to the number of words in a child's utterance:

Stage I: One-word level
Stage II: Two-word level
Stage III: Three-word level
Stage IV: Four-and-more-words level

If the child's utterance contains two or more clauses, we refer to:

Stage V: Compound sentence level
Stage VI: Narrative level

We follow both the continual process of language development, and the fact that lower-level syntactic means are present in more syntactically developed speech as well; however, their use is determined by discourse rules.

To characterize particular stages of development, we analysed the sentence elements structure of a child's utterance (in LARSPe 'clause' and 'phrase'), based on primary and secondary sentence elements. The basic sentence-forming act is the predication act, relating subject (S) and predicate (P) within a certain temporal and modal framework. Other sentence elements are: object (O), adverbial modifier (A), attribute (ATR)[4] and complement (C).[5]

A more detailed specification of the basic sentence structure enables us to distinguish between simple predicate and complex predicate, which may be either verbal (VVP) or verbo-nominal (VNP). Direct object (Od) and indirect object (Oi) are also distinguished.

Table 3.1 shows the developmental trajectory of syntactic structures in Slovak, providing examples as recorded in transcripts of longitudinally observed children.

Morphosyntactic structure (in LARSPe – Word)

Unlike LARSPe, we did not record specific morphemes at particular developmental stages, but noted specific morphological or morphosyntactic categories. From the perspective of the morphological character of Slovak, these categories were divided into nominal and verbal categories.

Nominal categories

In the nominal categories, we noted case (nominative, genitive, dative, accusative, locative, instrumental), number (singular, plural) and nominal agreement in gender, number and case. Specifically, we studied the occurrence of prepositions as the lexical means used to express a syntactic relationship, because using a preposition is at the same time an indicator of development. These categories are noted for nouns, adjectives and pronouns.

When adapting LARSP to Slovak, the developmental trajectory of nominal categories was determined from both the longitudinal observation of three children and from TEKOS II: Words and Sentences. We recorded the following: the age (in months) when a particular category was first produced by a child during the longitudinal observation, and for TEKOS II: Words and Sentences, the age when the child first produced a particular category, and also the age when more than 50% or more parents noted a particular category for the first time. However, in relation to TEKOS II we did not record all case forms observable during the longitudinal research.

TEKOS II was administered to record the following categories (see Appendix for abbreviations): Nsg., Npl., Gsg.+PREP *do*, Dsg., Dsg.+PREP *k*, Acsg., Acsg.+PREP *pre*, Acpl., Lsg.+PREP *na, o, vo*, Isg., Isg.+PREP *s, pod, pred, za*. The collected data were combined. Months of age at which a particular category was produced provide additional information about the procedural progression of morphosyntactic category acquisition. The gradual occurrence of particular categories is important, as, for instance, it has been shown that children first produce noun cases

Table 3.1 Developmental trajectory of syntactic structures based on the longitudinal observation of three children and complemented by examples of the first production of each structure

Syntactic structure	Age of first occurrence	Stage	Example of first occurrence	Word-by-word translation
SUB	0;9	I	*Tato.*	Daddy.
PRONdem	0;11	I	*Tu.*	Here.
A(PRONint)X	1;0	II	*Kde je?*	Where is?
INT	1;0	I	*Bác.*	Boom.
P(Vf)	1;1	I	*Daj!*	Give!
ADVloc	1;2	I	*Hore.*	Up.
P-A	1;2	II	*Tam čistí.*	There cleans.
P-Od	1;2	II	*To daj!*	It give!
PRONint	1;2	I	*Kde?*	Where?
S-P-A	1;2	III	*Tata je tam.*	Daddy is there.
A+PART	1;3	II	*Nie tu.*	Not here.
PART	1;3	I	*Tak.*	So.
S-A	1;3	II	*Havo pápá (= preč).*	Doggie away.
Vfneg	1;3	I	*Neni.*	Is not.
P-Od-Oi	1;5	III	*Toto daj mne.*	This give me.
S-P	1;5	II	*Tato volá.*	Daddy calls.
ADJ	1;6	I	*Malá.*	Small.
ADVtemp	1;6	I	*Ešte.*	More.
O-A	1;7	II	*Ešte kvietok.*	More flower.
A+A	1;8	II	*Schodami dole.*	Staircase down.
INF	1;8	I	*Otvoriť!*	Open!
NUM	1;8	I	*Menej.*	Less.
PRONpos	1;8	I	*Moja.*	My.
VVP	1;8	II	*Hajať ide.*	Sleep goes.
S/O	1;8	I	*Toto nie.*	This not.
A+INT	1;9	II	*Bum tam.*	Boom there.
ATR	1;9	II	*Obúvam druhú.*	Put (I) other.
O+	1;10	III	*Idem ti toto.*	Goes you this.
P-O-A	1;10	III	*Tak chytí traktor.*	So catches tractor.
S-C	1;10	II	*Maťko sám.*	Maťko alone.
S-VNP	1;10	III	*To je auto.*	It is car.
P-A-A	1;11	III	*Tu kde je?*	Here where is?
S-P-O	1;11	III	*Krája Maťko papriku.*	Chops Maťko pepper.
S-VVP	1;11	III	*Zatvorený je čajník.*	Closed is tea-pot.

(*Continued*)

Table 3.1 *(Continued)*

Syntactic structure	Age of first occurrence	Stage	Example of first occurrence	Word-by-word translation
P-A	1;11	IV	*Mohol liezť na dom.*	Could (he) climb on house.
S+	2;0	III	*Tuto ka (= kakao) moje.*	Here cocoa my.
P-Oi	2;0	II	*Daj mi!*	Give me!
A(+)	2;1	III	*Tu je mamiky.*	Here is mummýs.
P-K	2;1	II	*Sama budem.*	Alone will be (I).
S-P-O-A	2;1	IV	*Dedo opraví takto postieľku.*	Grandpa repairs so bed.
P-A-A-A	2;3	IV	*Ešte idem tam s ujom. Toňom.*	Just go (I) there with uncle Toňo.
S-P-A	2;3	IV	*Ja idem k tebe.*	I go to you.
S-P-O-O	2;3	IV	*Ktorý mi môže vidieť knihu?*	Which me can see book?
S-P-A-A	2;5	IV	*Potom pôjde Ninka tam.*	Then will go Nina there.
P-O-C	2;6	III	*Máš ich boľavé.*	Have (you) them aching.
S-P-O-O-A-A	2;6	IV	*Ujo tak dal si tam kartu.*	Uncle so gave there himself card.
P-O-O-A	2;6	IV	*Nechám ho tu vysušiť.*	Let (I) him here dry.

without a preposition, and later, the prepositional ones. Table 3.2 summarizes the gradual occurrence of the first production of particular nominal categories during longitudinal observation. Table 3.3 shows the first occurrences of particular nominal categories, and the age of the child when parents noted the use of each category in more than 50% of the children included in the sample of 1012 children. Table 3.4 combines and offers a review of development, which formed the basis for a more detailed characterization of particular stages of LARSPsk. [6]

Similar findings were reported by Kesselová (2014b), who, however, did not observe singular and plural forms of case and focused more on case semantics: 'According to parental observations, 90% of children younger than three years of age used all case forms in the singular, and nominative/accusative also in the plural. However, case meanings are acquired selectively. Preferred semantic specifications are formed in four semantic categories: locationality, objectness, sociativity and benefitiality' (Kesselová, 2014b: 86).

A relevant syntactic means is the category of nominal agreement. For nominal parts of speech (nouns determined by adjectives and adjective pronouns), we refer to agreement in gender, number and case. On average, this occurs for the first time at the age of 23 months.

Table 3.2 Developmental trajectory of nominal categories based on longitudinal research

Case	Number	Preposition	Age of first occurence	Child
N	sg		0;11	M
Ac	sg		1;01	M
N	pl		1;03	N
L	sg		1;08	M
I	pl		1;08	M
I	sg		1;08	M
L	pl		1;10	N
D	pl		1;10	Z
G	pl		1;10	N
G	sg		1;10	N
D	sg		1;10	N
Ac	pl		1;10	Z
G	sg	PREP	1;11	M
L	sg	PREP	1;11	M
Ac	sg	PREP	2;00	M
D	sg	PREP	2;02	Z
Ac	pl	PREP	2;02	Z
I	pl	PREP	2;02	Z
I	sg	PREP	2;04	Z
D	pl	PREP	2;06	N
G	pl	PREP	2;07	Z
L	pl	PREP	3;02	Z

For adjectives and adverbs, we noted the lexical-grammatical category of gradation. Longitudinal observation showed minimal occurrence of this category. A comparative form was produced by a 20-month-old child and a superlative form was produced by a single child at the age of 39 months.

Verbal categories

In verbal categories, we observed person (1st, 2nd, 3rd), number (singular, plural), tense (present, preterite, future; for perfectives, future present was distinguished because forms of these verbs are present, but their meaning denotes future), mood (indicative, imperative, conditional), voice (active, passive), for past tense also gender (masculine, feminine, neuter) and agreement in person and number, and for preterite also in gender. When analysing non-finite forms, we observed the developmental trajectory of infinitives and participles.

Table 3.3 Developmental trajectory of nominal categories based on cross-sectional research TEKOS II: Words and Sentences

TEKOS II	Age of first occurence	Age of 50 % production		Age of first occurence	Age of 50 % production
Acsg	1;5	1;9			
Acpl	1;5	1;11			
Gsg + *do*	1;5	1;11			
Dsg + *k*	1;5	1;11			
Npl	1;5	2;0			
Isg	1;5	2;0			
Isg + *s, pod*	1;5	2;0	**Isg** + *pred, za*	1;5	1;10
Acsg + *pre*	1;5	2;1			
Lsg + *na, o*	1;6	2;1	**Lsg** + *v*	1;5	2;0
Dsg	1;7	2;3			

Table 3.4 Developmental trajectory of nominal categories based on the combination of longitudinal research and data from TEKOS II: Words and Sentences

Age	Case	Number	Preposition
0;11	N	sg	
1;5	Ac	sg	
1;7	N	pl	
1;8	L	sg	
1;8	I	pl	
1;8	I	sg	
1;9	Ac	pl	
1;9	G	sg	PREP
1;9	L	sg	PREP
1;10	L	pl	
1;10	D	pl	
1;10	G	pl	
1;10	G	sg	
1;10	Ac	sg	PREP
1;10	D	sg	PREP
1;10	I	sg	PREP
1;11	D	sg	
2;2	Ac	pl	PREP

Observation of the developmental trajectory of verbal categories was similar to that of nominal categories. In addition to data collected via longitudinal observation, we also observed age (in months) when the child first produced a particular category, and for data from TEKOS II: Words and Sentences the age when a particular category first occurred and the age of the child when 50% or more parents noted a particular category for the first time. For verbal categories, all categories found via longitudinal observation were not recorded via TEKOS II. We observed the following categories: 1st, 2nd and 3rd person singular; 1st, 2nd and 3rd person, plural, present, indicative, active; preterite, future present, analytical future tense, imperative, conditional, negation, and analytical resultative construction. The findings from both data sources were combined, as with those for nominal categories.

The categories of infinitive and passive participle were recorded at 21 months of age and at 27 months of age, respectively.

Table 3.5 Developmental trajectory of verbal finite forms based on longitudinal research according to first occurrence of a particular category and cross-sectional research TEKOS II: Words and Sentences

Person	Number	Tense	Mood	Negation	Voice	Age of first occurence longitude	Age of first occurence TEKOS II	Age of 50 % production TEKOS II
2	sg		imp		act	0;11	1;5	1;8
3	sg	present	ind	neg	act	1;2	1;5	1;9
3	sg	present	ind		act	1;2	1;5	1;8
3	sg	preterite	ind		act	1;7	1;7	2;2
3	pl	preterite	ind		act	1;8		
1	sg	present	ind		act	1;9	1;5	1;11
1	sg	future	ind		act	1;10		
3	sg	present/ future	ind		act	1;10		
3	pl	present	ind		act	1;10	1;5	2;2
3	pl	present/ future	ind		act	1;11		
2	sg	future	ind		act	1;11		
2	sg		imp	neg	act	1;11		
1	pl	present/ future	ind		act	1;11	1;5	2;0
3	sg	future	ind		act	1;11		
1	sg	present/ future	ind	neg	act	2;0		
1	sg	preterite	ind		act	2;0		
1	pl	present	ind		act	2;1		

(Continued)

Table 3.5 *(Continued)*

Person	Number	Tense	Mood	Negation	Voice	Age of first occurence longitude	Age of first occurence TEKOS II	Age of 50 % production TEKOS II
1	sg	present	ind	neg	act	2;1		
2	sg	present	ind		act	2;1	1;5	2;2
2	sg	present	ind	neg	act	2;1		
2	pl	present	ind	neg	act	2;3		
2	sg	preterite	ind	neg	act	2;4		
1	pl	present/ future	ind	neg	act	2;4		
1	pl	preterite	ind		act	2;5		
1	sg	present	cond		act	2;5	1;7	3;0
2	pl		imp		act	2;6		
3	sg	preterite	ind		act	2;7		
3	pl	preterite	ind		pas	2;7		
1	pl	present	ind	neg	act	2;7		
2	pl	present	ind		act	2;7	1;5	2;3
2	sg	preterite	ind		act	2;7		
1	pl	present	cond		act	3;2		
3	sg		imp		act	3;3		
2	sg	present/ future	ind		act	3;5		

For verbal categories, we noted agreement between the subject noun and predicative verb in number, and for preterite also agreement in gender. The category of nomino-verbal agreement in number was first observed at 17 months of age (*Tato volá* 'Daddy calls'), and in number and gender at 27 months of age (*Neopravila mama auto* 'Not repaired mummy car').

Unlike LARSPe, we did not specify negation within sentence elements structure because in Slovak negation is not expressed by special syntactic structures. To include this syntactic component of child's utterance in the clinical profile, we recorded it separately in the morphosyntactic category at stage II. We also took into consideration both negation expressed by a modifying morpheme in form of a prefix, and negation expressed by a specific word.

Comments on the Slovak Adaptation of LARSPsk

In this section, comments are provided on the chart, which is an adaptation of the original English chart used to determine the clinical grammatical profile found in studies dealing with LARSP in English e.g. Crystal, 1979, 1992; Crystal *et al.*, 1989; Boehm *et al.*, 2005).

Data about name, age, sample date and type of dialogue as well as data about total number of sentences, mean number of sentences per turn, and mean sentence length remain the same as in the English version. Also, sections A–D remain the same (Unanalysed, Responses, Spontaneous, Reactions).

The pragmatic character of children's utterances is presented before their grammatical characteristics.[7] We have preserved the structure of LARSPe – commands, questions and statements. These are very important to obtain information about the language level of Slovak-speaking children from a pragmatic but not grammatical point of view. In Slovak, questions are not formed by using a separate morphosyntactic apparatus, but are rather based on word order and intonation – they have the same syntactic structure as non-interrogative utterances. Similarly, commands show identical syntactic structure to that of statements, and the fact that in both commands and statements the subject is not expressed lexically under certain conditions is grammatically irrelevant. Despite this, the pragmatic dimension remains important because questions and commands are shorter on average, being frequently expressed by a single word, and syntactically simpler. Not distinguishing between questions and commands could affect the overall profile of a child's syntactic development. During the stage when children use single-word utterances, the production of interrogative pronouns signalling questions is especially important as a relevant form of utterance within a discourse.

Stages of development are proposed according to data collected from Slovak-speaking children (both longitudinal and cross-sectional) as follows:

Stage I: 0;9–1;2
Stage II: 1;3–1;8
Stage III: 1;9–2;2
Stage IV: 2;3–2;8
Stage V: 2;9 and more

Minor structures, similarly to LARSPe, represent utterances with no potential for syntactic development: yes/no responses, vocatives by names or family positions (*mama* 'mum', *tata* 'daddy'), and other textual, numeral, social, and play routines. Major structures were assessed on the level of sentence elements structure, and morphosyntactic structure.

Stage I: One-word level

The grammatical quality of one-word sentence structures is noted from both the point of view of (i) sentence elements structure and (ii) word class and form structure. If an utterance is expressed by a finite verb, it is classified as a predicative structure from the perspective of sentence elements structure. If an utterance is expressed by a different word class (non-predicative utterances), or a non-finite verb form, it is referred to as the so-called sentence equivalent.[8] From a developmental point of view, we may refer to one-word developmental sentence equivalents, which are the result of neither actual ellipsis nor of the maxim of quantity, but are developmentally determined – a child is unable to produce an utterance consisting of more than one word (e.g. due to limited syllable capacity – cf. Fečková & Slančová, 2001). At the higher stage of language acquisition, we may refer to one-word sentence equivalents that are determined pragmatically. One-word sentence structures are found in children's speech also during the period when children produce two- or multiple-word sentence structures. Similarly to fully developed adult speech, their occurrence is determined by the communication context (most often when answering questions, etc.).

A one-word sentence equivalent may be expressed by a noun, adjective, pronoun, infinitive, adverb, numeral, particle or interjection. At the one-word level the grammatical profile chart shows the following sentence structure:

P(Vf) – predicate expressed by a finite verb
SUB – sentence equivalent expressed by a noun
PRON – sentence equivalent expressed by a pronoun
ADV – sentence equivalent expressed by an adverb
Other

At the one-word level, the clinical grammatical profile chart shows the level of abstraction corresponding to the two above-mentioned perspectives, namely sentence elements structure and word class and form structure. At lower levels of abstraction, a more detailed word-class, semantic and grammatical specification at the one-word level revealed: a predicate expressed by a finite verb, as well as by a verb without identifiable morphological categories, the finite verb in the positive and negative form; a sentence equivalent expressed by a pronoun in the form of an interrogative pronoun in questions, by a demonstrative pronoun, and by a possessive personal pronoun; a sentence equivalent expressed by an adverb of place or adverb of time. Among other sentence equivalents were interjectional, particle, adjectival, and numeral equivalents; however, such equivalents are not further specified in the profile chart.

Unlike LARSPe, at the level of one-word utterances we also studied gestures, which are considered to be the precursor of syntactic development (Capirci *et al.*, 1996; Kapalková, 2008, 2018; McEachern & Haynes, 2004), and also one of the syntactic means (Slančová & Sokolová, 2012; Slančová & Kičura Sokolová, 2018). Developmentally, a distinction is made between two types of connections. A complementary connecting of a gesture with a word is developmentally a simpler type of connection. This means that within a single utterance a child expresses the same semantic or pragmatic meaning by using both word and gesture. For instance, a child uses the gesture of opening and closing the palm when saying *daj* 'give'. More developmentally complex, and closer to two-word utterances, is the type of supplementary connection: in a single utterance a child produces a word to express one meaning but uses a gesture to expand the meaning of the word. For instance, when saying *daj* 'give', a child points a finger at a glass of juice. LARSPsk denotes morphosyntactic structure by Nsg., and imperative in 2nd person sg. With regard to the prediction of syntax, supplementary connection seems more relevant (Kapalková, 2018).

Stage II: Two-word level

When determining two- and multiple-element structures, we did not take into consideration word order, which has no grammatical function in Slovak. Addressing a person followed by a sentence structure is also understood and evaluated as two separate utterances: *Mama daj* 'Mummy give', *Ujo podaj* 'Uncle pass', *Tatino pod'* 'Daddy come'.

The grammatical quality of two-word sentence structures is studied by combining: (i) the perspective of basic sentence element structure and its specification and (ii) the perspective of two-word sentence equivalents. Within the basic structure of sentence elements, we identified the predicate structure P(X), i.e. a predicate or a predicate combined with another sentence element: subject (S-P), object (P-O), adverbial (P-A). All other structures fall into the category Other (1). The occurrence of attribute ATR-[9] is noted separately.

When specifying syntactic structure, we identified a predicate expressed by a finite verb (Vf) in the analytical grammatical form and complex verbal predicate (VVP), direct object (Od) and indirect object (Oi) within object structure, and adverbial structure expressed by an interrogative pronoun in connection with another sentence element. In this case, we respect the pragmatic division of utterances, because the structure A(PRONint)X is an interrogative syntactic structure.

A two-word sentence equivalent is expressed by the structure A+, i.e. an adverbial expressed by two words, mostly a preposition + another word (noun or pronoun), or particle + another word (noun or pronoun); and adverbial + another sentence element: adverbial + subject (S-A), object (O-A), attribute (A-ATR) and combination of two adverbials (A+A). All other structures are classified as Other.

At stage II, we noted structures determined by the syntagmatic connection of two autosemantic words as well as two-word single-element structures. Two-word expression of syntactic structures with a single sentence element is determined by:

- a sentence element in the analytical (two-word) grammatical form: *Syčať bude* 'Fizz (it) will' (PVffut), an analytical verbal and verbo-nominal predicate: *Hajať ide* 'Sleep goes' (Vflimit+INF), *Čítať musím* 'Read (I) must' (Vfmod+INF), *Je otočené* 'Is (it) turned' (Vfcop+PARTpas);
- prepositional case of the word functioning as a sentence element: *Na rádio* 'On radio', *Na posteľ* 'On bed', *Do roboty* 'To work' (PREP+SUB);
- connecting an autosemantic word as a sentence element and a synsematic word having no sentence element function: *Už dosť* 'Already enough' A(PART+ADVmod), *A vstáva* 'And gets up' (CON+Vf).

At a lower level of abstraction, more detailed form and semantic specification may reveal a greater variety of syntactic structures. Predicate structure in the following forms may serve as an example:

P(Vf) – predicate expressed by a finite verb in the analytical grammatical form – *Syčať bude* 'Fizz (it) will'.
CON+P(Vf) – conjunction + predicate *A vstáva* 'And gets up'.
P(VVP) – complex verbal predicate in the form of:
- VVP(Vfmod+INT) – modal verb + interjection: *Chcem hopi* '(I) want *hopi*' (interjection denoting activity – to sit);
- VVP(Vfmod+INF) – modal verb + infinitive: *Môžu ísť* '(They) can go', *Chceš papať?* 'Want (you) eat?'
- VVP(Vflimit+INF) – limiting verb + infinitive: *Hajať ide* 'Sleep goes';
- VVP(Vfcop+PARTpas) copular verb + passive participle: *Je otočené* 'Is (it) turned';
- VVP(Vfmod+PARTpas) modal verb + passive participle: *Mám nabité* '(I) have charged';
- VVP(Vfmodneg+PARTpas) negated modal verb + passive participle: *Nemám napísané* '(I) do not have written'.

All these forms and semantically specified structures fit into the predicative two-word structure.

The variability of syntactic structures, of course, increases at the next levels of the grammatical profile. At this stage, with respect to morphosyntactic structure, we expect the following nominal and verbal categories: nominal categories Npl., Acsg., Isg., Ipl.; verbal categories 3rd person sg., 3rd person pl., 1st person sg. present, present/future, preterite, negation *ne+* ; indicative, agreement.

Stage III: Three-word level

The grammatical quality of three-word sentence structures is expressed by combining: (i) the perspective of basic sentence elements structure and its specification and (ii) the perspective of three-word sentence equivalents.

Within the basic structure of sentence elements we identified the predicate structure P(X), i.e. predicate or predicate with another sentence element: subject (S-P), object (P-O), adverbial (P-A). Among other syntactic structures produced at this stage are: predicate and two objects (P-O-O), predicate–object–adverbial (P-O-A), predicate and two adverbials (P-A-A), subject–predicate–object (S-P-O), and subject–predicate–adverbial (S-P-A). The occurrence of attribute ATR- is noted separately. All other structures fall into the category Other.

When specifying the syntactic structure we identified a predicate expressed by a finite verb (Vf), complex verbal predicate (VVP) and complex verbo-nominal predicate (VNP); in object structures we identified direct object (Od) and indirect object (Oi).

Three-word sentence equivalents are expressed by structures S+ (subject + another sentence element/other sentence elements), O+ (object + another sentence element/other sentence elements) and A+ (adverbial + another sentence element/other sentence elements).

At the three-word level, we identified structures determined by the connection of three autosemantic words as well as three-word two-element structures.

Expressing three-word syntactic structures with one sentence element is determined by:

- the analytical expression of a corresponding grammatical category: *Nech sa varí* 'Let (it) cooks'. This refers to the imperative in the 3rd person sg. using the particle *nech* and the form of the reflexive passive *sa varí*;
- the connection of an autosemantic word functioning as a sentence element, which in its analytical grammatical form is expressed by two words, and a synsemantic word without a sentence element function: *Alebo budem variť* 'Or (I) will cook' P: CON+Vffut; *Preto budú zatepľovať* 'Because (they) will heat clad' P: CON+Vffut;
- the connection of an analytical form of predicate and a synsemantic word without a sentence element function: *Lebo chce hajať* 'Because wants sleep' P: VVP: CON+VVP(Vfmod+INF).

Expressing three-word syntactic structures with two sentence elements is determined by:

- the analytical form of the predicate: *Čo je to?* 'What is it?' S-P: S-VNP: S(PRONdem)-VNP(Vfcop+PRONint); *To je auto* 'It is car' S-P:

S(PRONdem)+VNP(Vfcop+SUB); *Ty si veľká* 'You are big (feminine)' S-P: S(PRONper)-VNP(Vfcop+ADJ); *Džíp je pokazený* 'Jeep is broken' S-P: S(SUB)-VVP(Vfcop+PARTpas); *Maťko otočiť chce* 'Maťko (= name) turn wants' S-P: S(SUB)-VVP(Vfmod+INF); *Toto otočiť chcem* 'This turn want (I)' P-O: VVP-Od: VVP(Vfmod+INF)-Od(PRONdem);

- the prepositional case of one of the sentence elements: *Na cintorín nepôjdeme* 'At the cemetery (we) will not go' P-A: P-Aloc: P(Vfneg)-Aloc(PREP+SUB); *Ku zajkovi dáme* 'To bunny (we) give' P-A: P(Vf)-Aloc (PREP+SUB);
- connecting autosemantic words functioning as sentence elements and a synsematic word without a sentence element function (CON, PART): *Preto robí bubu* 'That is why does *bubu*' (= interjection of fear) CON+P-O; *Aj džúsik piť* 'Also juice drink' CON+P(0+INF)-Od; *A tatinka kresliť* 'And daddy draw' CON+P(0+INF)-Od; *Asi idem okolo* 'Maybe (I) go around' PART+P(Vf)-Aloc(ADVloc);
- the analytical expression (two-word) of a corresponding grammatical category of one of the sentence elements: *Ja kresliť budem* 'I draw will' S-P: S(PRONper)-P(Vffut).

With respect to nominal categories, this stage is characterized by the occurrence of at least one case structure: Dsg, Dpl, Acpl, Gsg, Gpl, Lsg, Lpl. At the same time, cases associated with prepositions occur: G+, L+, Ac+, D+, I+, agreement. In the verbal categories, 2nd person sg., 1st person pl., future tense, and passive participle (in the resultative construction) occur. As for prepositions, we expect occurrences of the prepositions *na, do, s, pre* and *v*.

Stage IV: Four-and-more-words level

The grammatical quality of four-word and multi-word sentence structures was determined from the perspective of the sentence elements structure and its specification with the proportion of the following structures:

One-element structure: P;
Two-element structure: P-O, P-A, S-P;
Three-element structure: P-O-O, P-A-A, P-O-A, S-P-O, S-P-A;
Four-element structure: P-A-A-A, P-O-O-A, P-O-A-A, S-P-A-A, S-P-O-A[10]

The occurrence of attribute ATR- and coordinative syntagmas (X(+)X) is noted separately.

All other structures are classified as Other. Four-word and multi-word expression of syntactic structures by one, two and three sentence elements is analogous to that for three-word structures. We also expect the production of other prepositions (*o, k*), as comparative and superlative occur among nominal categories, and of the conditional as a new development within verbal categories.

Stage V: Compound sentence level

The grammatical quality of compound sentence structures was determined with reference to basic sentence structures. We distinguish between simple compound and complex compound sentences according to the number of clauses. A simple compound sentence consists of two clauses, and according to the syntactic relationship is classified into paratactic (HV-HV) and hypotactic (HV-VV) types (cf. Ivanová, 2011; Kočiš, 1973; Nižníková, 1994). A complex compound sentence consists of three clauses, and according to the syntactic relationship we distinguish between a paratactic compound sentence (HV-HV-HV), a hypotactic complex sentence (HV-VV-VV) and a mixed (paratactic-hypotactic) compound sentence (HV-VV-HV).

We specify basic syntactic structure according to the content relationships between clauses and according to the nature of the connectives. Paratactic compound sentences may be divided into copulative complex sentences (KOP), adversative complex sentences (ADZ), disjunctive complex sentences (DIZ) and gradational complex sentences (GRA). For hypotactic compound sentences, dependent clauses are classified according to the sentence element expressed by the object clause (vvO), the adverbial clause (vvA) and the attributive clause (vvATR). More rarely occurring types of compound sentence constructions are classified as Other.

Despite the fact that the first occurrences of both coordinative and subordinative connectivity expressed by conjunctions are found at earlier stages of syntactic development, conjunctions and other connecting means become indicators of connection at the level of two and more clauses. According to Ivanová (2011), clauses may be connected asyndetically within paratactic compound sentences. As reported by Kesselová *et al.* (2013: 202–203), 'in communication, conjunctions *a*, *aj*, *ale*, *lebo*, *aby*, *že* form the most frequently used core of the conjunction subsystem; idiolect of particular children contains also other conjunctions and relatives such as *či*, *ako*, *čo*, *keď*, *alebo*.' In verbal categories we expect an active participle. At the level of two and more clauses we identify syntactically correct and syntactically incorrect utterances.

Stage VI: Narrative level

Narrative refers to a connection of three and more utterances related by a temporal or logical and causal relationship (Owens, 2001). This stage is evaluated via other diagnostic tools; therefore this stage is not presented in the chart. The narrative level only indicates further progression in language and syntactic development. What is becoming an important part when evaluating narratives is the assessment of a story's microstructure (cf. Gagarina *et al.*, 2012; Kapalková *et al.*, 2016), which tends to be expressed via a variety of grammatical and/or lexical means.

Formal Design of the LARSPsk Chart[11]

Sections A–D are identical to those in LARSPe (English terms are translated into Slovak).

For minor syntactic structures, the types of utterances are identical to those in LARSPe.

On a separate line, the pragmatic characteristics of the utterances are recorded (English terms commands, questions, statements are translated into Slovak).

For major syntactic structures, respective grammatical categories and their representatives are noted in the following columns:

Stages I–V (*Úroveň* I–V);
At stage I–IV, column labelled *Vetnočlenská štruktúra* (sentence elements structure);
At stage I, column labelled *Slovnodruhová a tvarová štruktúra* (word class and form structure);
At stage I, column labelled *Neverbálna štruktúra* (non-verbal structure), *Gesto* (gesture) with complementary (KG) and supplementary (SG) connections of gesture and word;
At stages II–V, a column labelled *Spojky* (conjunctions): used conjunctions are recorded;
At stages II–IV, columns labelled *Základná* (basic) and *Špecifická* (specific) sentence elements structure;
At stages II–III, a column labelled *Vetný ekvivalent* (sentence equivalent);
At stages II–IV, a separate line for recording attribute (ATR-);
At stage IV, a separate line for recording coordinative syntagma (X(+)X);
At stage V, compound sentences are noted in the column labelled *Súvetná štruktúra* (complex compound sentence structure): columns *Základná* (basic) and *Špecifická* (specific) complex compound sentence structure;
At stage V, a separate line for recording correctly (+) and incorrectly (-) produced syntactic constructions;
At stage I–V a column labelled *Morfosyntaktická štruktúra* (morphosyntactic structure). In the column labelled *Menné kategórie* (nominal categories) and in the column labelled *Slovesné kategórie* (verbal categories), we recorded the occurrence of the corresponding category together with frequency of occurrence. Unlike LARSPe, the production of grammatical meanings within morphosyntactic categories is noted from the one-word level;
At stages III–V, a separate column labelled *Predložky* (prepositions).

Meno	Vek	Dátum	Druh rozhovoru

A	Neanalyzované			Problémové		Rutinné
	Nezrozumiteľné	Interjekcie	Odchýlky	Neúplné	Nejednoznačné	

B	Odpovede dieťaťa	Opakovania	Bežné odpovede				Nie bežné odpovede		Problematické
			Produktívne			Neproduktívne	Štruktúrne	Nulové	
	Všetky		Celé	Redukované	Eliptické				
					1				
	Typ podnetu terapeuta				2				
	Otázky				3+				
	Iné								
C	Spontánne výpovede								

D	Reakcie partnera	Opakovania	Všeobecné	Štruktúrne	Nulové	Iné	Problematické
	Direktívy		Otázky			Referencie	
Neproduktívne			Oslovenia		Problémové		

Úroveň	Spojky	Základná	Špecifická	Vetný ekvivalent	Neverbálna štruktúra / Predložky	Menné kategórie	Slovesné kategórie
Úroveň I (0;9-1;2) 1 slovo	Produktívne: Vetnočlenská štruktúra: P(Vf)	Slovnodruhová a tvarová štruktúra: SUB	PRON	ADV, Iné	Neverbálna štruktúra: Gesto: KG, SG	Morfosyntaktická štruktúra: Menné kategórie: Nsg	Slovesné kategórie: imp
Úroveň II (1;3 - 1;8) 2 slová	Spojky: a aj	Vetnočlenská štruktúra – Základná: P S-P P-O P-A Iné	Špecifická: Vf VVP Od Oi A(PRONin)X ATR-	Vetný ekvivalent: A+ Iné Problémové		Asg Npl Isg Ipl	3sg 3pl 1sg préz sfut prét ind inf ne+ zhoda
Úroveň III (1;9 - 2;2) 3 slová	a aj alebo preto lebo	Základná: P S-P P-O P-A P-O-O P-O-A P-A-A S-P-O S-P-A Iné	Špecifická: Vf VVP VNP Od Oi ATR-	Vetný ekvivalent: O+ S+ A+ Problémové	Predložky: na do s pre v	Dsg Apl Dpl Gpl Lsg Lpl G+ L+ A+ D+ I+ zhoda	2sg 1pl 2pl fut part/pas
Úroveň IV (2;3 - 2;8) 4 a viac slov	a ale a potom aj-aj aby pretože lebo	Základná: P P-O P-A S-P P-O-O P-A-A P-O-A S-P-O S-P-A P-A-A-A P-O-O-A P-O-A-A S-P-O-O S-P-A-A S-P-O-A S-P-O-O-A-A Iné	Špecifická: Vf VVP VNP Od Oi ATR- X(+)X	Problémové	o k	komparatív superlatív	kondicionál
Úroveň V (2;9 +)	a ale a potom aj-aj aby pretože lebo že kde čo	Súvetná štruktúra – Základná: 2 klauzy HV-HV HV-VV 3 klauzy HV-HV-HV HV-VV-VV HV-HV-VV	Špecifická: KOP ADZ GRA DIS Iné vvO vvA vvATR Iné		Iné		part/akt
	(+) syntakticky správne výpovede				(-) syntakticky nesprávne výpovede		
Celkový počet výpovedí		Priemerný počet výpovedí v replike			Priemerná dĺžka výpovede v slovách		

Figure 3.1 LARSP chart for Slovak

An Example of the Use of the Profile Chart

In Slovakia, several assessment methods and procedures are used to determine the current communication level of children in early speech-language intervention. Among the primarily used, internationally known and standardized methods in Slovakia are the Slovak adaptation of the MacArthur-Bates CDI (Test komunikačného správania TEKOS – Kapalková *et al.*, 2010) and the adaptation of Margaret Lahey's model (Lahey, 1988; Mikulajová & Kapalková, 2002). Both approaches are applied to determine the childreńs communication level from several perspectives – lexical-semantic, morphological-syntactic and pragmatic. They also partially describe the capacity of Slovak children to use grammatical patterns. The LARSP approach represents a systematic and simplified form of grammatical development placing emphasis on the analysis of syntactic components present in children's grammar. This aspect is important to children in early intervention. Their characteristic feature is the fact that their speech development does not correspond to their chronological age. When compared to their peers, these children do not speak at all or speak a lot less (Rossetti, 2001).

To verify LARSPsk we studied a language sample produced by a 39-month-old child.[12] The child's parents consulted a speech therapist because of concern about their child's development and also because their child spoke less than his peers. The child was raised in a complete family, was not diagnosed with a hearing disorder, mental disability or neurological disorder.

A language sample was collected during a standardized screening of the child in the counselling centre, resulting in 66 utterances which met the requirements for further analysis. The majority of the child's utterances were assigned to stage II. Within the sentence elements structure, we found that all expected structures except attribute were used. At the same time, however, we noted other relatively frequently occurring structures, within which the child connected predicate or subject with an interjection (*Mama fúfú* 'Mummy *fúfú*' – interjection of blowing, *Stalo bum* 'Happened *boom*'). The child did not express all defined case constructions within nominal categories, but did express almost all verbal categories typical for the given stage.

The sample also included four three-word utterances. Again, however, we noted other occurrences, where the child replaced the predicate by an interjection (*Tam ocko pá* 'There daddy' – *pá* is an interjection denoting 'away') or completely omitted the predicate (*Tam ocko preč* 'There daddy away'). There was no prepositional connection in the sample. In terms of given structures, the child was assigned to stage II (1;3-1;8), despite its chronological age of 3;3 years, when the first narrative structures are expected. The detailed clinical sample chart is presented in Figure 3.2.

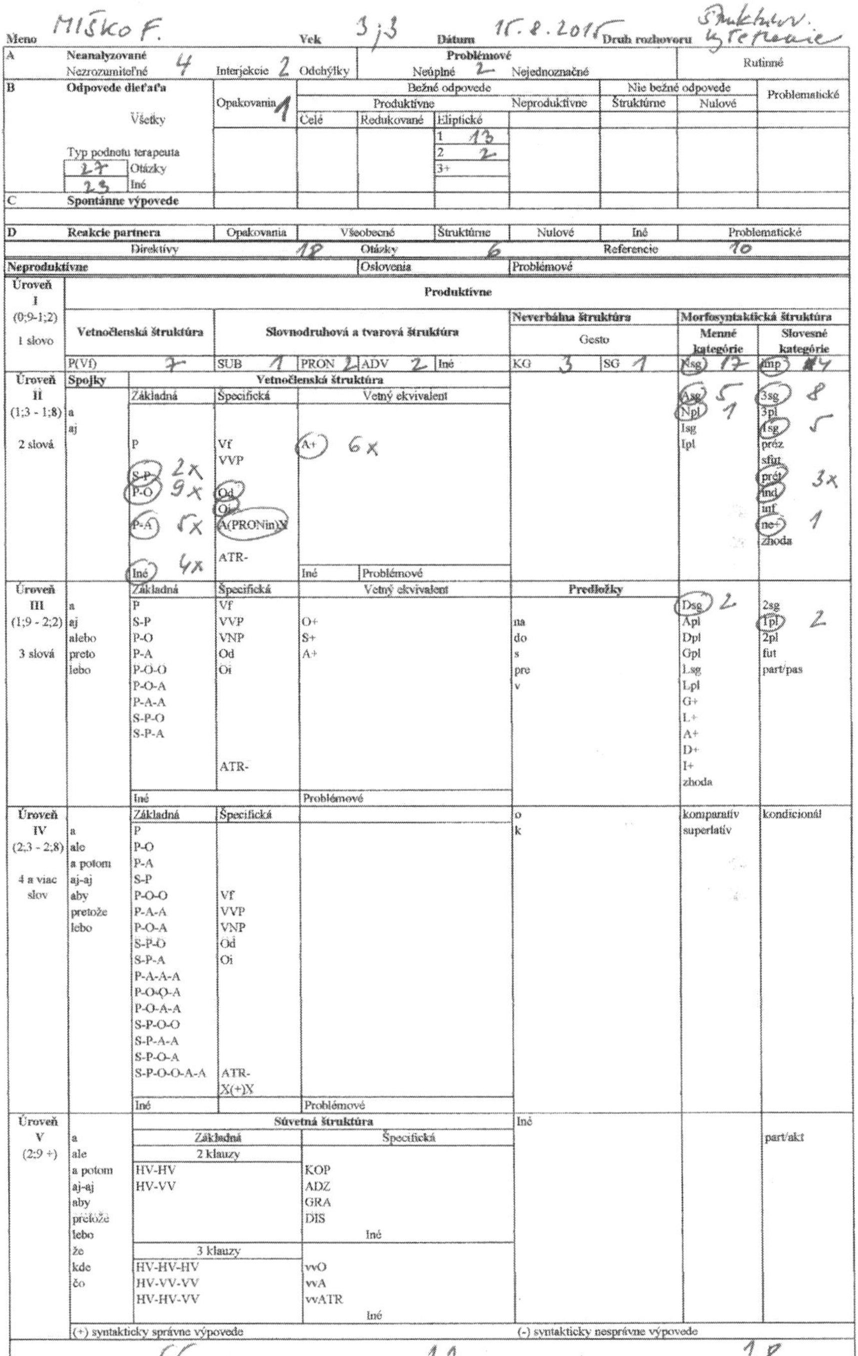

Meno MIŠKO F. Vek 3;3 Dátum 15.8.2015 Druh rozhovoru

A Neanalyzované: Nezrozumiteľné 4; Interjekcie 2; Odchýlky. Problémové: Neúplné 2; Nejednoznačné. Rutinné

B Odpovede dieťaťa: Všetky. Opakovania 1. Bežné odpovede: Produktívne (Celé, Redukované, Eliptické: 1 13, 2 2, 3+); Neproduktívne. Nie bežné odpovede: Štruktúrne, Nulové. Problematické

Typ podnetu terapeuta: 27 Otázky; 23 Iné

C Spontánne výpovede

D Reakcie partnera: Opakovania, Všeobecné, Štruktúrne, Nulové, Iné, Problematické. Direktívy 18; Otázky 6; Referencie 10

Neproduktívne: Oslovenia; Problémové

Produktívne

Úroveň I (0;9-1;2) 1 slovo: Vetnočlenská štruktúra: P(Vf) 7. Slovnodruhová a tvarová štruktúra: SUB 1, PRON 2, ADV 2, Iné. Neverbálna štruktúra – Gesto: KG 3, SG 1. Morfosyntaktická štruktúra – Menné kategórie: Nsg 17; Slovesné kategórie: imp 14

Úroveň II (1;3-1;8) 2 slová: Spojky: a, aj. Vetnočlenská štruktúra – Základná: P, S-P 2x, P-O 9x, P-A 5x, Iné 4x; Špecifická: Vf, VVP, Od, Oi, A(PRONin)X, ATR-; Vetný ekvivalent: A+ 6x; Iné; Problémové. Menné kategórie: Asg 5, Npl 1, Isg, Ipl. Slovesné kategórie: 3sg 8, 3pl, 1sg 5, préz, sfut, prét 3x, ind, inf, ne+ 1, zhoda

Úroveň III (1;9-2;2) 3 slová: Spojky: a, aj, alebo, preto, lebo. Základná: P, S-P, P-O, P-A, P-O-O, P-O-A, P-A-A, S-P-O, S-P-A; Špecifická: Vf, VVP, VNP, Od, Oi, ATR-; Vetný ekvivalent: O+, S+, A+; Iné; Problémové. Predložky: na, do, s, pre, v. Menné kategórie: Dsg 2, Apl, Dpl, Gpl, Lsg, Lpl, G+, L+, A+, D+, I+, zhoda. Slovesné kategórie: 2sg, 1pl 2, 2pl, fut, part/pas

Úroveň IV (2;3-2;8) 4 a viac slov: Spojky: a, ale, a potom, aj-aj, aby, pretože, lebo. Základná: P, P-O, P-A, S-P, P-O-O, P-A-A, P-O-A, S-P-O, S-P-A, P-A-A-A, P-O-O-A, P-O-A-A, S-P-O-O, S-P-A-A, S-P-O-A, S-P-O-O-A-A; Špecifická: Vf, VVP, VNP, Od, Oi, ATR-, X(+)X; Iné; Problémové. Predložky: o, k. Menné kategórie: komparatív, superlatív. Slovesné kategórie: kondicionál

Úroveň V (2;9 +): Spojky: a, ale, a potom, aj-aj, aby, pretože, lebo, že, kde, čo. Súvetná štruktúra – Základná: 2 klauzy: HV-HV, HV-VV; 3 klauzy: HV-HV-HV, HV-VV-VV, HV-HV-VV. Špecifická: KOP, ADZ, GRA, DIS, Iné; vvO, vvA, vvATR, Iné. Iné. part/akt

(+) syntakticky správne výpovede; (-) syntakticky nesprávne výpovede

Celkový počet výpovedí 66; Priemerný počet výpovedí v replike 1,1; Priemerná dĺžka výpovede v slovách 1,8

Figure 3.2 Clinical sample LARSP chart for Slovak

The exact definition of child's developmental level based on the acquired morphosyntactic structures enables the primary logopedig quantification and assessment of how much is the child behind his/her peers. The rate of the lag is important from the point of other diagnostic processes and can be easily combined with the classical method based on the model of Margaret Lahey, broadly used in Slovak logopedic intervention (Mikulajová & Kapalková, 2002). In the next step, the grammatical profile of a given child enables exact definition of the therapy targets, which are usually determined by the structures with the biggest developmental delay. Last but not least, it is important to consider the LARSPsk as a tool for measuring of the therapy effect, when during repeated re-diagnostic sessions enables the speech therapist to control the rate of improvement.

Notes

(1) As we have had the possibility to observe the given children growing (now they are 16 years old), we may conclude that our assumption proved to be correct.
(2) The examples come from transcribed recordings of children's utterances. The examples do not follow the pronunciation of the child, which is not consistent with the target words of adults. These examples are translated word-by-word.
(3) Based on the transcript, a word is defined as every sequence of morphemes separated by spaces – taking into account the so-called first words as well. According to Kesselová (2008: 131), first words are considered to be 'such sound complexes which in their sound form more or less differ from target words used by adults, but the child uses them repeatedly, however, with a fixed meaning. Such words are situationally interpretable by adults and the child accepts such interpretation by agreement or at least by not appealing such interpretation.'
(4) The position of attribute is different from the position of other sentence elements. Attribute, being dependent on the noun, is a sentence element that modifies the noun in any position within the sentence elements structure. Attribute is not a regular constitutive component of the sentence structure. According to form and position in the word order a distinction is made between congruent and non-congruent attribute.
(5) In the context of Slovak syntactic tradition, the complement is understood as a sentence element modifying noun, or pronoun, and predicative verb or adjective, where noun, or pronoun functions as subject or object within the sentence elements structure (Ivanová, 2011: 104; Kačala, 1971). The complement is a sentence element, which at the same time forms a complementary semi-predicative construction.
(6) Data in Table 3.4 were obtained by calculating the average of the month when the child used a particular category for the first time throughout the longitudinal observation, and when the category was first time noted via TEKOS II and when more than 50% of parents observed production of such category. With respect to cases not evaluated by TEKOS II, we took into account the data obtained throughout the longitudinal observation.
(7) A case study dealing with the development of pragmatic functions of utterances showed that basic syntactic structure in the early phase of development are formed especially in utterances with pragmatic functions of here and now statements, answers and prompting (Slančová & Sokolová, 2012; Slančová & Kičura Sokolová, 2018).
(8) 'Sentence equivalents are assessed as a separate syntactic form, not as a result of actual ellipsis. An argument in favour of such understanding is the fact that complementing a potential predicate would result in a redundant utterance, which would interfere with maxim of quantity within the cooperation principle.' (Ivanová, 2011: 62).

(9) Sign – refers to a syntactic relationship; sign (+) refers to coordination, sign + refers to (a) connection between a sentence element and synsemantic word not functioning as a sentence element; (b) any other syntactic structures based on sentence equivalents.
(10) This study revealed a single six-element structure (S-P-O-O-A-A): *Ujo tak dal si tam kartu* = Uncle so gave himself there card.
(11) The full LARSPsk chart is presented in Figure 3.1.
(12) The next pilot study (Bezáková, 2017) tested LARSPsk on three children with Developmental Language Disorder.

References

Bezáková, A. (2017) Pilotné overenie gramatického profilu u slovenských detí s vývinovou dysfáziou. [Master's thesis]. Bratislava: Pedagogická fakulta Univerzity Komenského.

Boehm, J., Daley, G., Harvey, S., Hawkins, A. and Tsap, B. (2005) *Language Assessment Remediation and Screening Procedure*. Users manual. La Trobe University.

Capirci, O., Iverson, J., Pizzuto, E. and Volterra, V. (1996) Gestures and words during the transition to two-word speech. *Journal of Child Language* 23 (3), 645–673.

Crystal, D. (1979) *Working with LARSP*. London: Edward Arnold.

Crystal, D. (1992) *Profiling Linguistic Disability* (2nd edn). San Diego: Singular Publishing Group. http://hdl.handle.net/10092/5510

Crystal, D., Fletcher, P. and Garman, M. (1989) *Grammatical Analysis of Language Disability* (2nd edn). London: Cole and Whurr. http://hdl.handle.net/10092/5583

Dale, P. and Penfold, M. (2011) *Adaptations of the MacArthur-Bates CDI into non-U.S. English languages*. http://mb-cdi.stanford.edu/documents/AdaptationsSurvey7-5-11Web.pdf

Dolník, J. (2000) Vývin morfológie súčasnej spisovnej slovenčiny. In J. Mlacek (ed.) *Studia Academica Slovaca* 29, 277–286.

Fečková Kapalková, S. (2002) Vytvorenie modelu jazykových schopností po slovensky hovoriacich detí na základe Laheyovej teórie. [Dissertation thesis]. Bratislava: Pedagogická fakulta Univerzity Komenského.

Fečková, S. and Slančová, D. (2001) K niektorým východiskám výskumu a modelovania rečového vývinu dieťaťa. In V. Lechta (ed.) *Logopaedica*, 4. Bratislava: Vydavateľstvo Liečreh Gúth, 38–45.

Gagarina, N.V., Klop, D., Kunnari, S., Tantele, K., Välimaa, T., Balčiūnienė, I. *et al.* (2012) MAIN: Multilingual assessment instrument for narratives. *ZAS Papers in Linguistics*, 56. Berlin: ZAS.

Ivanová, M. (2011) *Syntax slovenského jazyka*. Prešov: Vydavateľstvo Prešovskej univerzity.

Kačala, J. (1971) *Doplnok v slovenčine*. Bratislava: Vydavateľstvo SAV.

Kapalková, S. (2008) Gestá v kontexte psychického vývinu. In D. Slančová (ed.) *Štúdie o detskej reči* (pp. 169–211). Prešov: Filozofická fakulta Prešovskej univerzity.

Kapalková, S. (2018) Gesto ako prediktor gramatiky. In D. Slančová (ed.) *Desať štúdií o detskej reči* (pp. 424–445) Prešov: Filozofická fakulta Prešovskej univerzity v Prešove, Bratislava: Veda.

Kapalková, S., Slančová, D., Bónová, I., Kesselová, J. and Mikulajová, M. (2010) *Hodnotenie komunikačných schopností detí v ranom veku*. Bratislava: Slovenská asociácia logopédov.

Kapalková, S., Slančová, D., Kesselová, J., Bónová, I., Mikulajová, M. and Zajacová, S. (2011) Vývin gramatiky v detskej reči na základe priemernej dĺžky výpovede. In M. Ološtiak, M. Ivanová and D. Slančová (eds) *Vidy jazyka a jazykovedy*. (pp. 104–115). Prešov: Filozofická fakulta Prešovskej univerzity v Prešove. http://www.pulib.sk/elpub2/FF/Olostiak2/index.html

Kapalková, S., Polišenská, K., Marková, L. and Fenton, J. (2016) Narrative abilities in early successive bilingual Slovak-English children: A cross-language comparison. *Applied Psycholinguistics* 37 (1), 145–164.
Kesselová, J. (2008) Sémantické kategórie v ranej ontogenéze reči dieťaťa. In D. Slančová (ed.) *Štúdie o detskej reči* (pp. 121–168). Prešov: Filozofická fakulta Prešovskej univerzity.
Kesselová, J. and Slančová, D. (2010) Slovak. *Revue Belge de philologie et d'historie* 88 (2), 873–896.
Kesselová, J., Karpinský, P., Imrichová, M. and Podhajecká, K. (2013) *Spojky a spájacie prostriedky v slovenčine*. Bratislava: Veda.
Kesselová, J. (2014a) Ako sa rodí pád. In J. Kesselová, M. Imrichová and M. Ološtiak (eds) *Registre jazyka a jazykovedy*. II (pp. 22–34). Prešov: Filozofická fakulta Prešovskej univerzity v Prešove.
Kesselová, J. (2014b) *Funkčno-sémantická ktegória relačnosť v ranej ontogenéze reči dieťaťa hovoriaceho po slovensky*. Prešov: Prešovská univerzita v Prešove. http://www.pulib.sk/web/kniznica/elpub/dokument/Kesselova5
Kičura Sokolová, J. (2013) Vývin substantívnych vetných štruktúr v ranej syntaxi dieťaťa. In *Jazyk a kultúra* 4 (14). http://www.ff.unipo.sk/jak/cislo14.html
Kičura Sokolová, J. (2014) Pronominálne a adverbiálne jednoslovné vetné štruktúry a ich postavenie v ranom vývine detskej syntaxe. In *Jazyk a kultúra* 5 (19–20). http://www.ff.unipo.sk/jak/cislo19-20.html
Kočiš, F. (1973) *Zložené súvetie v slovenčine*. Bratislava: Vydavateľstvo SAV.
Lahey, M. (1988) *Language Disorders and Language Development*. New York: Macmillan Publ. Comp.
McEachern, D. and Haynes, W. (2004) Gesture-speech combination as a transition to multiword utterances. *American Journal of Speech-Language Pathology*, Aug; 13 (3), 227–235.
Mikulajová, M. and Kapalková, S. (2002) Terapia narušeného vývinu reči. In V. Lechta (ed.) *Terapia narušenej komunikačnej schopnosti* (pp. 23–58). Martin: Osveta.
Nižníková, J. (1993) *Praktická príručka slovenskej skladby*. Prešov: Slovacontact.
Novák, Ľ. (1977) Typologická charakteristika slovenčiny. In J. Mistrík (ed.) *Studia Academica Slovaca*, 6, 389–406.
Owens, R. (2001) *Language Development: An Introduction*. New York: Allyn and Bacon.
Rossetti, L.M. (2000) *Communication Intervention: Birth to Three*. Delmar Cengage Learning.
Slančová, D. (ed.) (2008) *Štúdie o detskej reči*. Prešov: Filozofická fakulta Prešovskej univerzity.
Slančová, D. (ed.) (2018) Desať štúdií o detskej reči. Bratislava, Prešov: VEDA, Filozofická fakulta Prešovskej univerzity v Prešove.
Slančová, D., Kapalková, S., Kesselová, J. and Zajacová, S. (2011) Mean length of utterance in morphemes, syllables and words in Slovak as a flective language – theory and practice. In *IASCL 2011. Montreal. The International Association for the Study of Child language. 12th Congress. 19–23 July, 2011, Montreal, Canada. Social, genetic and cognitive determinants in the acquisition and development of language.* (p. 192). Montreal: Université du Quebec à Montréal.
Slančová, D. and Sokolová, J. (2012) Vzťah syntaxe a pragmatiky v ranom vývine detskej reči. In R. Novák (ed.) *Slovo a obraz v komunikaci s dětmi. Svoboda jazyka – jazyk svobody* (pp. 27–37). Ostrava: Ostravská univerzita v Ostravě, Pedagogická fakulta, katedra českého jazyka a literatury s didaktikou.
Slančová, D. and Kičura Sokolová, J. (2018) Vývin syntaxe v ranom veku. In D. Slančová (ed.) *Desať štúdií o detskej reči* (pp. 508–626). Prešov: Filozofická fakulta Prešovskej univerzity v Prešove, Bratislava: Veda.
Sokolová, J. (2013) Východiská výskumu vývinu ranej syntaxe. In B. Bednaříková and P. Hernandezová (eds) *Od slova k modelu jazyka* (pp. 332–342). Olomouc: Univerzita Palackého v Olomouci.

Appendix

List of abbreviations

A	adverbial modifier
Ac	accusative case
act	active voice
ADJ	adjective
ADV	adverb
ADVloc	adverb of place
ADVmod	adverb of manner
ADVtemp	adverb of time
ADZ	adversative complex sentence
Aloc	adverbial modifier of place
ATR	attribute
C	complement
CON	conjunction
cond	conditional mood
D	dative case
DIZ	disjunctive complex sentence
G	genitive case
GRA	gradational complex sentence
HV	main clause
I	instrumental case
imp	imperative mood
ind	indicative mood
INF	infinitive
INT	interjection
KOP	copulative complex sentence
L	locative case
LARSPe	LARSP for English-speaking children
LARSPsk	LARSP for Slovak-speaking children
N	nominative case
neg	negation
NUM	numeral
O	object

Od	direct object
Oi	indirect object
P	predicate
PARact	active participle
PARpas	passive participle
PART	particle
pas	passive voice
pl	plural
PREP	preposition
PRON	pronoun
PRONdem	demonstrative pronoun
PRONint	interrogative pronoun
PRONper	personal pronoun
PRONpos	possessive pronoun
S	subject
sg	singular
SUB	noun
TEKOS	test of communicative behaviour
V	verb
Vf	finite verb
Vfcop	copula
Vffut	finite verb in future tense
Vflimit	limitative verb
VFmod	modal verb
Vfneg	finite verb in negative form
VNP	complex verbo-nominal predicate
VV	subordinate clause
vvA	subordinate adverbial clause
vvATR	subordinate attributive clause
vvO	subordinate object clause
VVP	complex verbal predicate

4 Croatian LARSP

Vesna Mildner, Vesna Stojanovik and Diana Tomić

Introduction

The aim of this chapter is to provide a pilot adaptation of a Croatian version of the Language Assessment, Remediation and Screening Procedure (LARSP). As far as we are aware, this is the first attempt to produce a LARSP in Croatian, and we expect that this first version will later be further adapted and refined. It is designed on the model of the English version of LARSP, developed by Crystal *et al.* (1989) and covers the grammatical development of Croatian between 10 and 36 months. This pilot version of the Croatian LARSP is based on the analysis of longitudinal data from three children in the Croatian corpus currently available on CHILDES and the data from four other children aged between 3;0 and 3;4 collected in 2015–2016 in Croatia. The proposed stages should be treated as approximate and future research should verify the reliability of the stages for a larger sample. Because of the small sample size, it is possible some structures currently featuring in specific stages should be moved to a stage above, or stage below the one they are currently in. The data for stages I, II, III and IV are based on entirely spontaneous productions. Hence, the absence of certain structures in specific stages may be due to the lack of data, rather than the fact that these structures may not have been acquired yet. The chapter is organized as follows: first we describe Croatian and its grammatical features, then we provide a description of grammatical development as it unfolds over five stages with illustrative examples. A copy of the proposed chart is found in Appendix 1 of this chapter.

Croatian is a Western South Slavic language (Indo-European language family), spoken by about 4 million people in Croatia and as many abroad. It is one of the official languages of the European Union. It uses Latin script (some letters include diacritics) and has shallow orthography, i.e. high degree of phoneme-to-grapheme correspondence (although due to assimilation processes, spoken language does not always preserve the written form).

Standard Croatian is a pitch-accent language. The full accent system comprises four accent types that combine stress (emphasis), duration (nucleus length) and tone (high tone on the stressed syllable or the one following it; low tone on others) with additional lengthening of unstressed post-accentual vowel in specific conditions, but the full distinction is not used in all dialects. Vowels and syllabic /r/ are accent carriers and accent position is free, with few exceptions (that are also violated in some dialects). Croatian is a syllable-timed language (like e.g. Spanish, French, Italian, Japanese), i.e. the length of unstressed syllables is not noticeably reduced as in stress-timed languages (like e.g. English, Russian, Swedish). Clitics do not have an accent of their own and share the stress of the word preceding them (enclitics) or following them (proclitics). Some types of stress from the lexical word may be transferred to a proclitic. Each of the three elements of the accent may change the meaning of the word on its own.

Croatian includes three groups of dialects that got their names based on the word for what: Chakavian (what = /tʃa/), Kaikavian (what = /kaj/) and Shtokavian (what = /ʃto/). Standard Croatian is Shtokavian.

Characteristics of Croatian Grammar

Word and phrase level

There are four inflectional word classes (nouns, verbs, adjectives, pronouns) and four non-inflectional (adverbs, prepositions, conjunctions, exclamations). Nouns, verbs, adjectives, adverbs and exclamations are lexical (open-class) words whereas pronouns, prepositions and conjunctions are grammatical (closed-class) words.

Nouns

Gender

Croatian nouns belong to one of three genders: masculine, feminine, neuter. As a rule, nouns that denote men and male animals share masculine gender, those that denote women and female animals are feminine, and nouns denoting children and young animals take neuter, but there are exceptions. Inanimate nouns can take any gender. Noun gender determines gender of its attributes (adjectives, numerals, pronouns) and some verb forms (e.g. participles in past tense and conditional). Exceptions aside, there are a few simple rules in recognizing noun gender from the ending in citation form (Jelaska, 2015) (vowel or consonant), which can be seen in Table 4.1.

Number

Nouns can have singular or plural form (with some exceptions). They differ in the number and type of suffixes. Gender and number agreement is obligatory when nouns are accompanied by adjectives, pronouns and numerals (see Table 4.2).

Case

Cases are important for expressing relationships within a sentence. Croatian has seven cases, summarized in Table 4.3. Plural is formed from

Table 4.1 Recognizing gender of Croatian nouns

Ending in citation form	Gender	Exceptions
-a	almost definitely feminine	very few masculine
-e	most likely neuter	proper names, loan-words (→masculine)
-o	probably neuter	proper names, loan-words (→masculine); derived from or alternating with –l (→masculine or feminine)
-i	masculine	foreign female names; *mati* ('mother'), *kći* ('daughter')
-C	most likely masculine	very few feminine

Table 4.2 Gender and number agreement of pronouns, adjectives and nouns

	FEM	MASC	NEUT
sg	*Ova dobra žena* 'this good woman'	*Ovaj dobar muškarac* 'this good man'	*Ovo dobro dijete* 'this good child'
pl	*Ove dobre žene* 'these good women'	*Ovi dobri muškarci* 'these good men'	*Ova dobra djeca* 'these good children'

Table 4.3 Summary of Croatian cases

Case	Role	Note
Nominative (NOM)	Subject (agent, patient) Noun predicate	
Genitive (GEN)	Missing subject Possession Part of whole Characteristics Adverbial of time	In nonstandard variants possession is sometimes expressed by adding *od* ('of') E.g. **kuća od moje bake* ('my granny's house')
Dative (DAT)	Receiver Direction	
Accusative (ACC)	Object	In singular, masculine nouns referring to inanimate objects take the nominative form and those referring to animate ones take the genitive form. In some nonstandard variants the distinction is not made and both take genitive form.
Vocative (VOC)		In nonstandard speech it is frequently replaced by nominative in singular (in plural that is standard).
Locative (LOC)	Place Topic of conversation	In singular, nouns in dative and locative have the same form. In plural, dative, locative and instrumental forms are the same.
Instrumental (INST)	Means Company	

Nominative (NOM) singular (sg) according to noun type. There are fewer different forms than in singular (2-4).

Adjectives

In addition to gender, number and case (determined by the noun), adjectives have indefinite and definite form. This is perhaps one of the most neglected features of Croatian and many native speakers do not apply (or are aware of) the difference. Part of the problem may lie in the fact that the two differ in writing only in the singular of masculine adjectives whereas the rest rely on prosodic differences that have been lost in many variants. Also, some adjectives do in fact have only the definite form and some only the indefinite form. Ordinal numerals are definite adjectives. In everyday speech definite forms are used more frequently.

(a) *Attributive* adjectives typically precede the noun (though in the early stages of language acquisition, adjectives may follow the noun):

1. *Odjenula je* *izgužvanu* *suknju.*
 'She put on a creased skirt.'

They can follow the noun for stylistic purposes, or if they are part of an adverbial phrase:

2. *Odjenula je* *suknju* *izgužvanu do neprepoznatljivosti.*
 'She put on a skirt creased beyond recognition.'

(b) *Predicative* adjectives are conjoined with the verb 'to be' (*biti*). In that case the indefinite form is obligatory:

3. *On* *je visok.* (not **visoki*)
 'He is tall'.

(c) *Nominal* adjectives are similar to nouns in their form and function. They are used to refer to the previously mentioned noun or as a mass noun/plural count noun. Note the use of the definite form here:

4. *Dvojica su* *mladića* *u teretani.* *Visoki* *je košarkaš.* (not **visok*)
 'There are two young men in the gym. The tall one is a basketball player.'

Comparison

Comparative is typically formed by adding *–ij* to the stem followed by the appropriate ending with respect to gender, number and case. Gender and number endings correspond to definite adjective endings: e.g. *zelen + ij + i = zeleniji* ('greener'-MASC NOMsg). Some adjectives, however, do not form comparatives by the same pattern, as illustrated by these examples in MASC NOMsg: e.g. *jak → jači* ('stronger'); *lak → lakši* ('easier'); *težak → teži* ('heavier'); *dalek → dalji* ('more distant'). There are also a small number of irregular comparatives, which are in fact found in some of the most frequent adjectives: *dobar → bolji* ('good → better'); *loš/zao → gori* ('bad/evil → worse'); *malen → manji* ('small → smaller');

velik → *veći* ('big → bigger'). Superlatives are formed by prefixing the comparative by *naj-* (*naj* + *manji*).

Possessive adjectives

Possessive adjectives are formed by two suffixes added to the noun stem. Suffix –*in* is used for feminine nouns (preceded by dropping the final *a*), e. g. *žena* + *in* → *ženin* ('woman's'). Suffix –*ov*/-*ev* (depending on stem final consonant) is used for masculine and neuter nouns: *muž* + *ev* → *mužev* ('husband's'); *brat* + *ov* →*bratov* ('brother's).

Numerals

Whereas ordinal numerals are definite adjectives and have to agree with the noun in number, gender and case, not all cardinal numerals behave the same. Numeral 'one' (*jedan*) behaves like an adjective. Numeral 'two' has different forms for feminine (*dvije*) and masculine/neuter nouns (*dva*). Numerals 'three' and 'four' (*tri*, *četiri*) have the same form for all genders. The noun following numerals 'two', 'three' and 'four' has the same paucal case. Numerals from 'five' up are unchangeable (followed by adjectives and nouns in GENpl). In spoken language numerals 'two', 'three' and 'four' are frequently not declined either.

Pronouns

The form of *personal* pronouns is determined by person (1st, 2nd, 3rd), number (singular or plural), gender (with the 3rd person; in case of mixed genders masculine form is used), case and formality (in formal address, 2nd person singular is replaced by plural). In addition to long forms, most have short, unstressed forms (in NOM, GEN and DAT). These are clitics and they share the stress of the word they precede or follow. They are used in all situations except at the beginning of a sentence, after prepositions and for emphasis. Croatian is a pro-drop language. *Interrogative* and *relative* pronouns are the same items with two functions (relative pronouns are obligatory in connecting the dependent and the main clause). The ACC of *čiji* ('whose') and *koji* ('which') take the form of NOM in case of inanimate objects and GEN in case of animate ones. There is only one *reflexive* pronoun (long form: *sebe*; short form: *se*) that is used regardless of number, gender or person. It is declined as feminine nouns ending in –a. The stem of *possessive* pronouns is determined by the gender and number of the possessor whereas the ending is determined by the gender and number of the possessed. They are declined in accordance with the gender of the noun. These pronouns may replace possessive adjectives. The *reflexive-possessive* pronoun *svoj* is perhaps the most difficult to use correctly (i.e. when something belongs to the subject of the sentence). It can be used for any person, singular or plural, but it is frequently replaced by possessive pronouns:

5. *Oprala sam* ***svoj*** *auto.* vs *Oprala sam* ***moj*** *auto.*
   I washed my car.
6. *Jesi li oprao svoj auto?* vs *Jesi li oprao tvoj auto?*
   Have you washed your car?

In 3rd person singular and plural, this replacement can affect the meaning. In other instances, it is just nonstandard use:

7. *Je li Boris oprao svoj auto?* vs *Je li Boris oprao njegov auto?*
   Did Boris wash his (own) car? Did Boris wash his (e.g. John's) car?

The degree of proximity is reflected in the three *demonstrative* pronouns (increasing in distance from the speaker): *ovaj, taj, onaj*. They have different forms for all genders. Some speakers have only *ovaj* or *taj* for the meaning of 'this' and *onaj* for 'that'. Demonstrative pronouns that refer to size or kind behave as adjectives. As many other languages, Croatian has universal, assertive existential, elective existential and negative *indefinite* pronouns. Multiple negatives in a sentence are obligatory:

8.	*Nigdje*	*nema*	*nikakvog*	*hlada.*
(literally:	*Nowhere	there isn't	no	shade.)
	'There is no shade anywhere.'			

Verbs

Along with its main (lexical, full) verbs, Croatian has two auxiliaries: *biti* ('to be') and *htjeti* ('to want'). They can also be main verbs. Verbs express grammatical categories by conjugation for tense, person, number, mood and voice. There is obligatory agreement in gender (FEM, MASC, NEUT), number (sg, pl) and person (1st, 2nd, 3rd) with the subject. This is achieved by an elaborate inflectional system whose details are beyond the scope of this chapter. More information can be found in e.g. Jelaska (2015) and Silić and Pranjković (2005).

Tense

Croatian has four past tenses, one present tense and two future tenses, summarized in Table 4.4.

In everyday use, past is commonly expressed by Perfect and future by Future I.

Voice

Croatian has active and passive voice. Passive is formed by adding a suffix (-t, -n or -en) to the infinitive or present form of transitive (very rarely intransitive) verbs. Gender suffixes are attached after that., e.g. *pjevati* ('to sing') → *pjeva + n + a* (FEM form) ('sung').

Transitivity

Transitive verbs are used with the (direct) object in accusative. Intransitive verbs have no direct object. Reflexive verbs contain the

Table 4.4 Summary of Croatian tenses

Time reference	Tense	Formation	Note
Past	Perfect	PRES of the short form of 'to be' + active past participle of the main verb	In case of null subject the order is reversed, i.e. the auxiliary follows the main verb
Distant past	Pluperfect (past perfect)	PAST of 'to be' + active past participle of the main verb	Used in complex sentences
	Aorist	Main verb	only perfective verbs
	Imperfect	Main verb	only imperfective verbs
Present	Present	Main verb	Only imperfective verbs
Future	Future I	PRES of the short (enclitic) form of 'to want' + INF of the main verb	In case of a 0 subject the order is reversed: INF of the main verb + short form of 'to want'
Precise point in the future	Future II (future perfect; future exact)	PERF of 'to be' + active past participle of the main verb	Used in complex sentences (temporal, conditional); only imperfective verbs

obligatory reflexive particle/pronoun *se*. The intransitive and reflexive alternatives have different meaning (see examples below).

9. *Zahvaljujem se na pozivu.* vs *Zahvaljujem na pozivu.*
   'Thank you for the invitation (but no, thanks).' 'Thank you for the invitation.'

Some verbs may occur in all three uses:

10. *Ana se igra s prijateljicama.* (reflexive)
    'Ana is playing with her friends.'
11. *Ana igra košarku.* (transitive)
    'Ana plays basketball.'
12. *Ana igra prljavo.* (intransitive)
    'Ana plays dirty.'

Aspect

Croatian verbs have two aspects: perfective (clear beginning and/or end of action) and imperfective (actions that are incomplete, ongoing, habitual, reversed or repeated). Some verbs have only one aspect, a few are biaspectual. From the same root (im)perfective verbs are formed by prefixation or suffixation:

13. *Kup-ov-a-ti* (imperfective) vs *kup-i-ti* (perfective)
    'To be (in the process of) buying' ('to buy')

14. *Kup-ov-a-ti* (imperfective) vs *na-kup-ova-ti* (perfective)
'To be (in the process of) buying' ('to buy (a lot)')

Verbal prefixes include 15 prepositions and additional five non-prepositional suffixes.

Finiteness

Finite verbs can stand on their own, whereas non-finite ones must be accompanied by auxiliary or a modal. There are three non-finite conjugation groups: infinitive, gerund and participle. Most Croatian verbs in the infinitive form end in *–ti* (some in *–ći*).

Modality

Modality can be expressed by lexical, morphological and other means. Modals can be used to request help or make suggestions. Most modals can have more than one meaning (see 15 and 16 below).

15. *Mora da si umorna.* 'You must be tired.'
16. *Moraš se odmoriti.* 'You must get some rest.'

Mood

Croatian has indicative, imperative and conditional mood (rarely optative as well). The tenses summarized in Table 4.4 are in indicative. Imperatives for 2nd person singular as well as for 1st and 2nd person plural are simple, morphological imperatives, consisting of a single word. For 1st person singular, a compound imperative consisting of the particle *da* + present tense:

17. *Da vidim!*
'Let me see!'

In 3rd person singular and plural, the particle *neka* + present tense are used.

18. *Neka vide!*
'Let them see!'

Negative imperatives can be expressed in two ways – (a) is direct prohibitions, or (b) as polite, indirect prohibitions:

19(a) *Ne gledaj!* 19(b) *Nemoj gledati*!
Don't look!

Conjugations

Main verbs are conjugated depending on the class they belong to. Most Croatian verbs are thematic (regular). Athematic (irregular) verbs frequently form the past tense with different stems. Auxiliaries *biti* ('be') and *htjeti* ('have') as well as the modal *moći* ('to be able to') have special conjugations in the present tense. Other modals and main verbs are conjugated in accordance with the general rules. The present form of *biti* has a long form (used for emphasis, some questions, single-word answers) and a short form (more common). The perfective form of *biti* is used to make Future II, and its past form is used in the conditional. The auxiliary *htjeti* also has a long and a short form. The long form is used for emphasis and at the beginning of the sentence.

Uninflected word classes have only one form – they do not decline or conjugate – but some have phonological alternatives, for ease of pronunciation and/or avoidance of double consonants or clusters:

20.	*s Matom*	but	*sa Sašom*
	'with Mate'		'with Saša'

Prepositions

A noun or a pronoun preceded by a preposition always takes one of the oblique cases. Most prepositions take only one case (the majority of them appear with GEN). Some of the most frequent prepositions in Croatian can appear with two cases, which changes their meaning (a different case would be translated e.g. in English with a different pronoun):

- GEN (coming down from a place) or INST (accompaniment) – *s(a)* ('from' / 'with')

21. *Nakon 2 godine sišao*	*je s vrha*	*sa svojim psom.*
	-MASC,GEN	*-MASC,INST*
'After 2 years he came	from the top	with his dog.'

- ACC (goal of action/direction of motion) or LOC (place of action) – u ('into' /'in'), na ('to' / 'on'), po ('to' / 'on'), o ('against' / 'about')
- ACC (goal of action/direction of motion) or INST (specific place relations) – *pred* ('in front'), *pod* ('under'), *nad* ('above'), *među* ('between'), *za* ('for')

Adverbs

Adverbs modify/qualify mostly verbs, but also other adverbs, adjectives or clauses with respect to place and motion, time, frequency, manner, degree or any other aspect contained in the verb(phrase). They are typically placed immediately before the words they modify/qualify. Some adverbs are very similar to adjectives, some to pronouns. Adverbs can be derived from adjectives, nouns or adjectives that have been derived from nouns. There are three adverbs in Croatian that are frequently problematic for native speakers – in nonstandard use the distinction between them is lost (e.g. all three may be used to denote goal or *gdje* covers first two meanings, whereas the phrase *kojim putem* (literally 'which way') is used to cover the third):

22. *Gdje si?* (denoting place)
    'Where are you'?
23. *Kamo ideš?* (denoting goal of movement)
    'Where are you going'?
24. *Kuda ideš?* (denoting route)
    'Which way are you going'?

Conjunctions

As many other languages, Croatian distinguishes between coordinating conjunctions, e.g. *i* ('and'), *ali* ('but'), *ili* ('or') and subordinating ones, e.g. *da* ('that'), *ako* ('if'), *jer* ('because').

25. *Otišao je na dopust **i** pošteno se odmorio.*
    'He took his vacation and had a really good rest.'
26. *Ako ode na dopust, pošteno će se odmoriti.*
    'If he takes his vacation, he'll have a really good rest.'

Sentence level

In expressing relationships within a sentence, Croatian is a synthetic language as it relies on inflections and function words to indicate grammatical relations. Word order is not critical/fixed, however SVO is the unmarked order and other alternatives are considered to be marked and have stylistic value.

Declarative sentences (statements) typically follow SVO. The Subject is frequently omitted as it is implied from the form of the predicate. The direct object takes accusative case, and if there is an indirect object, it follows the direct object (and is usually in dative case).

An example of a declarative sentence with unmarked word order (27).

27.	*Baka Ana*	*često*	*peče*	*fine palačinke sčokoladom*	*svojoj maloj unuci*
	S	A	V	Od	A
	NP(NN)	AP(A)	VP(V)	NP (Adj N PP)	NP (Det Adj N)

'Grandma Ana frequently makes tasty pancakes with chocolate for her little granddaughter'

Interrogative sentences (questions) can be formed in several ways:

- Using a question word (Wh-questions)

  28. *Što* *čitaš?*
      What read-2nd person sg. PRES
      'What are you reading?'

- Declarative word order with rising intonation

29. *Čitaš* *knjigu?* (with rising intonation)
read-2nd person sg. PRES book-FEM,ACC
'Are you reading a book?'

Depending on sentence stress, the above question can be understood as asking:

(a) whether the person is in fact **reading** the book (rather than just looking at it) – stress on *čitaš*, or
(b) whether the person is reading the **book** (not a magazine) – stress on *knjigu*.

- Changes in word order and/or prosody, depending on what the topic of the question is.
  Emphasis on the object (book) can also be expressed by reversing the word order, i.e. OV (as in 30 below). In all examples there is null subject.

30. *Knjigu* *čitaš?*
book-FEM,ACC read-2nd sg. PRES
'Is it a book you are reading?'

- Yes/no questions with the use of the particle 'li' (not so frequent in spoken language)

31. *Čitaš li knjigu?*
'Are you reading a book?'

Commands are typically formed by the verb in imperative form followed by optional elements, e.g. direct object, indirect object, adverbials

32. *Stani!*
Stop- 2ndsg.IMP
'Stop!'
33. *Zadrži* *onu knjigu koju sam ti posudila lani.*
Keep-2nd sg.IMP the book I loaned you last year.

In spoken language *elliptical* sentences are quite common – especially in response to questions or in warnings, commands etc (see 34 for an example).

	Question	**Answer**
34.	*Koga čekate?*	*Prijatelja.*
		friend-MASC,ACC
	'Who are you waiting for?'	'My/A friend.'

Sentences can be simple or multiple. Multiple sentences contain more than one clause. There are three types of multiple sentences:

(1) compound (when two independent clauses are linked with a coordinator such as 'i' (and), 'ali' (but), 'or' (ili); though sometimes there is no coordinator and in writing punctuation is used). Traditional Croatian grammar books tend to classify these clauses into additive, alternative, inclusive, sequencing, contrastive. Additive, sequencing and contrastive are acquired before the age of 5.
(2) complex, in which clauses are linked by subordination. The subordinate clause may expand different part of the sentence (its subject, object, complement or adverbial). Those expressing causality using the subordinator 'jer' (because), goal using the subordinator 'da' (to) and temporal relationship using adverbs of time such as 'had' (when) are typically acquired before age 5.
(3) It is possible for coordination and subordination to occur in the same sentence and these are compound complex sentences.

More information on sentences and syntax in general can be found in Silić and Pranjković (2005).

Data Analysis

The data for the Croatian LARSP come from two sources: for children aged between 10 months and 3 years of age, the data come from the CHILDES database. The children were videotaped in naturalistic situations at home, interacting with family members and engaging in play activities. For children aged between 3;0 and 3:6 the data were collected as part of a larger project following a protocol. The sessions consisted of two parts: a 15 minute quasi-spontaneous conversation in which children talked about everyday situations, e.g. animals, fruits, vegetables they love/hate, where they like to play, who their friends are etc., and a more structured part (also approximately 15 minutes or longer) in which children were shown pictures of three family scenes (in the kitchen, in the living room, in the yard) and asked to talk about them as if they were happening in the past, present or future, respectively. When necessary they were prompted with questions in order to elicit as much language material as possible. The picture depicting a doctor's office was used to elicit general statements like When you go to the doctor's what do you do, what does the doctor do etc. Prepositions and oppositions (e.g. on, above, in front-behind, up-down) were elicited by asking questions about objects in different spatial relations presented in a drawing. All interviews were audiotaped at children's homes, by interviewers who were familiar to the children.

The A and B parts of the chart, which focus on interaction variables has been adopted from the English version of LARSP (Crystal *et al.*, 1989) and from the InuLARSP (Allen, Dench and Isakson, this volume). This section focuses on the types of responses that the child has produced and the way the responses were elicited.

Section A

This section of the Croatian LARSP is very similar to LARSP profiles for other languages (see Figure 4.1). It provides information about the child's name, date of birth and age, date of assessment, name of speech and language therapist and any other relevant information. This section also records the number of utterances which remained unanalysed because they were unintelligible, contained only a symbolic noise or were deviant. It also records the number of utterances which are problematic for analysis due to being incomplete, ambiguous and stereotypical. These have all been defined in the LARSP revision (Crystal, 1982: 16).

SECTION A	
Unanalysed 1 Unintelligible 2 Symbolic Noise 3 Deviant	**Problematic** 1 Incomplete 2 Ambiguous- 3 Stereotypes

Figure 4.1 Section A

UNANALYSED

1. An utterance is classed as **Unintelligible** if it is not possible to figure out its exact meaning and hence it is not possible to classify it into a grammatical category.
2. An utterance is classed as **Symbolic Noise** if it consists of an onomatopoeic noise representing a noise an animal would make (e.g. 'moo'), or the noise made by an object (e.g. 'wroom wroom')
3. An utterance is classed as **Deviant** if is structurally ungrammatical.

PROBLEMATIC

1. An utterance is coded as **Incomplete** if it was not finished
2. An utterance is coded as **Ambiguous** when it was possible for an utterance to be interpreted in two different ways and both would be correct
3. An utterance is coded as a **Stereotype** if it denoted a fixed phrase such a greeting ('bye-bye'), learnt utterances such as 'all gone', nursery rhyme lines.

Section B

We reduced section B to mark only the total number of utterances produced by the child and the number of utterances which were used for analysis (see Figure 4.2).

SECTION B **Total number of utterances** ___________	**Analysed utterances** __________

Figure 4.2 Section B

Developmental Analyses

The Croatian LARSP focuses on three levels of grammatical analysis: clause, phrase and word levels. The Croatian LARSP profile covers five stages as specified below.

Stage I [0;10-1;5] – one-element stage
Stage II [1;6-2;0] – two-element stage
Stage III [2;1 -2;6] – three-element stage
Stage IV [2;7-3;0] – four-element stage
Stage V [3;1-3;6] – complex sentences

Stage I

This stage in Croatian is similar to other languages, in that the majority of children's utterances contain a single element or word. The data presented for this stage come from 3 different children whose transcripts are on the CHILDES database-Croatian (MacWhinney, 2000). There were two female and one male child. In order to cover the range between 0;10 and 18 months, the transcripts were put together into one 'corpus'. A total of 663 utterances were included for analysis.

Working across the profile chart, we identify three types of utterances: Command-Type, Question-Type and Statement-Type. The Command-Type utterances usually contain directional verbs (e.g. *daj* 'give'). The Question-Type usually contain a question word (e.g. *što* 'what'). Children's statements are classified into: (1) **'N'** or noun-like responses. These are utterances which usually consist of a noun, such as for example, *mama* 'mummy'. The nouns do not usually include case marking at this stage, but they may be inflected for plural or they are 'pluralia tantum' nouns; (2) **'V'** or verb like responses, such as, for example, *igrati* 'play'). The verbs are usually not inflected for person, number or gender at this stage; they tend to be either in the infinitive form (e.g. *igrati* 'play') or in the neutral 3rd person sing form (*igra* 'play'); and (3) **Other** which contain adjectives (e.g. *velika* 'big'), adverbs (e.g. *tamo* 'there') or onomatopoeia (when the child produced the noise which an object or an animal makes).

As an illustration of what stage 1 may look like for a typically developing child, see Table 4.5 below. This is based on an audio recording of a girl aged 17 months, 16 days while interacting with her parents in her own home. A total of 160 utterances were transcribed, of which 138 are included in the analysis. The remaining 22 are either babbling or

Table 4.5 Stage I – Typically developing child – Child M, female, age 17 months

Major				
Command	**Question**	**Statement**		
'V'	'Q'	'N'	'V'	Other
5	1	155	12	10

unintelligible. There were four minor utterances: one was a yes/no response and there were three vocatives.

Statements

The predominant category of words used at this stage are nouns, which is common in many languages – though not universal (Nelson *et al*., 1993). It was often the case that the child repeated the same noun a number of times within the same turn (e.g. *mama, mama, mama, mama* 'mummy, mummy, mummy, mummy). Some of the nouns the child used were marked for case. For example, nine nouns were in the accusative case. Examples are provided in 35 below:

35. **Adult:** *joj kako lepu loptu si nacrtala*
('what a beautiful ball you have drawn')
Child: ***otu***[:loptu]
ball -ACC,FEM
'ball' (M, 17 months)

However, some nouns were incorrectly inflected for accusative case as well, suggesting that the child is still acquiring the system as in 36 below, in which the child uses the accusative form of the noun when they should use the nominative form.

36.
Adult: *šta je to?*
'what's this'
Child: *emu*[:kremu]
*cream-ACC,FEM
'cream' (M, 17 months)

Of the nine nouns which were produced in the accusative case, only five were used correctly.
There was one noun in the dative case as in 37 below.

37.
Adult: *šta radi tamo M (child's name)*?
'what is M (child's name) doing there?
Child: *mami*
mummyDAT
'to mummy' (M,17 months)

Adult: *mami daš, hvala*
'you give it to mummy, thank you'

There were 12 verbs used as statements and these were either in the infinitive or 3rd person singular.

38.
Child: *pisati*
Write-INF
'to write'
Adult: crtati. Šta da mama nacrta M (child's name)ini?
'to draw. What should mummy draw for M(child's name)?' (M, 17 months)

Of the 138 utterances, there were four examples of the child putting two elements together, two within the Phrase level (NN or AdjN) and two at clause level (SV).

39.
beba meda
'baby bear' (M, 17 months)
veika *lota* [:velika lopta]
big-Adj FEM ball-N FEM
'big ball' (M, 17 months)

Questions

There were few questions at this stage and although these were single words mainly, there was an attempt to use two words and the adult recasts the child's utterance.

40.
Child: *a*[:sta] *to*?
What this?
'what is this'?
Adult: *sta je to*?
'what is this'? (M, 17 months)

Commands

These were also mainly single words.

41.
Child: *otoli* [:otvori]
open-2ndsg IMP
'open' (the child is asking the mother to open something)
(M, 17 months)

Stage II (1;6-2;0)

This stage is characterized by the start of combinatorial structures and the child's use of predominantly two-element utterances. The data for this level come from the Croatian Corpus on CHILDES. The data from two children (both female, M and A) were used for whom there were available transcripts from age 18 months to 24 months and over 500 hundred utterances were analysed.

Clause level

At the level of the clause, there is evidence of the child being able to use a variety of two-element structures.

Statements

Within the category of statements, children produce two-clause elements including: Subject Verb (SV/VS), Verb Object (VO/OV), Verb Complement (VC), Verb Adverbial/Adjunct (VA/AV), Subject Complement (SC), or an Adverbial or Verb and another element (VX/AX). Given the generally free word of Croatian, there is flexibility as to how the clause elements are ordered. Because Croatian is a pro drop language, the subject is not obligatory in all contexts and this is indicated with 'Null V' where Null indicates that there is no overt subject but the features of person, number and gender are specified in the verb inflection. Below are a few examples of each of these two-element utterances.

42.

(a) SV

bebica	*papa*	
baby	eat3rd sg PRES	
'the baby eats'		(M, 20 months)

(b) VO

vozi	*cikl* [:bicikl]	
ride-3sg PRES	bike- ACC	
'rides a bike'		(M, 20 months)

(c) OV

**sireka*	*papati*	
cheese –ACC	eat-INF	
'to eat cheese'		(M, 22 months)

*It should be noted this is an example of regional use of accusative – instead of the direct object in nominative form that is standard for inanimate nouns (i.e. *sirek*), the child uses genitive form that is supposed to be used for animate direct objects (see Table 4.5).

(d) AV

gore	*je*	
upstairs	is (BE-3rdsg PRES)	
'he is upstairs' (referring to her father)		(A, 19 months)

(e) Null subject + V
zvoni
ring- 3rdsgPRES
'it rings' (A, 19 months)

(f) XV
ova[:ovako] *bacimo*
like this throw -1st pl PRESENT
'we throw like this' (A, 19 months)

It is relevant to note that the children at this stage were combining two verbs (an auxiliary and/or modal) and the infinitive form of a lexical verb. In 43b, the child uses Future I.

43.

(a) *moraš* *ići* *doktorici*
must-2nd sg IMP go- INF doctor-LOC,FEM
'you must go to the doctor's' (A, 23 months)

(b) *ja* *ću* *pjevati*
I will-enclitic1stsgFUT I sing-INF
'I will sing' (A, 23 months)

Commands

Commands within this stage should contain two elements, a Verb V and another element. However, it was also noticeable that both children still used one-element commands in this stage, which mainly contained a single verb. There were hardly any examples of commands in the transcripts, hence we are unable to provide an example.

Questions

Questions at this stage contain two words: a question word and a verb(QV). There was already some evidence of occasional use of three-element commands, but the predominant pattern was two-element questions.

44.

(a) *gde* *je*
where be-3rd sg PRES
'where is it' (referring to a sweetie) (A, 21 months)

(b) *kome* *bacim*
whom-DAT throw-1st sg PRES
'who should I throw to' (A, 21 months)

Phrase level

There is a wider variety of phrases at this stage. Within the NP, the children are using a variety of two-element combinations, including

Adjective Noun (AdjN), Noun Noun (NN), Determiner Noun (DN/ND). Adjectives and determiners agree with the noun in number, gender and case. Also there is evidence of prepositional phrases (PPs) containing a preposition (Prep) and an N (Prep N).

45.

(a) *mala* *curica*
little –FEM girl-FEM
'little girl'
Adj N (M, 22 months)

(b) *u* *kadi*
in bath-LOC,FEM
'in the bath'
Prep N (M, 22 months)

(c) *baka* *Ana*
grandma- FEM Ana- FEM
'Grandma Anna'
N N (A, 19 months)

(d) *curica* *jedna*
girl-FEM one-FEM
'One girl' (A, 23 months)

Also, there is evidence of the use of some personal pronouns as well as other pronouns (interrogative, indefinite).

Within the Verb Phrase (VP), there is evidence of the use of more complex VPs consisting of an auxiliary (including modal) + infinitive. The most common infinitive inflection is 'ati', 'iti' or 'eti' depending on the verb ending, though there are exceptions. There are occasions when the children omit the auxiliary clitic and only use the infinitive in this stage.

46.

rukice *brisati* (auxiliary is missing)
hands-pl wipe-INF
'to wipe hands' (M, 22 months)

The verb BE has a number of forms: full forms, enclitics and negated forms, and there is evidence of use of all of these forms. It combines to form the Perfect Tense (be+ L participle), which is commonly used in spoken language (examples will be provided in the Word Level section below). The participle agrees in number and gender with the Subject.

Word level

The data show approximately 75% correct use of accusative, dative and locative for each child. There were few examples of genitive and instrumental. There were also not many examples of vocative use, apart from when the children were calling one of their parents.

As an illustration of what stage II may look for a typically developing child, see Table 4.6. The analysed data are taken from CHILDES, and are based on one session with a 19-month-old girl. The child was audio recorded by her mother and the interaction involves the child and two adults (the child's mother and her grandmother). There was a total of 150 utterances, of which five were unintelligible and 38 were minor utterances, hence the analysis is based on the remaining 107 major utterances.

As evident from Table 4.6, the child's predominant clause structure is the one with a null subject and a verb. In terms of phrase structure, there are a few personal pronouns and one of these is in the accusative case (*ga* –'him'). There were only two examples of a two-element noun phrase in this specific sample.

At the level of the word, 3rd person singular dominates, which is not surprising given the context (the child talks about other people or objects). Two verbs were produced in the past tense. With regard to nominal inflections, the predominant case was vocative, which is not surprising given the young age of the child (she was calling her mother quite often, although the mother was in the same room). Nominative was the next most commonly used case, especially in one-word noun utterances and there was some evidence of the use of accusative, locative and genitive case.

Table 4.6 Typical stage II profile, Child A (19 months, 15 days)

STAGE II					
CLAUSE		**PHRASE**		**WORD**	
Commands		**NN**	**Prep N** 1	**Verb inflections**	
**VX(XV)*				1st sg 2	1st pl 2
		DetN/N Det) 1	**AdjN**	2nd sg 1	2nd pl
Questions				3rd sg 12	3rd pl
QV 1	VA	**Pro P** 5 1(ga);1(ti);3(ja)			
Statements				Perfect Tense (be + L part) 1	
		Pron O 1(kome)			
SV 3	XV 3			**Noun/pronoun inflections**	
(Null S)V 8 1	VO/OV			NOM 8	VOC 21
				GEN 1	INST
VA (AV) 3	VC			DAT	LOC 3
AX 2	Other			ACC 6	
*the italicised words mean that there were no examples in the sample					

There were also stage I utterances in the sample and also some from stage III. For example, the child was already showing evidence of using a negated verb followed by an accusative clitic (47a) and A(Null S)VA (47b).

47.

(a)	*nema*	*ga*		
	neg-have-3sg PRES	him (clitic)-GEN		
	'He is not there'			
(b)	*tamo*	*je*	*u*	*parku*
	there	BE-3rdsg PRES	in	park-LOC
	'he is there in the park'			

A few errors also occurred occasionally. For example, the child omitted the 1st person inflection on the verb as in 48. The child uses the 3rd person singular form, which is more neutral. Also the verb is transitive and the child has omitted a direct object.

48. *ja pima* [:prima]
I host-3rdsg PRES (in the context of hosting her uncle)
'I am hosting'.

Stage III (2;1-2;6)

This is a stage which is characterized by mainly three-element units (within clauses and phrases). For this stage, the CHILDES (Croatian) sample was used. There are 38 recordings covering the age 24 to 30 months. The first child (V) was audio recorded 20 times over a period of 6 months (the recordings are 10 to 14 days apart). The second child (A) was audio recorded 18 times within the same period of 6 months. Both transcripts and audio files were available on CHILDES.

The category of pronouns has also been included again in this stage, as their use is much more frequent and the children use a wider variety of pronouns. Within the category Word, the same verb and noun inflections are included, and also we added Comparative and Superlative for Adjectives, because there was evidence in the corpus that children begin to use the comparative and superlative forms of adjectives.

Clause level

Statements

At the level of the Clause, there are a number of different structures being used to express statements. These include Subject Verb Object (SVO), Subject Verb Complement (SVC), Subject Verb Adverbial (SVA). Because Croatian is a null subject language, we have included the following as well: (Null S) V O/OV, (Null S) V A, (Null S) V C/CV, (Null S) Verb. Because of the relatively free word order in Croatian, there is often flexibility in the ordering of clause elements, as some of the examples below show. Examples of stage III clause structure for statements.

49.

(a) SVO

ja imam	*c(r)venu*	
I have-1st sg PRES	red – FEM,ACC	
'I have the red (one)' (in the context of blocks)		(A, 28 months)

(b) (Null S)VO

upalio	*sam*	*svijetlo*	
switch-MASC sg L-part	be-1st sg PRES	light-NEUT,ACC	
'I have switched the light on'			(V, 28 months)

(c) SVC

ovo	*su*	*kojači* [: kolači]	
this	be-3rd pl PRES	cakes-MASC,NOM	
'These are the cakes'			(A, 28 months)

(d) (Null S)VC/(Null S)CV

siguran	*sam*	
sure-MASC	be-1st sg PRES	
'I am sure'		(V, 26 months)

(e) SVA

kamion	*je*	*tu*	
lorry-NOM	be-3sg PRES	here	
'The lorry is here'			(V, 26 months)

(e) A (Null S) V

sada će	*kopat*
now will-3rd sg FUT I	dig-INF
'Now it will dig'	

(f) A (Null S) V A

sad	*ću*	*još*	
now	will-1stsg FUT I	more	
'I will (do) more'			(V, 26 months)

There were a few examples of two Adverbials being used in the same clause; because adverbials are optional, these are marked as A+.

(g) A (Null S) VAA

onda	*moja* [: mora]	*ići*	*sad*	*u bo(l)nicu*	
then	must-3sg	go-INF	now	in hospital-FEM,ACC	
'Then he/she must go to hospital now'					(A, 30 months)

Questions

Similarly to the statements, the Questions are more complex now containing three elements (and some questions more than three).

Questions can take different syntactic form. Several question words, such as *zakaj* or *zašto*, meaning 'why' (depending on the regional dialect), *kuda* meaning 'where', *kak(o)* meaning 'how' are being used. The children are also using a 'Verb first' utterance. Two examples of questions are listed below:

50.

(a) Q XV
zakaj je *tu* *doš(a)o?*
why be-3rd sg here come-MASC sg L-participle
'Why has he come here?' (A, 30 months)

(b) VXY
je *ova* *bojesna* [bolesna]?
be-3rd sg this-FEM,NOM ill-FEM,NOM
'Is this one ill? (referring to a dolly) (A, 30 months)

(c) Q (Null S)V
kaj *neće*
why Neg-want 3sg
'why wouldn't it go? (in the context of a toy car) (A, 30 months)

Commands

Commands at this stage also contain three elements, though there is a wide variation in that children continue to use two-element commands, but they also include utterances which are more complex and contain more than three elements. There is evidence of use of the particle *da* ('let's') for commands as well.

51.

(a) *daj* *mi Blazeka* [:Blaženka] *dohvati*
come on me-DAT Blaženka- FEM,VOC reach-2nd sg, IMP
'come on, Blaženka, reach for me' (V, 26 months)

(b) *da* *vidimo* *još*
let's see-1st pl more
'let's see more' (A, 28 months)

Phrase level

At the level of the phrase, there are expansions. There is evidence of the use of three-element phrases, containing Noun Preposition Noun (N Prep N), or coordinated nouns using the coordinator *i* ('and'). Pronouns are more frequently used and there is a wider range including both personal and other pronouns. Within the Verb Phrase, there is a productive use of auxiliary (including modal) enclitics + infinitive and negated auxiliary enclitics + infinitive. Examples of NPs are provided below. Also, there is the emergence of use of Future II as a regional feature instead of Future I. This is made by using a form of the auxiliary BE ('budem/budeš/bude/budemo, budete, budu) and the L-participle.

52.
N Prep N

(a)	*kamion*	*za*	*smeće*	
	lorry-NOM	for	rubbish-ACC	
	'bin lorry/garbage truck'			(V, 26 months)

NcN

(b)	*daj*	*mi*	*Jenatu* [: Renatu]	i	*Anu*
	give-2nd sgPRES	me-DAT	Renata-ACC	and	Anna-ACC
	'give me Renata and Anna'				(A, 29 months)

Examples of VPs
Auxiliary Enclitic + infinitive

(c)	*ja*	*ću*	*s(l)ožiti*	*tu*	
	I(NOM)	will(aux)3sg FUT	make-INF	this-ACC	
	'I will make this one' (in the context of a puzzle)				(A, 29 months)
(d)	*ne*	*mogu*	*sad*	*ići*	*u školu*
	Neg	can(aux)1stsgPRES	now	go-INF	to school-ACC
	'I can't go to school now'				(A, 29 months)

Future II

(e)	ja se	budem	digija[:dignula]	
	I reflex.pr	be-1stsgFUT II	get-up-FEM, sing,L-part	
	'I will get up'(she gets up from the chair)			(A, 29 months)

Word level

At the level of the word, there are more case inflections used at this level. There are more examples of use of Instrumental and Genitive case at this stage. Also there is evidence of use of plural markers and a few examples of comparative of adjectives. There was evidence of use of possessive determiners/pronouns, which are made by adding *-ov* for masculine zero-ending or *o* / *e* nouns, *-ev* for the same after palatal consonants, and *-in* for a nouns ('*tatino*' meaning daddy's).

Errors of over-generalization are common. For example, the child uses the infinitive inflection '*iti*' which is very frequent with a verb which takes the less frequent one, '*ići*'.

53.

ja mojam [: moram]	*si*	*mavo* [: malo]	*jegiti* [:legiti]	
I must-1stsg PRES	refl	a bit	lie down-INF	
'I must lie down a bit'				(A, 28 months)

As an illustration of what stage III grammatical profile may look for a typically developing child between the ages of 2;1 and 2;6, see Table 4.7 below. The analysed data are taken from CHILDES, and are based on one session with a 26-month-old girl. The child was audio recorded while playing with her mother. There were a total of 258 utterances of which 90 were minor, four were unintelligible, ten were stereotypical, two were deviant and seven were incomplete. Hence the analysis is based on the remaining 145 major utterances.

As Table 4.7 below shows, the majority of clause structures contain three elements, although the child continues to produce two-element clauses as well. At the phrase level, there are many more pronouns being used at this stage, both personal and others. Also, the child readily uses auxiliary enclitics + infinitive constructions to express immediate future and is starting to use another form of Future tense, i.e. Future II. Past tense was marked using the Perfect tense. It is obvious from the word section that the child's inflectional morphology is much richer and the child inflects verbs for person and number. There are no examples of 2nd person plural inflections, but there was no relevant context for these to be produced. Also there was evidence of case marking, nominative and accusative case being the most commonly used.

The child also produced seven clauses which were longer than three elements; one included coordination of two clauses (54a) and one included a non-finite subordinate clause in object position (54b).

54.

Coordination: S V O c S V O

(a) *ja imam*	*vejiki [: veliki], a*	*ti*	*imaš*	*maji [: mali]*	
I have-1stsg PRES	big-MASCsg c-but	you	have-2ndsg PRES	small-MASC sg	

'I have the big one, but you have the small one'

Subordination: X OiSVOd (the direct object is a subordinate clause)

(b) *daj*	*mi*	*ti*	*reci*	*da*	*možemo*	*ići*
come on	to me	you	tell-2ndsgPRES	that	can-1stpl PRES	go-INF

'Come on tell me that we can go'

Stage IV (2;7-3;0)

Stage IV is characterized by the child's ability to use clauses and phrases which contain four or more elements. Children also start producing sentences which may be more complex and contain more than one clause, with coordination and subordination emerging in spontaneous speech. The phrase level is also more complex with coordination of different types of phrases as well as post modification of phrases by other phrases or clauses. Coordinators and subordinators are also being used. At the word level, comparative and superlative being used more

Table 4.7 Typical profile (Child A, 26 months)

<table>
<tr><td colspan="3">Minor</td></tr>
<tr><td>Responses</td><td>Vocatives</td><td>Other</td></tr>
<tr><td colspan="3">Major</td></tr>
<tr><td>Command</td><td>Question</td><td>Statement</td></tr>
<tr><td colspan="3">STAGE I 0;10;1;5</td></tr>
<tr><td>‘V’ 3</td><td>‘Q’ 8</td><td>‘N’ 7 ‘V’ Other 1</td></tr>
<tr><td colspan="3">STAGE II 1;6-2;0</td></tr>
<tr><td>CLAUSE</td><td>PHRASE</td><td>WORD</td></tr>
<tr><td>Commands
VX(XV) 2

Questions
QV QX 7

Statements

SV(VS) 5 XV (Null+V) 3

VO/OV VA(AV)1

(Null S)VC1

AX 4 Other 4</td><td>NN Prep N
3

DetN/N Det 3 AdjN

Pro^P 15

$Pron^O$ 33</td><td rowspan="3">Verb inflections
1st sg 13
2nd sg 8
3rd sg 35
1st pl 8
2nd pl
3rd pl 2

Past Tense
Perfect Tense (be + L part)
5

Noun/pronoun inflections
NOM 23
GEN 3
DAT 3
ACC 20
VOC 1
INST
LOC

Plural
-i- 1
e- 3
a-

Possessive</td></tr>
<tr><td colspan="2">STAGE III 2;1-2;6</td></tr>
<tr><td>Commands

VXY 1 VXY+

Da+VX 1

Questions

QVS(QVX) 5 QXY+

Q(Null S)V 1

Statements

SVO 12 SVC 13 SVA 1

(Null S)VO 6 (Null S)AV
6 (Null S) VC 1
A(Null S)VA 4
(Null S)VV 3 Other1</td><td>NcN 1 cX 3

N Prep N

Aux + Infinitive 9

NegAux+Infinitive 1

Neg V 7</td></tr>
</table>

frequently, both with adjectives and with adverbs. For this stage, transcripts from the Croatian corpus on CHILDES were used. We analysed over 1800 utterances from three children, taken at various points between ages 2;7 and 3;00.

Clause level

Statements

There were four-element clauses used including the following structures: XSVO (or SVOX), SVOdOi, SVOA /(Null S)VOA. There is also an example of use of Future I (55a).

55.

X SVO

(a)	*evo*	*ja*	*ću*	*to*	*s(l)ožiti*
	So	I	will (aux)+1stsgPRES	that-ACC	make-INF
	'So I will make that'				(A, 32 months)

S V Od Oi

(b) *ja sam*	*pusu*	*dala*	*pesiću*	
I be+1stsgPRES	kiss-FEM ACC	give-FEM sg L-part	doggie-DAT	
'I gave the puppy a kiss'			(A, 32 months)	

(Null S) V O A

(c) *bacio*	*ga*	*u mole [: more]*	
throw-3rdsg L-part	him-ACC MASC	in see-ACC	
'He threw him in the sea'			(V, 34 months)

Compared to stage III, there are many more examples of the children using multiple adverbials (mostly temporal) in the same clause.

All three children used a number of coordinate and subordinate clauses. Most coordinate clauses are linked with the conjunction *and*:

56.

(a) *ovo*	*je*	*k(r)avica,*	*a*	*ovo*	*je*	*pajcek*
this	be-3rdsgPRES	cow	and	this	be-3rdsg PRES	pig
'This is a cow and this is a pig'						(A, 31 months)

Subordinate clauses are used with different functions. The subordinate clauses play an adverbial/adjunct role (Sub A) or a complement role. Within the complement role, the most commonly found at this stage are subordinate clauses which have an object role (Sub O). Subordinate clauses are introduced either with the subordinator *da* ('to'), or other subordinators such as *kada* ('when'), the form '*je li*', or a 0 subordinator. See examples below under commands.

Commands

Commands are also more complex at this stage and include four-element simple clauses, usually starting with a verb, or complex clauses with subordination or coordination, also starting with a verb. In example 57a) the child uses the enclitic form of the pronoun (*mi*) whereas in 57b) the child uses the full form of the same pronoun (*meni*).

57.

V Oi Od A

(a) *daj* *mi* *još jedan* *tanjurčić* *za ovo*
give-2ndsgIMP me-DAT another one-MASC ACC plate-ACC for this-ACC
'Give me another plate for this' (M, 35 months)

V Oi Od +A sub clause

(b) *daj* *meni* *vodicu* *da si ja* *opejem* [:operem]
give-2ndsgIMPme-DAT water-ACC to refl-DAT wash-1stsgPRES

juke *tu* *u čašicu*
hands-ACC,pl here in glass-ACC
'Give me water for me to wash my hands here in the glass' (A, 32 months)

They may also include a subordinate clause in the role of direct object:

(c)

čekaj *da vidim* *kaj* *piše*
wait-2ndsgIMP to see-1stsgPRES what write-3rdsgPRES
'Let me see what is written' (A,32 months)

Questions

Questions at this stage consist of either four elements (if they are a simple clause) or can include more than one clause.

58.

4-element clause c QVAO

(a) *a* *di [: gdje]* *su* *sad* *one*
and where be-3rdpl PRES now they-FEM 3rd pl NOM
'And where are they now?' (V, 34 months)

Question with subordinate clause (Q V+ A sub clause)

(b) *zakaj* *se* *smiješ* *dok* *ja p(r)ičam* *abesedu*
Why se-refl laugh-2ndsgPRES while I say-1stsgPRES alphabet-ACC
'Why are you laughing while I am saying the alphabet?' (A, 32 months)

Phrase level

At the level of the phrase, there is evidence of some four-element phrases such as: coordinated noun phrases, coordinated prepositional phrases P Adj c P Adj, or nouns being postmodified by another phrase (usually prepositional phrase) or using a relative clause. Examples:

59.

Prep Adj c Prep Adj

(a) *može* *sa* *p(l)avom* *i* *sa čvenom* [: crvenom]
can-3rd sg PRES with blue-INST,FEM c (and) with red-INST,FEM
'It is possible with the blue or with the red one' (A, 32 months)

N PP (Prep N N)

(b) plinceza [: princeza] na zlnu [: zrnu] glaška [: graška].
Princess-NOMsg on grain-LOCsg pea-GENsg
'The Princess and the Pea' (A, 32 months)

(c) Det Adj N Prep N
kakav *veliki* *sapun* *sa* *ruzicama*
what-MASC big-MASC soap-MASC with flowers-pl FEM,INST)
'what a big soap with flowers' (A, 32 months)

Postmodifying clause (relative clause)

(d) *i* *medića* *kaj* *je* *na s(l)adoledu*
c-and bear-ACC that be-3rdsg on icecream(LOC)
'And the bear that is on the icecream' (A, 32 months)

Word level

The most prominent development at word level at this stage is the children's use of comparative and superlative inflections for both adjectives and adverbs. Example 60a shows overuse of inflection. The child added an inflection marking case and gender on the adverb 'malo' (a little bit).

60.

(a) *a* *molam* [: moram] *maloga* *većega*
c-and need-1stsg little-ACC,MASC big-AA, MASC, COMP
'I need a little bigger one' (A, 32 months)

(b) *ja* *sam* *bolji* *od* *tebe*
I-NOM be-1stsg PRES good-NOM,MASC,COMP than you-GEN
'I am better than you' (V, 35 months)

The child made occasional case errors, possibly due to the fact that the word is often used in the genitive case, however this context requires nominative case.

61. *evo* *vi(di)š* *ovo* *ti* *je* *glaška* [:graška] (instead of GRAŠAK)
Here see-2ndsgPRES this you-DAT be-3rdsgPRES peas-GEN
'Here see this is peas' (A, 32 months)

There are also examples of the child overusing the 1st person sg inflection 'm' on verbs which are exceptions to the rule, such as the word 'htjeti' (want). There were several instances of the child using 'hoćem' to mean 'I want' instead of hoću.

Typical profile, Stage IV (M, 2;11)

This is based on 150 utterances produced by child M, in conversation with her mother. Of the 150 utterances, only 80 were suitable for analysis; the other 70 were either one word elliptical responses, minor responses, incomplete or stereotypical responses. As can be seen from the LARSP chart below, presented in Table 4.8, the majority of the child's utterances were in stage III; however, there were quite a few in Stage IV including several complex clauses including coordination and subordination. Most inflectional morphemes are present as well.

Stage V 3;1-3;6

The data from this stage come from a language acquisition project run at the University of Zagreb. Three children aged between 3;1 and 3;3 (two male; one female) were audio recorded for one session each. The session comprised two parts: free play and semi-structured elicited production using picture materials. Each child produced between 250 and 300 analysable utterances and the total number of utterances analysed for this stage was 879. Due to the nature of the child–adult interaction, the majority of utterances were statements, with few questions and commands. Also about 60% of utterances were elliptical, because the adult was mainly asking questions and the child responded. We will refer to the participants in this part as child M, child F and child X.

Clause level

Statements

There was a range of different syntactic structures produced and the majority were simple clauses including 2, 3 or 4 elements (many with null subjects), however the children were able to produce more complex syntactic structures including coordination and subordination. Hence this stage is similar to stage IV in the sense that there were hardly any structures at stage V which were not found in stage IV. A structure which did not seem to appear in stage IV, but was present in stage V was the use of the contrastive conjunction 'a' meaning *but*. This conjunction is used to express a contrast. Also, the use of the conjunction 'jer' meaning *because* is more commonly found at this stage. There were also a few examples of more complex use of syntax where the subordinate clause contained coordinated predicates, or two coordinated clauses, one of which contains a subordination.

Table 4.8 Typical profile for stage IV

Command	**Question**	**Statement**
STAGE I 0;10-1;5		
'V'	'Q'	'N' 'V' Other
STAGE II 1;6-2;0		
CLAUSE	**PHRASE**	**WORD**
Commands *VX(XV) 1* **Questions** QV 1 QX VA 1 **Statements** SV(VS) (Null S) V VO/OV 1 VA(AV) 1 (Null S)VC AX 1 Other 1	NN Prep N / DetN/N Det 1 AdjN 1 Pro^P 1 Pron^O 9	**Verb inflections** 1st sg 4 2nd sg/ 2 3rd sg 14 1st pl 3 2nd pl 3rd pl 4 **Past Tense** Perfect Tense (be + L part) 4
STAGE III 2;1-2;6		
Commands *VXY* *VXY+* *Da+VX* *Ajde XY 1* **Questions** QVS(QVX) 1 QXY+ 2 Q(Null S)V 2 **Statements** SVO 1 SVC 3 SVA 3 (Null S)VO2 (Null S)AV 4 (Null S) VC 1 A(Null S)VA (Null S)VV Other2	NcN 1 cX N Prep N Prep N N1 Aux + Infinitive 1 NegAux+Infinitive 1 Neg V 5 **Conn: i**	**Noun/pronoun inflections** NOM 12 GEN 3 DAT 1 ACC 5 VOC 1 INST 2 LOC 3
STAGE IV 2;7-3;0		
Commands *VXY+* VXY+clause 1 VOiOdA 1 **Questions** QVAO QV+Clause **Statements** XSVO 2 SVOdOi/SVOiOd (Null S) V O A Subordination A 1 A+ O 2 C S Coordination 2 Conn: i 1, da 1, kad, kaj	XP c XP DetAdjNPrep 1 DetAdjNPrepN 1 NP PP (P N N) 1 NP+clause Conn:	Plural -i- 1 e- 3 a-2 Possessive **Adjective and Adverbs** COMP 2 SUP

Example (62a) shows coordination using 'a'

62.

(a) *tu* *je* *jedna,* *a* *tu* *druga.*
Here be-3sgPRES one-FEM, NOM but here another one-FEM, NOM
'Here is one, but here is another one'. (M, 39 months)

Example (62b) shows 'jer' within a sentence structure Neg VA (A is sub clause)

(b) *ne više* *plivat* *jer* *je* *sad* *suho* *more*
no more swim-INF because be-1sgPRES now dry-NEUT,NOM sea-NEUT,NOM
'No more swimming because the sea is dry now' (M, 39 months)

Example (62c) shows coordinated predicates within a subordinate clause, hence a compound complex clause.

(c) *rekli* *su* *doktori* *da* *i* *su* *bolesni*
say-3rdpl, L-part be-3rdpl doctor-i pl that and be-3rdpl ill-3rdpl NOM

i *prehlađeni*
and cold-3rdpl,NOM
'the doctors said that they were ill and had a cold' (M, 39 months)

Example (62d) also shows a compound complex clause in which there are two coordinated clauses and the first one also contains an Object subordinate clause.

(d) *nekad* *volim* *da* *ima* *snijega,*
sometimes love-1stsgPRES that have-3rd sgPRES snow-GEN

a *nekad* *ne* *volim*
but sometimes no-neg love-1stsgPRES
'sometimes I love there to be snow, but sometimes I don't'. (F, 37 months)

Questions and commands

There were very few questions and commands in the transcripts and all the structures present were also present at stage IV. This is comparable to the English version of the LARSP as well.

Phrase Level

Similarly to the Clause Level, the phrase structure at this level contained the types of phrases already described at level IV. This is comparable to what we find in the LARSP for English.

Word Level

All infections are present at this stage and the children use them productively. There is evidence of some over-regularization and occasional errors with regard to tense marking, case marking, plurals. Examples of errors at this stage are presented below.

63.

Adult: *a* *kome će* *ova djevojčica* *dodati* *loptu?*
'to whom is this girl going to throw the ball?
Child: *nje**
her-GEN(error)
'her' (instead of 'to her') (X, 38 months)

The pronominal form the child uses is genitive and it should be dative.

Another example of an inflectional error, this time to do with the verb, is illustrated with the following example:

64.

sad	*iduju**	*svi*	*papat*
now	go-3rdpl	all-NOM,pl	eat-INF

'Now they will all go to eat'

The child uses the inflection for 3rd person plural *ju* which is used with some verbs in Croatian. The child combines a dialectal feature and overgeneralization. The standard form is *idu* and the dialectal form would be *ideju*.

Based on the analyses provided above, in Table 4.9 we add in details for stage V. In Figure 4.3 we propose a possible Croatian LARSP chart as the first attempt to provide a systematic analysis of grammatical acquisition in the first 3 years, up to age 3;6, with provisional suggestions for stage VI+.

Croatian Language Acquisition Beyond 3;6

Our data only covered ages 0;9 to 3;6. Although the basic language system is in place by the time the child reaches 3 years and 6 months, language development continues. Below are some further accomplishments up to age 7, reported in what little research into Croatian language acquisition is available (e. g. Čuturić, 1996; Kovačević *et al.*, 1996; Kuvač & Palmović, 2007), see also Figure 4.3 in Appendix 1.

In the period between 37 and 48 months, children use all word classes – in most instances correctly in terms of morphology (including agreement) but nouns and verbs are still dominant. They also use past and future tenses. *Kada* and *koliko* ('when, how much') are used in questions. Possession is still expressed predominantly by possessive genitive. This may be explained by the fact that it is morphologically simpler to form than possessive adjective (and it doesn't involve agreement issues) and the influence of adult models, who frequently (probably for the same reason of simplicity) prefer this alternative. Possessive pronouns are used on their own or in (nonstandard) combination with *od*: *torba od mene* (literally: 'bag of me') instead of the standard *moja torba* ('my bag'). This persists well into age 5, especially in case of 1st, 2nd and 3rd person plural (Kuvač & Palmović, 2007). Children who have not started using personal pronoun *ja* (I) earlier do so in this period.

The concept of comparison is acquired, but language lags a little, especially irregular forms *jak* > *jakiji* ('stronger'). Children use verbs to express wishes and commonly name the desired object (rather than just gesturing toward it). They tend to verbally resolve conflict with other children.

Table 4.9 Stage V added to chart

SECTION A		
Unanalysed 1 Unintelligible 2 Symbolic Noise 3 Deviant **Problematic** 1 Incomplete 2 Ambiguous 3 Stereotypes		
SECTION B		
Total number of utterances _____ **Analysed utterances** ______		
Minor Responses	**Responses to Questions**	**Vocatives** **Other**
Major Responses		
Command	**Question**	**Statement**
STAGE I 0;10-1;5		
'V'	'Q'	'N' 'V' Other
STAGE II 1;6-2;0		
CLAUSE	**PHRASE**	**WORD**
Commands *VX(XV)* **Questions** QV QX **Statements** SV(VS) XV (Null+V) VO/OV VA/AV (Null S)VC AX Other	NN PrepN DetN/N Det AdjN Pro^P $Pron^O$	**Verb inflections** 1st sg 2nd sg 3rd sg 1st pl 2nd pl 3rd pl **Past Tense**
STAGE III 2;1-2;6		Perfect Tense (be + L part)
Commands *VXY* *VXY+* *Da+VX* *Ajde XY* **Questions** QVS(QVX) QXY+ Q(Null S)V **Statements** SVO SVC SVA (Null S)VO (Null S)AV (Null S) VC A(Null S)VA (Null S) VV Other	NcN cX N Prep N PrepNN Aux + Infinitive NegAux+Infinitive Neg V	**Noun/pronoun inflections** NOM GEN DAT ACC VOC INST LOC **Plural** -i-
STAGE IV 2;7-3;0		e-
Commands *VXY+* VXY+clause **Questions** QVAO QV+Clause **Statements** X SVO SVOdOi/SVOiOd (Null S) V O A Subordination A A+ O C S Coordination 1	XP c XP NP PP (P N N) DetAdjNPrep DetAdjNPrepN NP+clause Conn: and	a- **Possessive** **Adjective and Adverbs** COMP SUP
STAGE V 3;1-3;6		
Statements Sub Clause (VP+VP) Coord 1+ Conn: but, because, when	Conn:but	

Sentences typically comprise more than three to four elements and children are capable of producing complex sentences. Compound sentences are usually combined by conjunction *i* ('and') which can serve several functions, e.g. opposition, cause-effect, time sequence.

Language is mostly grammatically correct. Children are aware of language as a system, which is reflected in overgeneralization, but during this period also in the interest in meaning of words, experimenting with prosody and plays on words. These are the beginnings of metalinguistic competence which fully develops around age 6 (earlier in bilingual children). Also, they adjust their language when talking to pets and smaller children. They understand and can retell long stories. They understand sentences that contain multiple terms and negations in complex questions. During this period, children become capable of imagining hypothetical situations and can respond to questions *Što ako...* ('What if...'). When encouraged they use *hvala, molim, izvoli, oprosti* ('thank you, please, here you are, I'm sorry').

Between 49- and 60-months sentence length and complexity increase. Children can tell long stories keeping to the topic and putting emphasis on important words. Sentences typically comprise 4 to 6 elements and contain more than one verb: *Znam kako se to radi* ('I know how this is done'). All words are used correctly but there may still be some agreement issues. In this period children use polite form of requests. By age five *jučer, danas, sutra, ujutro, navečer* (yesterday, today, tomorrow, in the morning, in the evening) are used correctly. Cause–effect relationships may still be a problem which is reflected in their language as well. Some aspects of phonological awareness are acquired by age five, but full range of phonological manipulation develops by age seven.

After age 5, speech is fluent and intelligible. Tenses as well as noun and verb inflections are correct. However, some children still have problems with some morphological aspects, e.g. obligatory sound changes or long/short plural, and some declension paradigms of masculine nouns by age six (Kuvač & Palmović, 2007). Metalinguistic competence develops and children can talk about language. They can also notice errors in the speech of others. Vocabulary keeps expanding and includes abstract notions such as happiness, wealth, love, hate. Children can name days of the week and seasons. They use complex sentence structures and express their thoughts and feelings with ease. Pragmatic skills are acquired.

Acknowledgements

The authors wish to thank students of phonetics at the Faculty of Humanities and Social Sciences, University of Zagreb, Ivana Božić, Elizabeta Kantoci, Bruno Tot and Tena Žganec for their diligent work in collecting data and their helpful insights. Sincere thanks to all parents and children who participated in the study.

References

Crystal, D. (1982) *Profiling Linguistic Disability*. London: Edward Arnold.

Crystal, D., Fletcher, P. and Garman, M. (1989) *The Grammatical Analysis of Linguistic Disability* (2nd edn). London: Edward Arnold.

Čuturić, N. (1996) *Psihomotorički razvoj djeteta u prve dvije godine života*. Jastrebarsko: Naklada Slap.

Jelaska, Z. (2015) *Basic Croatian Grammar: Sounds, Form, Word Classes*. Zagreb: HFD.

Kovačević, M., Jelaska, Z. and Brozović, B. (1996) Comparing lexical and grammatical development in morphologically different languages. In A. Aksu Koc, E. Taylan, S.A. Ozoy and A. Kuntay (eds) *Perspectives on Language Acquisition* (pp. 368–383). Istanbul: Bogazici University Printhouse.

Kuvač, J. and Palmović, M. (2007) *Metodologija istraživanja dječjega jezika* [Methodology of Research into Child Language]. Jastrebarsko: Naklada Slap.

MacWhinney, B. (2000) *The CHILDES Project: Tools for Analyzing Talk* (3rd edn). Mahwah, NJ: Lawrence Erlbaum Associates.

Nelson, K., Hampson, J. and Shaw, L. (1993) Nouns in early lexicons: Evidence, explanations and implications. *Journal of Child Language* 20 (1), 61–84. doi:10.1017/S0305000900009120

Silić, J. and Pranjković, I. (2005) Gramatika hrvatskoga jezika za gimnazije i visoka učilišta (Croatian language grammar for high-school and university students). Zagreb: Školska knjiga.

Appendix 1

<table>
<tr><td colspan="3">SECTION A</td></tr>
<tr><td colspan="3">Unanalysed
1 Unintelligible 2 Symbolic Noise 3 Deviant
Problematic
1 Incomplete 2 Ambiguous 3 Stereotypes</td></tr>
<tr><td colspan="3">SECTION B</td></tr>
<tr><td colspan="3">Total number of utterances _____ Analysed utterances ______</td></tr>
<tr><td colspan="3">Minor Responses Responses to Questions Vocatives Other</td></tr>
<tr><td colspan="3">Major Responses</td></tr>
<tr><td>Command</td><td>Question</td><td>Statement</td></tr>
<tr><td colspan="3">STAGE I 0;10-1;5</td></tr>
<tr><td>‘V’</td><td>‘Q’</td><td>‘N’ ‘V’ Other</td></tr>
<tr><td colspan="3">STAGE II 1;6-2;0</td></tr>
<tr><td>CLAUSE</td><td>PHRASE</td><td>WORD</td></tr>
<tr><td>Commands
VX(XV)
Questions
QV QX
Statements
SV(VS) XV (Null+V)
VO/OV VA/AV
(Null S)VC AX Other</td><td>NN PrepN

DetN/N Det

AdjN

Pro^P Pron^O</td><td rowspan="9">Verb inflections
1st sg
2nd sg
3rd sg
1st pl
2nd pl
3rd pl

Past Tense
Perfect Tense (be + L part)

Noun/pronoun inflections
NOM
GEN
DAT
ACC
VOC
INST
LOC

Plural
-i-
e-
a-

Possessive

Adjective and Adverbs

COMP

SUP</td></tr>
<tr><td colspan="2">STAGE III 2;1-2;6</td></tr>
<tr><td>Commands
VXY VXY+
Da+VX Ajde XY
Questions
QVS(QVX) QXY+
Q(Null S)V
Statements
SVO SVC SVA
(Null S)VO (Null S)AV
(Null S) VC A(Null S)VA
(Null S) VV Other</td><td>NcN cX

N Prep N PrepNN

Aux + Infinitive

NegAux+Infinitive

Neg V</td></tr>
<tr><td colspan="2">STAGE IV 2;7-3;0</td></tr>
<tr><td>Commands
VXY+ VXY+clause
Questions
QVAO QV+Clause
Statements
X SVO SVOdOi/SVOiOd
(Null S) V O A
Subordination
A A+ O C S
Coordination 1</td><td>XP c XP

NP PP (P N N)

DetAdjNPrep

DetAdjNPrepN

NP+clause

Conn: and</td></tr>
<tr><td>STAGE V 3;1-3;6</td><td></td></tr>
<tr><td>Statements
Sub Clause (VP+VP)
Coord 1+
Conn: but, because, when</td><td>Conn:but</td></tr>
<tr><td>STAGE VI+ 3;6+</td><td></td></tr>
<tr><td>Conditionals, cause-effect relationships, can answer questions beginning with ‘Što ako’, use of Kada, Koliko in questions, etc</td><td>Det+Noun agreement, use of 1st person pronoun ‘ja’ (I) etc</td></tr>
</table>

Figure 4.3 Croatian LARSP CHART (Stage VI+ is a preliminary approximation)

Appendix 2

List of abbreviations

A	adverbial
ACC	accusative
Adj	adjective
AP	adverbial phrase
Aux	auxiliary
c	conjunction
C –	consonant
C	complement (in sentence structure)
COMP	comparative
DAT	dative
Det	determiner
FEM	feminine
FUT	future
GEN	genitive
IMP	imperative
INF	infinitive
INST	instrumental
LOC	locative
MASC	masculine
N	noun
NEUT	T-neuterNeutral
NOM	nominative
NP	noun phrase
O	object
Od	direct object
Oi	indirect object
PERF	perfect
pl	plural
PP	prepositional phrase
Prep	preposition
PRES	present
Pro	pronoun
Q	question word
Refl	reflexive
S	subject
sg	singular
V	verb
VOC	vocative
VP	verb phrase

5 Slovenian LARSP

Darija Skubic, Ana Praprotnik, Tamara Sevšek and Martina Ozbič

Introduction

Speech-language therapists are frequently asked to determine whether or not a child has a language problem or to determine whether there is a language disorder or delay. Children with language impairment (LI) show difficulties in all language domains in all settings. The collection of language development data in children and adult speakers is done in different ways – sampling more or less spontaneous speech in a natural or semi-natural setting (narration, story retelling, explanation, during constructional games, etc.), administering tests in more structured contexts, or using checklists. In some circumstances, administering tests is not possible, due to inattention, shyness, age, etc., especially in preschoolers. In addition, a richer language sample can be obtained in a natural unstructured or structured setting. Although a large number of norm-referenced standardized tests in several languages have been developed, many young children cannot be tested using formal procedures. Further, some languages (among these, Slovenian) lack standardized tests or checklists and questionnaires about language in all age groups or in some of them. In this case, in the absence of tests or as a choice, the speech-language therapist can use language sample analysis as an alternative to standardized testing for evaluating expressive language (Eisenberg *et al.*, 2001). While such analyses may have lower reliability and validity than normed procedures, they can still be predictive and informative for practitioners. In this chapter, we introduce the Slovenian Language Assessment, Remediation and Screening Procedure (SLO-LARSP). The adaptation of LARSP to Slovenian was based on LARSP in English – LARSP-e (Crystal, 1992), adapted according to the typology of the Slovenian language and research findings on the language acquisition of Slovenian-speaking children (Fekonja *et al.*, 2005; Koltaj & Žagar, 2007; Kranjc, 1992, 1997, 1999, 2003; Marjanovič Umek *et al.*, 2004; Praprotnik, 2017; Sevšek, 2016; Žagar, 1993). As in other morphologically rich languages, so in Slovenian an additional morphological page and additional categories in the original LARSP chart were added and others deleted.[1]

The Slovenian Language

Slovenian is a fusional or inflected language, morphologically very rich. It allows a free word order, subject omission, transitive and intransitive verb valency (avalent, intransitive, transitive, ditransitive), perfective and imperfective aspects, three verb moods (indicative, imperative, conditional), active and passive voice, three genders, three persons and three (or four) tenses. The morphology of Slovenian is very rich and challenging for a developing child. In addition to the three word classes that decline – nouns, verbs and adjectives – there are six that do not decline: adverbs, prepositions, conjunctions, particles, predicatives and interjections (Kalin Golob *et al.*, 2007: 37–39). Descriptive references below are to Herrity (2000) or Toporišič (1992).

Nouns

There are two types of noun in Slovenian: proper and common. Proper nouns refer to a particular person, place or institution by name, whereas common nouns are either concrete or abstract. In declension (the fourth case), there is a distinction between animate and inanimate nouns, seen in the suffix for masculine nouns. Nouns do not have articles. Nouns are divided into three grammatical genders (masculine, feminine, neutral/neuter), have six cases (nominative, genitive, dative, accusative, locative, instrumental) and usually three numbers (singular, dual, plural), although Slovenian has singularia and pluralia tantum as well. The masculine and feminine genders have four declensions, and the neuter gender has three, in which the word ending is different. Words are arranged in declensions according to the gender and the genitive singular ending.

Adjectives

Adjectives denote a quality, relation or possession. They are divided into three types: qualitative, relational and possessive. As with nouns, adjectives in Slovenian distinguish gender, case and number, reflecting the gender, case and number of the noun they qualify, including the accusative singular masculine if the qualified noun is an animate/inanimate noun. Adjectival words have the same declensions as nouns, and agreement between the suffixes is required. Most adjectives denoting the quality of something can form comparatives, which may be used attributively or in the predicate as a complement after a linking verb. The comparative is formed either by means of the derivational suffixes *-ši, -ša, -še* (for m, f, n genders, respectively) or *-ji, -ja, -je* (m, f, n) or *-ejši, -ejša -ejše* (m, f, n). Alternatively, it is formed by analytical means using the comparative adverbial forms *bolj* (more) or *manj* (less) together with the positive form of the adjective. The superlative is derived from the comparative form by means of the prefix *naj-*. In the case of the comparative form by analytical means, the prefix *naj-* is added to the comparative adverbs *bolj* and *manj*, resulting in *najbolj, najmanj*.

Pronouns

Pronouns may be classified either as substantive (replacing nouns) or adjectival (behaving like adjectives and agreeing in gender, case and number with the noun they qualify). Types of pronouns are: personal, the reflexive *se* ('self'), possessive, the reflexive possessive *svoj* (one's own), demonstrative, interrogative, relative, indefinite, negative, evaluative, reciprocal and pronouns of totality. The empathic pronoun *sam* ('self') declines like an adjective and agrees with the noun or pronoun it qualifies.

Numerals

In Slovenian, there are cardinal, ordinal (ordinals except *prvi* 'first' and *drugi* 'second' are derived from cardinals), collective, differential with the aid of the suffix *-en* or from cardinal numerals with the suffix *-kraten,* multiplicative and adverbial numerals (adverbs of frequency and time, and indefinite adverbs expressing amount, measure). The cardinal numerals two, three and four distinguish gender in the nominative case, where they differentiate masculine from feminine or neuter. The other cardinal numerals (five, six, etc.) do not distinguish gender.

Adverbs

According to Toporišič (1992), Herrity (2000) and Greenberg (2006), Slovenian has: adverbs of time indicating the point in time when something happens, the frequency and the duration, adverbs of place/location indicating position; adverbs of manner denoting the way something is done, as well as the circumstances in which something is done rather than how it is done; adverbs of causality denote the cause of something that is done.

Verbs

The basic grammatical categories of the Slovenian verb are:

- aspect – perfective aspect indicates the completed action of the verb or its foreseen or expected completion, while imperfective aspect focuses on the action's progress, duration, frequency or repetition;
- transitivity – transitive verbs describe actions that must, in addition to the subject, involve someone or something else, while intransitive verbs describe an action that does not involve anyone or anything other than the subject;

- person – 1st, 2nd and 3rd persons in finite verbal forms, each of which occurs in singular, dual and plural;
- number – singular (involving a single participant or singularia tantum), dual (for two participants), and plural (signalling more than two participants or pluralia tantum in simple and compound tenses);
- gender – qualifies a person or object in terms of masculine, feminine and neuter categories;
- tense – present, future, perfect;
- mood – indicative, imperative, conditional, optative;
- voice – the active voice is more frequent than the passive voice, which is used to emphasise inverted roles.

The Slovenian verb distinguishes finite and non-finite verb forms. The finite forms indicating person (1st, 2nd, 3rd) and number (singular, dual, plural) are the present tense and the imperative, which are expressed synthetically, and the future, past, and pluperfect tenses, which are expressed analytically with the auxiliary verb *biti* ('to be'). Non-finite verb forms, which cannot be inflected for person, are the participles, the verbal adverbs (gerunds), the present and past conditional moods, the infinitive, the supine and the verbal noun.

The present and past active participles, as well as the past participle passive, decline like adjectives. The so-called resultative – *l* participle is also adjectival and is used to form the future, past, and pluperfect tenses as well as the present and past conditional. In the analytical construction, the – *l* participle is only used in the nominative case.

Prepositions

All Slovenian prepositions precede the word they govern, the only exceptions being the adverbial prepositions. The meanings and functions of prepositions are: spatial, temporal, causal, purpose or intention, means and manner, concession, quantifying and comparison.

Conjunctions

Slovenian conjunctions are divided into two types: coordinating, which are used to link words, word groups or clauses of equal importance, and subordinating, which join a subordinate clause to a main clause in order to develop some aspect of what is said in the main clause.

Particles

Particles are indeclinable words that impart additional nuances to other words, word groups, or whole clauses. They are mainly a feature of spoken language, where they are used to introduce additional information, to express a variety of subjective attitudes or assessments, to justify statements, to appeal for agreement, to add emphasis, to indicate possibility, etc. Particles may be divided into two types: primary (whose sole function is that of a particle) and secondary (not restricted to the role of particle, but may also function as adverbs or conjunctions).

Interjections

There are three types of interjections: emotive, onomatopoeic and appellative (imperative).

Language Development in Slovenian

The course of Slovenian language development is similar to other languages, and is summarized in Table 5.1. First, interjections occur, followed by nouns and verbs (telegraphic style as *Mama piti* 'Mummy, to drink'), and function words (conjunctions, prepositions, and particles), pronouns, adverbs and adjectives (Marjanovič Umek in Zupančič, 2013). S. Kranjc (1992) found that two word-clauses appear between 18 and 20 months of age, where nouns and verbs are used, whereas conjunctions, prepositions and particles are omitted. This telegraphic style disappears after age 2. Before achieving the competence to produce morphologically and syntactically correct clauses, children use some sentence patterns, e.g. *Kje Žan?* 'Where Žan?' for assertions, questions etc. In the two-word clause stage children can realize different communicative functions - request, negation, description, etc. The demonstrative pronoun is often first in a clause, followed by a noun, an adjectival word before noun, the owner before the ownership. In two-word sentences, children comply with the sentence stress (last word). Children aged 24 months rarely produce full sentences; they often omit subject, verb, or object, and pronouns are absent.

S. Kranjc (1996) found the following word frequencies in utterances from 14–23-month-old children: nouns 27.95%, interjections 25.21%, verbs 23.60%, pronouns (mainly demonstrative) 12.23%, adverbs (mainly of place and mode) 6.41%, particles 2.77%, adjectives 0.93%, numerals 0.67%, prepositions 0.16%, conjunctions 0.03%. Among 24–27-month-old children the frequency is: verbs 25.93%, interjections 22.47%, nouns 22.47%, pronouns 22.47%, adverbs 11.17%, particles 11.17%, adjectives 11.17%, numerals 11.17%, and prepositions 11.17%. There were no conjunctions.

In 28–31-month-old children the frequency was different: verbs 11.17%, nouns 11.17%, pronouns 16.35%, interjections 12.86%, particles 10.39%, adverbs 6.77%, adjectives 2.33%, numerals 1.36%, prepositions 0.27%, conjunctions 0.25%. Children tend to develop basic sentence structure. Three months later the frequency was: verbs 29.17%, nouns 21.27%, pronouns 14.17%, interjections 13.21%, particles 9.20%, adverbs

Table 5.1 A sketch of the stages of typical grammatical development in Slovenian children

6–9 months	first signs of language comprehension, contextualized.
9–12 months	language comprehension of simple structures.
10–12/14 months	first words (S,V, Adv, etc.). Prosodic sentences. Presence of gestures, deixis. Nouns: nom., acc.
From 16 months	first attempts to express past and future
20–24 months	expressive language: min. 50 words and two-word sentences (MLU) – VO, AdvS, SV, SO, etc. Children also achieve the level of a three-word sentence (SOV, SVO, OVS, etc., Adv.). Co-presence of gestures. First attempts to coordinate sentences. Emergence of pronouns, numerals, adverbs, adjectives. Verbs: fem., masc., neuter; 1st, 2nd, 3rd person, sing., dual, plur.; nouns: fem., masc., neuter, sing., dual, plur.; nom., acc., instr. frequent; dat., gen., loc. less frequent. Frequent hyper-regularity/overgeneralization (correct and incorrect) in language or comprehension, and use of exceptions (in verbs, adjectives, nouns).
30/36–48 months	expressive language: min. three-word sentence structure. Development of morphology and semantics, further syntax. Coordinate sentences, first attempts to subordinate structures. Presence of nouns, numerals, adverbs, adjectives. Less frequent incorrect hyper-regularity/overgeneralization. MLU: 4, from 2 to 5 in narration.
48 months	basic language knowledge; developing of morphology for less frequent and more complex and abstract concepts, development of pragmatic language skills, coherence and cohesion in narratives. MLU: 5, from 4 to 7 in narration. First attempts to express, describe mental states of others.
5 years	development of coordinate and subordinate structures in narration; decrease of one-clause sentences. Increase of subordinate conjunctions in narration, increase of change of prospective in narration, description of mental states.

7.98 %, adjectives 2.46%, numerals 1.72%, prepositions 0.76%, conjunctions 0.06%. Among verbs, aspect is not yet used (Kranjc, 1995/1996). The number of verbs increases at the expense of nouns; the increase of function words is linked to the appearance of multiword utterances (Kranjc *et al.*, 2006). The number of adjectives also increases, as the child increasingly wants to name the properties of the objects in the immediate environment (Kranjc, 1999) and the relationships between them.

When children make progress in acquiring grammar, they often add adjectival words describing the qualities of objects and their location (Marjanovič Umek, 1990). With the development of multi-word and ever more complex utterances they more frequently include conjunctions, prepositions, auxiliary verbs, adverbs and pronouns (Toporišič, 1992). As toddlers, children begin to form subordinate and coordinate clauses that contain verbs in the past or future tense (Fekonja, 2002).

S. Kranjc *et al.* (2006) studied language comprehension and expression, and the pragmatic use of language. The results highlight significant differences between three- and four-year-olds. Early childhood sees the continuing development of negative and interrogative statements, while children increasingly understand the meaning of auxiliary verbs and the use of negative verb forms such as *Nočem več pit* 'I don't want to drink any more'. They also use appropriate negative forms when the clause begins with words such as *nobeden* 'no-one' and *nikjer* 'nowhere' (Marjanovič Umek *et al.*, 2004). The number of interrogatives in child speech increases up to the age of five and then starts falling (Marjanovič Umek, 1990).

S. Kranjc *et al.* (2006) also studied the development of narration among 80 children, aged 3;1 and 4;1, with story-telling, prompted by pictures. The results were analysed in terms of grammatical structure and coherence. The criteria for the analysis of grammatical structure were based on the use of different kinds of words and grammatical rules: total number of nouns, number of different nouns, different nouns in dual number; total number of verbs, different verbs, verbs in the past tense, verbs in the future tense; total number of adjectives, different adjectives; total number of pronouns, different pronouns; subordinate and coordinate clauses; interrogative utterances, negative utterances, imperative utterances, and utterances in direct and indirect speech. The results show the great effect of children's age on the coherence and grammatical structure of the stories. Developmental changes were apparent in the much more complex grammatical structure of the stories. Changes to grammatical structure include the use of significantly more nouns and verbs, the use of different verbs, verbs in the past tense, the total number of adjectives, the use of different adjectives, the total number of pronouns, the use of different pronouns, multi-word, subordinate and coordinate clauses, and utterances in indirect speech. As reported by S. Kranjc *et al.* (2006), no significant differences, arose in the number of different nouns, the number of dual nouns, verbs in the future tense, or in the number of interrogative, negative or imperative utterances, or utterances in direct speech, as these were rarely used in the stories by children of either age. There were no significant differences between boys and girls with regard to age-related changes in the grammatical structure or coherence of their stories.

The results show that Slovene vocabulary and grammar develop rapidly in early childhood, while children's utterances become increasingly structured and similar to the grammatically correct utterances of adults. At the second assessment, when their average age was 4;1 years, children were more successful at carrying out tasks measuring their understanding of spatial relationships, properties, and grammatical roles. The two sets of results also point to changes in the children's level of language expression, shown in the scope of their vocabulary, the recognition and use of grammatical rules in the conjugation of verbs and the use of third person and past tense forms, in the use of the dual and plural or declensions, and the ability to repeat utterances.

The results also point out certain developmental changes in the grammatical structure of stories, which were largely comparable to changes in language development as measured by the relevant scale. Brown (1973, quoted in Kranjc *et al.*, 2006) claims that after the age of two children acquire additional grammatical rules, making correct use of adverbs and pronouns in their speech. At both stages children used pronouns in their stories, but their number did not change significantly. At the first assessment, they used fewer words that were often repeated. Siegler (1998, in Kranjc *et al.*, 2006) asserts that, in spite of the fact that they know more than one word with the same meaning, toddlers tend to use the ones that are easiest to pronounce. The findings indirectly support this, as four-year-olds, more often than three-year-olds, name the same objects with different words. Between the two assessments there was also an increase in the number of multi-word dependent clauses and coordinate clauses. Three-year-olds more often used the kind of one-word and two-word utterances characteristic of toddler speech. At the first assessment in particular there were examples of telegraphic speech characterized by the inclusion of only full lexical items but a word order similar to that children hear in adult speech (Bates & Goodman, 2001; Papalia *et al.*, 2001, in Kranjc *et al.*, 2006). The number of interrogative, negative, and imperative utterances, and examples of direct and indirect speech remained low, while the use of future-tense verbs occurred very infrequently. It seems that the frequency of use of particular kinds of utterance was influenced by the testing of storytelling, which to a limited extent encouraged the use of interrogative and imperative forms as well as the use of the future tense.

The Development of Slovenian LARSP

Allen and Dench (2015) claim that in SLI (Specific Language Impairment, now more commonly termed Developmental Language Disorder) children the specific structures that present difficulties vary in accordance with the typology of the language, and are often those structures that are also difficult for younger typically developing children (Leonard, 2014). For this reason, different languages cannot rely on English-tailored measures and tools, but have to develop their own methodology, meaningful for the language and its community of users. There is a lack of studies for many other languages, among these Slovenian, about both language measures like MLUm, MLUw, MLUsyll, as well as profiling and assessment tools. Additionally, there is a dearth of comprehensive studies about language development in Slovenian preschoolers and school-aged children in all language domains from birth to adulthood. Several studies (Fekonja *et al.*, 2003, 2004, 2005; Gnamuš, 1976; Kranjc, 1993, 1999, 2003, 2004; Kranjc *et al.*, 2006; Marjanovič Umek *et al.*, 2004, 2006; Žagar, 1961) focused on a single domain, such as storytelling or spatial concepts, or on a restricted age group. Among researchers, Kranjc, Marjanovič, Fekonja *et al.* in past decades have published some studies and developed tools relating to typically developing children. And there are a very limited number of studies in the domain of language impairment in Slovenian speakers.

For the assessment of language development in Slovenian some specific instruments were adapted, for example versions of the MacArthur-Bates CDI I, II and III, and story retelling. For earlier development in domains such as pragmatics and gesture, other questionnaires were adapted and some of them published, among them Wetherby and Prizant's (2001) Communication and Symbolic Behavior Scales – Developmental Profile (CSBS-DP) (http://firstwords.fsu.edu/), the Socio-Conversational Skills Questionnaire (Girolametto, 1997), and the Language Use Inventory (O'Neill, 2007). These are tools primarily focused on lexical, gestural and pragmatic domains, and they do not cover morphosyntactic development. To fill this gap, we have adapted LARSP for Slovenian, in line with what we know about the morphosyntactic development of Slovenian children. LARSP-SLO offers the potential for a deeper analysis, both quantitative and qualitative.

The Adaptation of LARSP into SLO-LARSP

To adapt LARSP for Slovenian we had to transform a tool constructed for an analytic language, English, to a fusional-inflected language. We preserved parts A, B, C and D as they are in LARSP-e, since they are not dependent on morphosyntactic features.

In the developmental part of SLO-LARSP we excluded age milestones for individual stages, since there is no research which would establish a correspondence between English and Slovenian developmental stages. At clause level, we added structures that express the subject of the clause indirectly through the morphological features of the verb (stage II: (S)V, (S)O, (S)C; stage III: (S)VC, (S)VO, (S)VA; stage IV: (S)VOA, (S)VCA, (S)VO$_d$O$_i$, (S)VOC) (e.g. *hoditi* 'to walk' → *hodi***m** 'I walk', *hodi***mo** 'we walk'). At phrase level, we added reflexive verbs in stage III (e.g. *spomniti* **se** 'to remember'), since they are expressed with a verb phrase and are quite frequent in Slovene. At stage III phrase level we also separated pronouns. We made two categories: personal pronouns and others.

At compound sentence level, we added an additional category for juxtaposition: a compound sentence that consists of a clause and apposition (e.g. ***Janez****, pridi sem* '**John**, come here' or ***Ja****, lahko to narediš* '**Yes**, you can do that'). We included three conjunctions (*in*, *ter*, *pa*) in place of the English conjunction *and*. In the bottom line, we preserved measures used in LARSP-e, and specified Mean Sentence Length as Mean Length of Utterance in Words (MLUw). The main profile is seen in Figure 5.1, and then in order to account for the full richness of morphological categories in the language, we added an additional page (see Figure 5.2).

Ime, priimek	Starost (leta, meseci)	Datum snemanja	Način interakcije	Trajanje

A	**Neanalizirani stavki**			**Problematični stavki**		
	1 Nerazu- mljivi st.	2 Simbolni zvoki	3 Nestan- dard. izj.	1 Nedo- končani st.	2 Dvo- umni st.	3 Stalne formule

B	**Odzivi**		Tipičen odziv						Netipičen odziv		
			Major								
			Reduciran st.			Negla- golski st.	Popoln st.		Strukt. nepri- meren odziv		
	Tipi dražljaja Skupaj Vprašanja Drugo	Pono- Vitve	1	2	3+			Minor		Ø	Teža-ve
C	**Spontane izjave**										
D	**Odzivi na otrokovo dejavnost**		Splošne	Strukt. pov.	Ø			Drugo	Težave		

Stopnja I	**Minor**	*Odgovori*			*Zvalniki*		*Drugo*		*Težave*		
	Major	*Ukazi* 'V'	*Vprašanja* 'Q'	*Trditve* 'V'	'N'		Drugo		Težave		
	Veznik	**Stavek**					**Besedna zveza**			**Beseda**	
Stopnja II		V*X*	Q*X*	SV SO SC Neg*X*	**(S)V** **(S)O** **(S)C**	A*X* VO VC Drugo	DN Adj N NN PrN	VV V part Int *X* Drugo		deležnik: - stanja - trpni d.	moški sp. srednji sp. ženski sp.
		X + S:NP	*X* + V:VP	*X* + C:NP			*X* + O:NP	*X* + A:AP		ednina	
Stopnja III		V*XY*	Q*XY* VS(*X*)	SVC SVO SVA Neg*XY*	**(S)VC** **(S)VO** **(S)VA**	VCA VOA VO_dO_i Drugo	D Adj N Adj Adj N Pr DN **Pron. – oseb.** **Pron. – drugi**	Cop Aux^m Aux^o **Povr. gl.** Drugo		dvojina množina sedanjik preteklik	3. os. ed. prvi sklon drugi skl.
		XY + S:NP	*XY* + V:VP	*XY* + C:NP			*XY* + O:NP	*XY* + A:AP		prihodnjik	tretji skl.
Stopnja IV		+ S V*XY*+	QVS Q*XY*+ VS(*X*+) tag	SVOA SVCA SVO_dO_i SVOC	**(S)VOA** **(S)VCA** **$(S)VO_dO_i$** **(S)VOC**	AA*XY* *Drugo*	NP Pr NP Pd D Adj N c*X* *X*c*X*	Neg V Neg *X* 2 Aux $_{(m,o)}$ Drugo		poved. n. velelni n. pogojni n.	četrti skl. peti skl. šesti skl.
Stopnja V	in,ter,**pa** s c Drugi	Prired. Drugo	Prired. Drugo	Prired. Podred. A S Primerjal. **Soredje**	1 1 C	1+ 1+ O	Oziralni stavek Dopolnit. fraza	1 1+	1+	nikalnice, zanikan glagol pomožni glagoli primerjal- nik presežnik - opisno - obrazilno prisl. nač. **členek**	svojilni rodilnik pomožni gl. biti copula – vez tvornik trpnik dovrš. nedovrš. prehod. neprehod. gl.

Figure 5.1 The SLO-LARSP profile – Analiza slovničnih zmožnosti slovenskih govorcev (2017)

	(+)			(-)				
	NP	VP	Stavek	Vezniki	Stavek	Besedna zveza		Beseda
Stopnja VI	Začetek Besede Razšir. st.	Večglag. st.	Pasivno Povedkovo dol. *Kako* *Kaj, kakšen*	in c s	Element Ø → ←	NP D Pr Pro^{p} D Ø Pr Ø D → Pr → ← ←	VP Aux^{M} Aux^{o} Cop Ø	N V *nepravil.* *pravil.*
	Drugo					*Dvoumni*		
Stopnja VII	*Diskurz*			*Skladenjsko razumevanje*				
	Adverbialna povezanost Komentarji Emfatični besedni red	Neosebna oblika Drugo		*Stil*				
	Skupno št. **povedi**		Povprečno št. **povedi** glede na izmenjavo			Povprečna dolžina **povedi (MLUw)**		

Figure 5.1 *Continued*

The Application of SLO-LARSP to Language Impairment (LI) in Children

S. Kranjc *et al.* (2003) published a study on story retelling and its use to determine language development in typical populations. Story retelling in LI children was studied by Grobler (2002), Grobler and Arapović (2007), Omahna (2011), Kovačič (2012) and Sevšek (2016), using tools developed by Marjanovič Umek *et al.* (2012). According to Grobler (2002), LI children have difficulties in inflections, the semantic linking of similar words, the use of suffixes, interfixes, and prefixes, and the use of function words and content/lexical words. In syntax, children with LI utter shorter utterances. We observe difficulties in the use of modal verbs, and in word and sentence order. Children with LI often reduce questions to the pivot word only, they use pronouns incorrectly, and they rarely use compound and complex sentences.

Grobler and Arapović (2007) analysed the narrations of 14 10-year-old Slovenian children with LI. Although their narration texts were acquired with unstructured encouragement, the data (total number of statements, number of compound sentences, number of connectors, and number of stimulations) are interesting. The study found statistically significant differences between the groups in narration text: shorter texts of lesser quality, with difficulties in structuring the narration into language form. Children with LI tended to have difficulties at multiple levels of oral language including phonology, syntax, vocabulary and pragmatics. Grammar, which integrates morphology and syntax, was the area where language difficulties and deficits were most expressed and visible.

Expressing and comprehending grammar is for some children the core of their deficit (Grobler, in Arapović, 2007). The typical deficit occurs in the agreement of sentence parts, in coordinate and especially subordinate relations, which are necessary for sentence interpretation and production. Deficits in the area of expression can be observed in the formation,

BESEDNA VRSTA	VRSTA	PODVRSTA	LASTNOSTI
samostalniška beseda	samostalnik	lastna imena nelastna – obča imena	**spol**: moški ženski srednji **1. podspol** (človeškost, nečloveškost) **2. podspol** (živo, neživo)
			sklon: 1. Imen. 2. Rod. 3. Daj. 4. Tož. 5. Mestn. 6. Orodn.
		Osnovna beseda Pomanjševalnica	**števílskost:** tri števila, eno samo število (redko dve)
			število: ednina dvojina množina edninski (skupna, snovna, pojmovna) množinski sam.
			sklanjatev: moška (1., 2., 3., 4.) ženska (1., 2., 3., 4.) srednja (1., 3. 4.)
			določnost: primarna določnost, nedoločnost se izraža posebej
	samostalniški zaimek	Osebni, nedoločni, povratno osebni, mnogostni, vprašalni, nikalni, oziralni, totalni, poljubnostni, kazalni	**spol:** vsi spoli za 1. in 2. os. ed. moški, ženski, srednji spol povratni zaimek sebe/se za vse spole
			število: ednina, dvojina, množina (os. z. in posam. z.) enoštevilski edninski, dvojinski, množinski nedoločno število
			sklon: 6 sklonov (razen povratno os. z., ki ima 5 sklonov)
			oseba: 3. oseba, razen os. z.
			sklanjatve: osebni za 1. in 2. os. ter povratni z. po a-jevski sklanjatvi, ostali po pridevniški sklanjatvi
	posam. prid. beseda		
pridevniška beseda		**spol:** moški ženski srednji	
		sklanjatev: 1. moška, ženska, srednja 2. moška, ženska, srednja	
		oseba: 1., 2. in 3. oseba	
		Določnost	
		števílnost: troštevilne prid. b., enoštevilne prid. b.	
		števílskost: ednina, dvojina, množina (razen vrste količinskih prid.)	
		stopnjevalnost: 1. tristopenjska (osnovnik, primernik, presežnik z desnim obrazilom s prislovom mere), 2. dvostopenjska (elativno stopnjevanje)	
	pridevnik	kakovostni in merni, vrstni, svojilni	
	števnik	Glavni, množilni, vrstilni, nedoločni, ločilni	
	prid. zaimek	lastnostni:	vprašalni, oziralni, nedoločni, poljubnostni, mnogostni, oziralnopoljubnostni, totalni, nikalni, drugostni, istostni, kazalni
		vrstni:	vprašalni, oziralni, nedoločni, poljubnostni, mnogostni, oziralnopoljubnostni, totalni, nikalni, drugostni, istostni, kazalni
		svojilni:	vprašalni, oziralni, nedoločni, poljubnostni, mnogostni, oziralnopoljubnostni, totalni, nikalni, drugostni, istostni, kazalni
		količinski:	vprašalni, oziralni, nedoločni, poljubnostni, mnogostni, oziralnopoljubnostni, totalni, nikalni, drugostni, istostni, kazalni
Glagol	**glagolski vid:** dovršni nedovršni		
	prehodnost: prehodni neprehodni		
	način: tvornik trpnik		
	glagolski naklon: povedni (3 os.) velelni (2 os.: 2. os. ed., 1. in 2. os. dv./mn.) pogojni (3 os.) naklonski glagoli *moči, morati, smeti*, povedkovnik *lahko, treba je*, členek *naj*		
	glagolski čas: sedanjik preteklik prihodnjik predpreteklik		
	glagolske os.: 1. os. (govoreči), 2. os. (ogovorjeni), 3. os. (neudeleženec dvogovora)		
	glagolsko št.: ednina, dvojina, množina		

Figure 5.2 Additional morphological page for Slovenian language

organization and ordering of the verbal message when children with LI are asked to tell a story, make a summary, describe an event, or form and give instructions. Children make pauses that lead to dysfluency; they frequently repeat words; the sequence of details might be unconnected; and they use short sentences or avoid speaking at all. Differences between groups of children with LI and typically developing children were

	neosebne gl. oblike: nedoločnik na -ati/-eti, -iti, V-ti, C-ti deležja na -č, -aje, -e, -ši deležnik na -č, -ši opisni deležnik na –l deležnik stanja na –l trpni deležnik na –n/-t in -oč/-eč se deležnik stanja na -n/-t namenilnik na -at, -it, -et ob glagolih premikanja ali za izražanje cilja drugih dejanj (gl. dati, poslati)		
prislov **stopnjevalnost:** osnovnik primernik presežnik	okoliščinski	prostorski mestovni:	vprašalni, oziralni, nedoločni, poljubnostni, mnogostni, oziralnopoljubnostni, celostni, nikalni, drugostni, istostni, kazalni
		prostorski ciljnostni:	Vprašalni, oziralni, nedoločni, poljubnostni, mnogostni, oziralnopoljubnostni, celostni, nikalni, drugostni, istostni, kazalni
		prostorski poti in razmeščenosti:	Vprašalni, oziralni, nedoločni, poljubnostni, mnogostni, oziralnopoljubnostni, celostni, nikalni, drugostni, istostni, kazalni
		časovni vrste kdaj:	Vprašalni, oziralni, nedoločni, poljubnostni, mnogostni, oziralnopoljubnostni, celostni, nikalni, drugostni, istostni, kazalni
		časovni vrste odklej	
		časovni vrste doklej	
	svojstvenostni	lastnostni kakovostni:	Vprašalni, oziralni, nedoločni, poljubnostni, mnogostni, oziralnopoljubnostni, celostni, nikalni, drugostni, istostni, kazalni
		lastnostni merni:	Vprašalni, oziralni, nedoločni, poljubnostni, mnogostni, oziralnopoljubnostni, celostni, nikalni, drugostni, istostni, kazalni,
		vzročnostni:	Zakaj, čemu, s kakšnim uspehom, kljub čemu, glede na kaj
	prislovni izrazi	Prostorski	
		Časovni	
		lastnostni:	načinovni, merni, zapovrstni
		Vzročni	
povedkovnik		povedkovniki, ki označujejo stanje narave	
		povedkovniki, ki označujejo stanje in razpoloženje doživljavca zunanjega in notranjega okolja	
		povedkovniki, ki označujejo vrednotenje	
Predlog		pravi, ki se uporabljajo kot predlogi	vezava z 1 sklonom ali 2 sklonoma: 1., 2., 3., 4., 5., 6. sklon
		nepravi, ki se uporabljajo kot prisl., sam. ali kaj drugega	
vezniška beseda	veznik	enodelni (enobesedni)	
		enodelni (večbesedni)	
		dvodelni vezniki: (ponovitev istega veznika v obeh delih besede ali v enem delu je en veznik, v drugem pa njegov soodnosni izraz)	
	soveznik	oziralni zaimki (sam., prid., prisl.)	
		vprašalni zaimki (sam., prid., prisl.)	
	Priredja: vezalno, stopnjevalno, ločno, protivno, vzročno, pojasnjevalno, sklepalno		
	podredja: osebkovo, povedkovo, predmetno, krajevno, časovno, načinovno, primerjalno, posledično, pogojno, dopustno, vzročno, namerno, prilastkovno		
Členek	a) pozivni:	Vprašalni, zahtevalni, ukazovalni, želelni, prepričevalni, zagotavljalni, nasprotovalni ,grozilni, očitalni	
	b) vrednotenjski:	– naklonski (gotovostni, primerjalni, popravljalni, domnevalni, merilni, poudarjalni) – vrednotenjski primerjalni – popravni – domnevalni (nečustvenostni, čustvenostni) – merilni (nepolnomerni, polnomerni, približne mere) – poudarjalni – čustvenostni	
		členki, ki členijo oz. hierarhizirajo besedilo oz. njegove dele:	– zaznamovanje začetka – premočrtno členitveno (naštevanje, opozarjanje) – sovsebnostni (s poudarjanjem nasprotja, z izbiro izrazov istega reda)
		Navezovalni, čustvovanja, poudarni, izvzemalni, presojevalni, dodajalni, zadržka, potrjevanja ali soglašanja, sovsebnostni (s poudarjanjem nasprotja, z izbiro izrazov reda, možnosti, verjetnosti, mnenja, domneve, vprašalni, spodbujalni, zanikanja in nesoglašanja	
Medmet		razpoloženjski	
		posnemovalni ali onomatopoejski	
		velelni	

Figure 5.2 *Continued*

statistically significant on three variables: the number of compound sentences, the number of conjunctions, and the number of stimulations needed to encourage narration. Without extensive support children with LI would not achieve the same length of utterance because they need far more encouragement than their peers. The authors suggest that language knowledge and the narrative abilities are strongly interdependent and positively correlated. The research into the narrative abilities of primary school children which was carried out for Croatian by Arapović (1996) reveals similar and in some cases equivalent results. Grobler's and Arapović's findings are that SLI children lag behind to a large extent in most of the characteristics of narration they analysed.

Having adapted the instrument LARSP-e into SLO-LARSP according to Slovenian linguistic features, and what is known about Slovenian language development, our aim then was to test the instrument on children with language impairment and typically developing (TD) peers. The sample consisted of 20 children, 11 males and 9 females, aged from 6 to 7 years. Half the children (5 males, 5 females) were TD, and the other half (6 males, 4 females) were diagnosed as LI without other developmental concerns and were receiving intervention from speech and language therapists. Language samples were collected from the children in a semi-structured activity, i.e. story retelling (Slovenian CDI III: Preizkus pripovedovanja zgodbe: *Žabji kralj/The Frog King*), by Marjanovič Umek *et al.* (2012), prompted by pictures. The requirements about sample size and sampling time in general were: a minimum of 50 utterances (gold standard 100 utterances) and 15 minutes of interaction (gold standard is 30 minutes), although there were some speakers where reaching this level was impossible. TD children, as seen in the results, reached this level. The samples were first analysed with the criteria defined in the test *Žabji kralj/The Frog King* (Marjanovič Umek *et al.*, 2012), and further, for this study, on the basis of the following variables:

- the number of clauses;
- the number of utterances;
- the total number of words;
- the mean length of clause in words;
- the MLU (mean length of utterances) in words;
- the clausal density;
- the average of total number of main clauses;
- the average of total number of subordinates;
- the proportion of main clauses out of all clauses;
- the proportion of subordinate clauses out of all clauses.

Comparing Typically Developing Children and Children with LI

To determine whether the language measures discriminate TD and LI children aged 6–7 years, we first analysed measures of language productivity, syntactic complexity, and hierarchical complexity, as listed above.

As Table 5.2 illustrates, in general, the TD group show higher productivity and complexity. The children with LI on average produce more utterances, but fewer clauses and words, lower clausal density, lower mean length of clauses in words, lower MLU in words, and fewer main clauses and subordinate clauses. The percentage of main (simple) clauses out of

Table 5.2 Descriptive statistics of language measures for TD and LI groups, Test of Homogeneity of Variances, and Robust Tests of Equality of Means (Welch) for variables of language productivity, complexity and hierarchy

		Mean		SD		Min		Max		Range		Test of Homogeneity of Variances				Robust Tests of Equality of Means (Welch)			
	GROUP	TD	LI	TD	LI	TD	LI	TD	LI	TD	LI	Levene Statistic	df1	df2	Sig	Statistic	df1	df2	Sig
Language productivity	N of clauses	33.2	29	14.65	12.55	19	15	64	60	45	45	0.451	1	18	0.511	0.437	1	17.485	0.517
	N of utterances	12	14.7	8.27	6.91	4	7	32	25	28	18	0.000	1	18	0.984	0.627	1	17.449	0.439
	total N of words	5.01	4.03	0.55	0.88	4.24	2.16	5.91	4.95	1.67	2.79	0.116	1	18	0.738	2.021	1	17.959	0.172
	mean length of clause	16.59	8.912	7.09	3.6	8.47	2.16	27.86	14.29	19.39	12.13	2.551	1	18	0.128	8.873	1	14.566	0.010*
	MLU	164.8	120.4	71.49	68.15	101	47	330	287	229	240	5.205	1	18	0.035	9.311	1	13.347	0.009*
Syntactic complexity	Clausal density	3.33	2.16	1.4	0.79	1.53	1	5.67	3.86	4.13	2.86	6.807	1	18	0.018	5.246	1	13.964	0.038*
Hierarchical complexity	total N of main clauses	28.2	25.8	9.91	10.71	17	14	51	52	34	38	0.006	1	18	0.939	0.271	1	17.893	0.609
	total N of subordinates	5	3.2	5.91	2.62	0	1	18	8	18	7	3.492	1	18	0.078	0.776	1	12.400	0.395
	% of main clauses out of all clauses	87.9	89.61	10.22	6.51	64.71	78.26	100	96.43	35.29	18.17	.404	1	18	0.533	0.026	1	15.581	0.875
	% of subordinate clauses out of all clauses	15.4	12.16	15.71	8.63	0	3.7	54.55	27.78	54.55	24.07	.886	1	18	0.359	0.327	1	13.978	0.576

all clauses is higher in the LI group than in the TD group, but the percentage of subordinate clauses out of all clauses is lower in the group with LI than in the TD group.

In a similar result to that of Khan *et al.* (2016), the total words in the samples vary between 364 and 375.

Language productivity

These measures offer a quantitative measure for language. Although we know that the quantity of language does not necessarily define the quality, we can state that, in story retelling, children with LI show lower means in quantity of clauses, utterances, and words, except in number of utterances. In the TD group the mean N of clauses is higher ($M = 33.2$, $SD = 14.65$) compared to the LI group ($M = 29.2$, $SD = 12.318$). In the TD group the mean of number of utterances is lower ($M = 12.0$, $SD = 8.273$) compared to the LI group ($M = 14.700$, $SD = 6.913$). In the TD children, the mean of total number of words is higher ($M = 164.800$, $SD = 71.492$) compared to the LI group ($M = 120.400$, $SD = 68.150$). The TD group shows a higher MLU ($M = 16.586$, $SD = 7.092$) than the LI group ($M = 8.912$, $SD = 3.599$). The same advantage is shown in mean length of clause (TD, $M = 5.010$, $SD = 0.547$; LI $M = 3.994$, $SD = 0.929$). Although the LI group produce more utterances (mono-, bi- and multi-clausal), they use fewer words and their utterances tend to be shorter. Both MLC and MLU are lower in the LI group than in TD group.

Syntactic complexity

Language impairment has an influence not only on language productivity, but on language complexity too, in the measure of clausal density, i.e. the number of clauses by total number of C or T units (Nippold, 2014). Clausal density is on average 2,753 ($SD = 1.250$), from 1.00 to 5.67. But TD children produce a greater clausal density (TD $M = 3.331$, $SD = 1.40$, LI $M = 2.174$, $SD = 0.768$). Children with LI show lower clausal density, although they produce more utterances.

Hierarchical complexity

In the LI group it was evident that, despite the number of clauses produced, hierarchical complexity is low: there are many coordinate clauses, with listing/itemizing and adding, but not many subordinate clauses. The mean of the total number of main clauses in the TD group is higher ($M = 28.200$, $SD = 9.908$) compared to the LI group ($M = 25.800$, $SD = 10.706$). In the TD group the mean of the total number of subordinates is higher (TD $M = 5$, $SD = 5.907$, LI $M = 3.200$, $SD = 2.616$). The mean proportion of main clauses out of all clauses in the TD group is lower (TD $M = 87.895$, $SD = 10.218$, LI $M = 88.513$, $SD = 6.737$). The mean of the proportion of subordinate clauses out of all clauses in the TD group is higher (TD $M = 15.397$, $SD = 15.705$, LI $M = 12.157$, $SD = 8.627$). The TD group show more main and subordinates (tot, sub1, sub 2) clauses compared to the LI group. In terms of proportion, the LI group show a higher percentage of main clauses out of all clauses than the TD group, but fewer subordinate clauses. To test the differences among groups, a Test of Homogeneity of Variances and Welch's Robust Tests of Equality of Means were carried out. As seen in Table 5.4, the two groups show statistically significant differences in means of MLCw, MLUw and CD (sig. >0.05), i.e. in a measure of language productivity and of syntactic complexity. The differences in variances show us that the two groups belong to two different populations in terms of language use and development.

Case Studies: SLO-LARSP in children with language impairment aged 6–7 years

To illustrate the application of SLO-LARSP in detail we have chosen four children from the full sample (2 TD and 2 LI). The children selected were those with the lowest scores in their respective groups in MLUw, MLCw and clausal density measures. Brief samples from each child were analysed according to SO-LARSP to illustrate profile differences.

Child 25, age: 6–7 years, typical language development

In a 3-minute sample Child 25 produced 19 sentences. All sentences were spontaneous and all were part of a story narration, supported by illustrations. All sentences were intelligible. All of the child's sentences were grammatically correct; the analysis of the transcription also showed the semantic correctness of the child's speech. The child's sentences are spread from stage I to stage V in the developmental part of the SLO-LARSP profile. MLUw for this sample is 9.32. The majority of the sentences in the sample are statements in the indicative or conditional mood. Five commands and one question are found in the sample. In the recorded sample the child produces only active sentences. Child 25 often combines two or more clauses in coordinate or subordinate sentences by using the conjunction *in* ('and') or other coordinate conjunctions with coordinate clauses (seven times) or different subordinate conjunctions with subordinate clauses (e.g. *dokler, če, da* 'until, if, that'). The majority of sentences consist of verb and subject; the subject is expressed directly (e.g. ***Princeska** se je igrala z žogo* 'Little princess (herself) was playing with the ball') or indirectly (e.g. *Nato ji je padla v vodo* 'then (the ball) fell her into the water' ['then it fell into the water']). The child expands verb phrases with the auxiliary verb 'to be' (e.g. ***je** jokala* 'she was crying'), with modal verbs (e.g. *on je* **hotel** 'he really wanted') or with a reflexive verb (e.g. *se je igrala* 'she played (herself)'). The correct negation of verbs is presented in the recorded sample. Noun phrases are expanded mostly by adding prepositions or determiners to nouns (e.g. ***v** vodo,* **tvoj** grad 'in the water, your castle'). He often uses personal pronouns (e.g. *jaz, ji, te, me* 'I, her, you, me') – there are 24 in the recorded sample. Five sentences start with a conjunction *in* 'and' or *ampak* 'but' (cX-structure). Morphological analysis of the recorded sample shows that he uses all three grammatical genders, five of the six cases (based on the recorded sample, which is very short), singular, dual, and plural, and past and present tense. The SLO-LARSP profile shows no deviations in this child's grammatical development. His sentences are structurally and semantically adequate (see Figure 5.3).

Child 19, age: 6–7 years, with language impairment

In a 1.5-minute sample Child 19 produced eight grammatically correct sentences. All were spontaneous and part of a story narration, supported by illustrations. All were intelligible. Three sentences were eliminated: two of them included symbolic noise; one sentence was deviant. The narration was poorly coherent and incomprehensible without the support of illustrations.

Child 19's sentences are spread from stage I to stage V in the developmental part of the SLO-LARSP profile (two clauses in stage I, one clause in stage II, two clauses in stage III, three clauses in stage IV and one sentence in stage V). MLUw for this sample is 3.5. Sentences are short, semantically poorly connected, and in three cases the verb is omitted. Two thirds of the sentences in the sample are statements, one is a command and three are questions. In the recorded sample, he produces only active sentence types. He connects two clauses in a subordinate sentence, using the subordinate conjunction *če* ('if') in one case.

He does not expand verb phrases. There is one case of copula use (*Zdaj mi je pa dovolj* 'but now it's enough for me'). The subject is expressed directly (e.g. *Nekoč je živel* **kralj** 'once upon a time there lived a king') or indirectly (e.g. *Vse ti obljubim* 'I promise you everything'). A noun phrase is presented once – he adds a preposition to a noun (***v** posteljo* 'to bed'). He often uses personal pronouns (e.g. *mi, ti, me, te* 'me, you, me, you') – there are nine in the recorded sample. Morphological analysis of the recorded sample shows that he uses feminine and masculine grammatical gender, first, fourth and fifth case, and singular (based on the recorded sample, which is very short). He uses only the present tense.

The SLO-LARSP profile (see Figure 5.4) shows structural and semantic weaknesses in this child's language: clause structure is poor, some elements are often omitted (e.g. verbs), and there are very few phrase expansions. A longer interaction sample is recommended for further diagnostics of his language.

SLO-LARSP – analiza slovničnih zmožnosti slovenskih govorcev (verzija 17/b)

Dr. Martina Ozbič, dr. Jerneja Novšak Brce, dr. Damjana Kogovšek, dr. Darija Skubic, Ana Praprotnik
Univerza v Ljubljani Pedagoška fakulteta

Ime, priimek	Starost (leta, meseci)	Datum snemanja	Način interakcije	Trajanje
25- brez SGJM	6-7 let			3 min

A	**Neanalizirani stavki**			**Problematični stavki**		
	1 Nerazu-mljivi st.	2 Simbolni zvoki	3 Nestan-dard. izj.	1 Nedo-končani st.	2 Dvo-umni st.	3 Stalne formule

B	Odzivi		Pono-vitve	Tipičen odziv						Netipičen odziv		Teža-ve
				Major					Minor	Strukt. nepri-meren odziv	Ø	
				Reduciran st.			Negla-golski st.	Popoln st.				
	Tipi dražljaja	Skupaj Vprašanja Drugo		1	2	3+						
C	**Spontane izjave**											
D	**Odzivi na otrokovo dejavnost**			Splošne	Strukt. pov.	Ø		Drugo		Težave		

Stopnja I	**Minor**	*Odgovori*		*Zvalniki*		*Drugo* 1	*Težave*
	Major	*Ukazi*	*Vprašanja*	*Trditve*			
		'V' 2	'Q'	'V'	'N'	Drugo 1	Težave

	Veznik	**Stavek**					**Besedna zveza**		**Beseda**
Stopnja II		V*X*	Q*X*	SV 3 SO SC Neg*X*	(S)V 7 (S)O (S)C	A*X* VO VC Drugo	DN 1 Adj N 1 NN PrN 8	VV V part Int *X* Drugo	deležnik: - stanja - trpni d.; moški sp. srednji sp. ženski sp.; ednina dvojina množina; 3. os. ed.; prvi sklon drugi skl. tretji skl. četrti skl. peti skl. šesti skl.
		X + S:NP 1	*X* + V:VP 8	*X* + C:NP		*X* + O:NP		*X* + A:AP 1	
Stopnja III		V*XY* 2	Q*XY* 1 VS(*X*)	SVC SVO 2 SVA 3 Neg*XY*	(S)VC (S)VO 2 (S)VA 3	VCA VOA VO$_d$O$_i$ Drugo 1	D Adj N Adj Adj N Pr DN 1 **Pron.** – oseb. 24 **Pron.** – drugi 1	Cop Aux^m 7 Aux^o 25 **Povr. gl.** 5 Drugo 2	sedanjik preteklik prihodnjik; pove. n. velelni n. pogojni n.; svojilni rodilnik
		XY + S:NP	*XY* + V:VP 7	*XY* + C:NP		*XY* + O:NP 1		*XY* + A:AP 3	nikalnice, nanikan glagol; pomožni gl. biti; copula – vez
Stopnja IV		+ S V*XY*+	QVS Q*XY*+ VS(*X*+) tag	SVOA 1 SVCA SVO$_d$O$_i$1 SVOC	(S)VOA4 (S)VCA (S)VO$_d$O$_i$ 3 (S)VOC	AA*XY* 1 *Drugo* 2	NP Pr NP Pd D Adj N c*X* 5 *X*c*X* 1	Neg V 4 Neg *X* 2 Aux (m,o) Drugo	pomožni glagoli; tvornik trpnik; primerjalnik presežnik
Stopnja V	in,ter,**pa** 7 s 6 c 5 Drugi	Prired. 1 Drugo	Prired. Drugo	Prired. Podred. A S Primerjal. **Soredje**	1 5 1 4 C	1+ 2 1+ O 4	Oziralni stavek 1 1+ Dopolnit. fraza 1+		- opisno - obrazilno; dovrš. nedovrš.; prisl. nač.; prehod. neprehod. gl.; členek

Stopnja VI	(+)			(-)				
	NP	VP	Stavek	Vezniki	Stavek	Besedna zveza		Beseda
	Začetek Besede Razšir. st.	Večglag. st.	Pasivno Povedkovo dol. *Kako* *Kaj, kakšen*	in c s	Element Ø → ←	NP D Pr Pro$^?$ D Ø Pr Ø D → ← Pr → ←	VP Aux^M Aux^o Cop Ø	N V *nepravil.* *pravil.*
	Drugo					*Dvoumni*		

Stopnja VII	*Diskurz*		*Skladenjsko razumevanje*
	Adverbialna povezanost	Neosebna oblika	
	Komentarji		*Stil*
	Emfatični besedni red	Drugo	

Skupno št. **povedi** 19	Povprečno št. **povedi** 19 glede na izmenjavo	Povprečna dolžina **povedi (MLUw)** 177/19=9,32

Figure 5.3 Child 25

Child 27, age: 6–7 years, typical language development

In a 3-minute sample Child 27 produced 16 sentences. All sentences were spontaneous and were part of a story narration, supported by illustrations. All sentences were intelligible; all were grammatically correct; and the analysis of the transcription also showed semantic correctness. Sentences are spread from stage II to stage V in the developmental part of the SLO-LARSP profile. MLUw for this sample is 7.88. Sentences in the

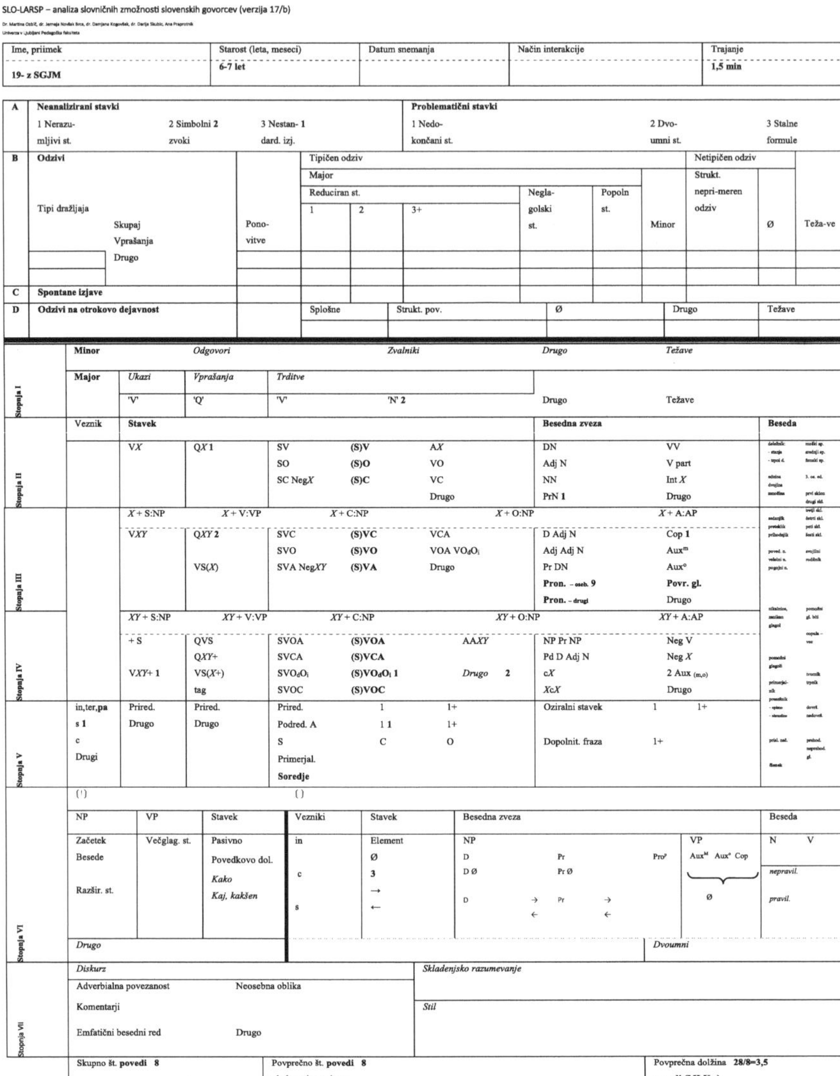
SLO-LARSP – analiza slovničnih zmožnosti slovenskih govorcev (verzija 17/b)
Dr. Martina Ozbič, dr. Jerneja Novšak Brce, dr. Damjana Kogovšek, dr. Darija Skubic, Ana Praprotnik
Univerza v Ljubljani Pedagoška fakulteta

Ime, priimek	Starost (leta, meseci)	Datum snemanja	Način interakcije	Trajanje
19- z SGJM	6-7 let			1,5 min

A Neanalizirani stavki: 1 Nerazu-mljivi st.; 2 Simbolni zvoki 2; 3 Nestan-dard. izj. 1
Problematični stavki: 1 Nedo-končani st.; 2 Dvo-umni st.; 3 Stalne formule

B Odzivi: Tipi dražljaja; Skupaj; Vprašanja; Drugo; Pono-vitve; Tipičen odziv; Major; Reduciran st.: 1, 2, 3+; Negla-golski st.; Popoln st.; Minor; Netipičen odziv; Strukt. nepri-meren odziv; Ø; Teža-ve

C Spontane izjave

D Odzivi na otrokovo dejavnost: Splošne; Strukt. pov.; Ø; Drugo; Težave

Stopnja I
Minor: Odgovori; Zvalniki; Drugo; Težave
Major: Ukazi 'V'; Vprašanja 'Q'; Trditve 'V' 'N' 2; Drugo; Težave

Stopnja II
Veznik; Stavek; Besedna zveza; Beseda
VX; QX 1; SV (S)V AX; SO (S)O VO; SC NegX (S)C VC; Drugo
DN VV; Adj N V part; NN Int X; PrN 1 Drugo

Stopnja III
X + S:NP; X + V:VP; X + C:NP; X + O:NP; X + A:AP
VXY; QXY 2; VS(X); SVC (S)VC VCA; SVO (S)VO VOA VO_dO_i; SVA NegXY (S)VA Drugo
D Adj N Cop 1; Adj Adj N Aux^m; Pr DN Aux^o; Pron. - oseb. 9 Povr. gl.; Pron. - drugi Drugo

Stopnja IV
XY + S:NP; XY + V:VP; XY + C:NP; XY + O:NP; XY + A:AP
+ S; VXY+ 1; QVS; QXY+; VS(X+); tag; SVOA (S)VOA AAXY; SVCA (S)VCA; SVO_dO_i $(S)VO_dO_i$ 1 Drugo 2; SVOC (S)VOC
NP Pr NP Neg V; Pd D Adj N Neg X; cX 2 Aux (m,o); XcX Drugo

Stopnja V
in,ter,pa s 1; c; Drugi
Prired. Drugo; Prired. Drugo
Prired. 1 1+; Podred. A 1 1 1+; S C O; Primerjal.; Soredje
Oziralni stavek 1 1+; Dopolnit. fraza 1+

Stopnja VI
(!) ( )
NP: Začetek Besede; Razšir. st.
VP: Večglag. st.
Stavek: Pasivno; Povedkovo dol.; Kako; Kaj, kakšen
Vezniki: in; c; s
Stavek: Element; Ø; 3; →; ←
Besedna zveza: NP: D, Pr, Pro; D Ø, Pr Ø; D → Pr →; ← ←
VP: Aux^M Aux^o Cop; Ø
Beseda: N V; nepravil.; pravil.
Drugo; Dvoumni

Stopnja VII
Diskurz: Adverbialna povezanost; Neosebna oblika; Komentarji; Emfatični besedni red; Drugo
Skladenjsko razumevanje
Stil

Skupno št. povedi 8; Povprečno št. povedi 8 glede na izmenjavo; Povprečna dolžina povedi (MLUw) 28/8=3,5

Figure 5.4 Child 19

sample are all statements in indicative or conditional mood – no commands or questions are presented. In the recorded sample, there are only active sentence types. He combines two or more clauses in coordinate or subordinate sentences by using the conjunction *in* with coordinate clauses (three times) or different subordinate conjunctions with subordinate clauses (e.g. *da, potem ko* 'that, after'). The majority of sentences consist of verb and subject; the subject is mostly expressed directly (e.g. ***Žogica*** *ji je padla v vodo* 'the ball dropped her into the water'), but in a fourth of the sentences

SLO-LARSP – analiza slovničnih zmožnosti slovenskih govorcev (verzija 17/b)

Dr. Martina Ozbič, dr. Jerneja Novšak Brce, dr. Damjana Kogovšek, dr. Darija Skubic, Ana Praprotnik
Univerza v Ljubljani Pedagoška fakulteta

Ime, priimek	Starost (leta, meseci)	Datum snemanja	Način interakcije	Trajanje
27- brez SGJM	6-7 let			3 min

A	**Neanalizirani stavki**			**Problematični stavki**		
	1 Nerazu-mljivi st.	2 Simbolni zvoki	3 Nestan-dard. izj.	1 Nedo-končani st.	2 Dvo-umni st.	3 Stalne formule

B	**Odzivi**		Tipičen odziv						Netipičen odziv		
			Major								
			Reduciran st.			Negla-golski st.	Popoln st.		Strukt. nepri-meren odziv		
	Tipi dražljaja: Skupaj / Vprašanja / Drugo	Pono-Vitve	1	2	3+			Minor		Ø	Teža-ve
C	**Spontane izjave**										
D	**Odzivi na otrokovo dejavnost**		Splošne		Strukt. pov.		Ø		Drugo	Težave	

Stopnja I	**Minor**	*Odgovori*			*Zvalniki*		*Drugo*	*Težave*		
	Major	*Ukazi*	*Vprašanja*	*Trditve*						
		'V'	'Q'	'V'	'N'		Drugo	Težave		
Stopnja II	Veznik	**Stavek**					**Besedna zveza**		**Beseda**	
		V*X*	Q*X*	SV **1** SO SC Neg*X*	**(S)V 1** **(S)O** **(S)C**	A*X* VO VC Drugo	DN Adj N NN PrN **4**	VV V part Int *X* Drugo	deležnik: - stanja - trpni d.	moški sp. srednji sp. ženski sp.
		X + S:NP	*X* + V:VP **4**	*X* + C:NP		*X* + O:NP		*X* + A:AP	ednina	3. os. ed.
Stopnja III		V*XY*	Q*XY* VS(*X*)	SVC SVO **3** SVA **6** Neg*XY*	**(S)VC** **(S)VO 2** **(S)VA 1**	VCA VOA VO_dO_i Drugo **1**	D Adj N Adj Adj N Pr DN **4** **Pron. – oseb. 8** **Pron. – drugi 2**	Cop **1** Aux^m **1** Aux^o **21** **Povr. gl. 4** Drugo	dvojina množina sedanjik	prvi sklon drugi skl. tretji skl. četrti skl.
		XY + S:NP	*XY* + V:VP **7**	*XY* + C:NP		*XY* + O:NP		*XY* + A:AP **4**	preteklik	peti skl.
Stopnja IV		+ S V*XY*+	QVS Q*XY*+ VS(*X*+) tag	SVOA **1** SVCA **1** SVO_dO_i SVOC	**(S)VOA 1** **(S)VCA** **(S)VO_dO_i1** **(S)VOC**	AA*XY* **3** *Drugo*	NP Pr NP Pd D Adj N c*X* **2** *X*c*X* **2**	Neg V Neg *X* 2 Aux $_{(m,o)}$ Drugo	prihodnjik poved. n.	šesti skl. svojilni
Stopnja V	in,ter,**pa** **4** s **3** c Drugi	Prired. Drugo	Prired. Drugo	Prired. Podred. A S Primerjal. **Soredje**	1 **2** 1 **2** C	1+ **1** 1+ O **1**	Oziralni stavek Dopolnit. fraza	1 1+ 1+	velelni n. pogojni n. nikalnice, zanikan glagol pomožni glagoli primerjal-nik presežnik - opisno - obrazilno prisl. nač. členek	rodilnik pomožni gl. biti copula – vez tvornik trpnik dovrš. nedovrš. prehod. neprehod. gl.

Figure 5.5 Child 27

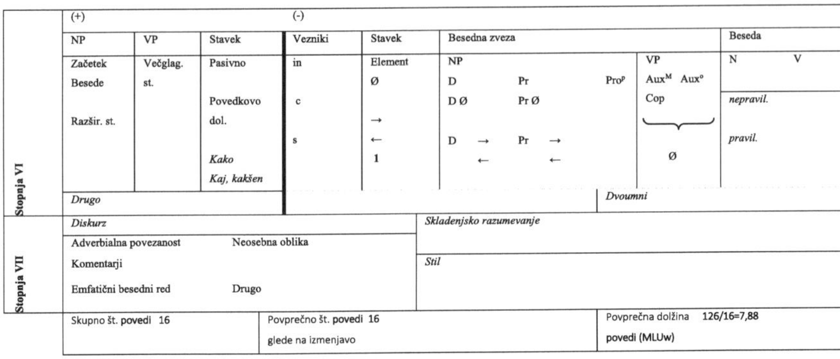

Figure 5.5 *Continued*

it is expressed indirectly (e.g. *Nato je jokala* 'then (she) was crying'). Verb phrases are expanded with the auxiliary verb 'to be' (e.g. ***je*** *padla* 'fell ') or with a reflexive verb (e.g. *so* **se** usedli 'they sat down (themselves)' ['they sat down']). Noun phrases are expanded mostly by adding propositions or determiners to nouns (e.g. ***k*** *mizi,* **v njeno** hišo 'to the table, into her house'). He uses personal pronouns (e.g. *mu, ji, ga* 'him, her, him') – there are eight in the recorded sample. Morphological analysis of the recorded sample shows that he uses all three grammatical genders, all six cases, singular, dual and plural. Only past tense is used in the recorded sample, which is probably the consequence of narration. There is one case of copula use (*In princesa* **je bila spet vesela** 'and the princess was happy again') and one case of modal verb use (*ne* **sme** hoditi 'is not allowed to walk'). In one case, he changed the position of the reflexive verb and the auxiliary verb (*je se poročila* 'was she married' instead of **se je** poročila 'she was married').

The SLO-LARSP profile (see Figure 5.5) shows no deviations in this child's grammatical development. His sentences are structurally and semantically adequate.

Child 57, age: 6–7 years, with language impairment

In a 2-minute sample Child 57 produced 22 sentences. All sentences were spontaneous and part of a story narration, supported by illustrations. All were intelligible. Three sentences were eliminated: one of them included symbolic noise, one sentence was deviant and one was ambiguous. The narration was poorly coherent and incomprehensible without support of illustrations.

This child's sentences are spread from stage I to stage IV in the developmental part of the SLO-LARSP profile (see Figure 5.6). The majority of sentences have stage I and stage II structure. MLUw for this sample is 2.0. Sentences are short, semantically poorly connected and clause or phrase

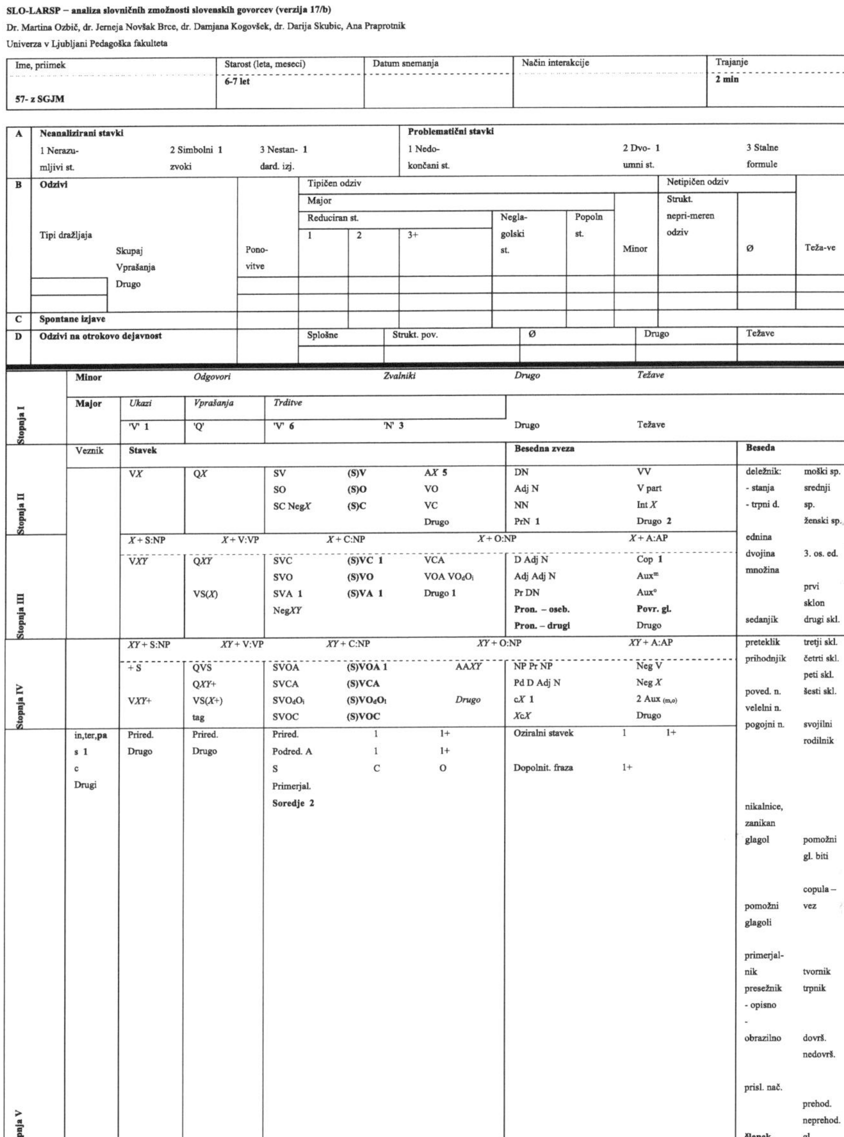

Figure 5.6 Child 57

elements are often omitted. The sentences in the sample are statements in indicative mood; one sentence is a command. In the recorded sample, he produces only active sentence types. He uses only one-clause sentences. In a clause, he often (in six cases) omits the verb (e.g. *Potem žabica not* 'then the little frog into'). He does not expand verb phrases; all verbs are in the present tense. There is one case of copula use (*Zato ker* **je grda** 'because

	(+)			(-)				
	NP	VP	Stavek	Vezniki	Stavek	Besedna zveza		Beseda
Stopnja VI	Začetek Besede Razšir. st.	Večglag. st.	Pasivno Povedkovo dol. *Kako* *Kaj, kakšen*	in c s	Element Ø **6** → ←	NP D Pr Pro^P D Ø Pr Ø **3** D → Pr → ← ←	VP Aux^M Aux^o Cop Ø	N V *nepravil.* *pravil.* **2**
	Drugo						*Dvoumni*	
Stopnja VII	*Diskurz*				*Skladenjsko razumevanje*			
	Adverbialna povezanost Komentarji Emfatični besedni red		Neosebna oblika Drugo		*Stil*			
	Skupno št. **povedi 22**		Povprečno št. **povedi 22** glede na izmenjavo				Povprečna dolžina **44/22=2,0** **povedi (MLUw)**	

Figure 5.6 *Continued*

it's ugly'). The subject is sometimes expressed directly (e.g. *Potem* **žoga** greje 'then the ball goes') or more often indirectly (e.g. *Joka* 'cries'). A noun phrase is presented once – he adds a preposition to noun (*v poslico* 'in the little bed'). In three cases the preposition is omitted (e.g. *Not hišo* instead of *Not* **v** hišo 'into the house'). He does not use any pronouns. In two cases, he declines verbs incorrectly (*greje* instead of *gre* 'goes', *hoja* instead of *hodi* 'walks'). Morphological analysis shows that he uses feminine grammatical gender, first and fourth case, and singular. This profile shows structural and semantic weaknesses in his language: clause structure is poor, elements are often omitted (e.g. verbs, prepositions), there are very few phrase expansions, and he does not connect clauses. A longer interaction sample is recommended for further diagnostics of this child's language.

Conclusion

Language measures and sampling natural language are the best way to get real language data; their weakness is that they are influenced by the speakers/participants, setting, material and activity. Sampling language is very useful when standardized tests are not available, when the child is very young, or when the person cannot collaborate as required by the structured tool, or finally, as a choice. When we adapt the setting (eliciting material, tempo, methods) according to the speaker's needs and competences, we improve the reliability of the data. According to Kranjc *et al.* (2006), the development of a child's vocabulary does not proceed separately from the development of the grammar (Tomasello & Bates, 2001). Many scholars (Caselli *et al.*, 2001; Karmiloff & Karmiloff-Smith, 2001; Kranjc, 1999) agree that as the child's grammatical acquisition progresses, there is also an increased use of adjectival words that describe the qualities of objects and the relations between them, as well as function words such as conjunctions and prepositions. Children understand the meaning of a greater number of words relating to the properties of objects and describing spatial relationships. As they grow, children master significantly more grammatical rules, such as conjugation and declension, so they are more able to complete tasks on subscales of verbal expression that demanded the use of verbs in the third person or the past tense and the use of declensions or the dual and plural. The acquisition of rules relating to verb conjugation is probably also connected to the growing number of verbs in the child's vocabulary (Kranjc, 1999; Owens, 1996, in Papalia *et al.*, 2001; Kranjc *et al.*, 2006).

According to Kranjc *et al.* (2006), between the age of three and four differences arise in the coherence of stories that children tell prompted by a picture book, from stories involving simple descriptions of people, objects, or illustrations, simple temporal stringing together of events, stories with no structure, and naming of people and objects. Stories at age three rarely had a beginning that acted as an introduction to the continuing events, but more often began with a description of the illustration on the first page of the picture book. Nor did they usually involve a problem or a connecting theme that determined events and the outcome or solution. The stories of four-year-olds usually already follow narrative conventions. The stories of 4-years olds more often had a beginning that introduced the continuing events, and also had a clear and logical ending.

In our sample, 6–7-year-old children with LI show similar narration skills, i.e. immature narration skill linked to the immediate environment, and naming of people and objects. The stories include simple descriptions and are to a great extent linked directly to their own perceptions. Typically developing children tell ever more structured, decontextualized, well-formed stories. These stories are not simply a string of utterances connected to a greater or lesser degree, as we can observe in children with LI.

The features are visible in the profiles, too. Well-formed stories in TD children are morphologically rich, whereas stories of LI children are poor.

LI children produce poorly coherent narration, incomprehensible without the support of illustrations. Their sentences are spread from stage I to stage IV or V in the developmental part of the SLO-LARSP profile. MLUw for the two children with LI that we discussed above is low (2–3.5). Sentences are short, semantically poorly connected, and clause or phrase elements are often omitted. They do not expand verb phrases, and subjects are expressed directly or indirectly. Noun phrases are presented rarely. Morphological analysis of the recorded samples show that they use feminine and masculine grammatical gender, first, fourth and fifth case, and singular. The use of tenses is limited. The SLO-LARSP profile shows structural and semantic weaknesses in the language of children with LI: clause structure is poor, some elements are often omitted (e.g. verbs, prepositions), there are very few phrase expansions, and there can be a limited connection between clause.

TD children produce more sentences; they are part of a story narration; and the speech shows semantic correctness. Their sentences are spread from stage I or II to stage V. MLUw is higher in the two TD children than in the LI pair, i.e. 9.32/7.88. The sentences in the sample are statements in the indicative or conditional mood. Commands and questions are found. They often combine two or more clauses in coordinate or subordinate sentences by using the conjunction *in* or other coordinate conjunctions with coordinate clauses (seven times) or different subordinate conjunctions with subordinate clauses. The majority of sentences consist of verb and subject; the subject is expressed directly or indirectly. TD children expand verb phrases with the auxiliary verb *to be*, with modal verbs, or with a reflexive verb. Correct negation of verbs is presented. Noun phrases are expanded mostly by adding prepositions or determiners to nouns. They often use personal pronouns. Morphological analysis shows that they use all three grammatical genders, five or six cases, singular, dual, and plural. They use past and present tense, and modal verbs. The profile shows no deviations in their grammatical development. Sentences are structurally and semantically adequate.

In conclusion, we can say that quantitative language measures can describe the children's linguistic proficiency, but a profile tells us more about morphosyntactic development, especially in languages that are as morphologically rich as Slovenian. Applying SLO-LASRP to typically developing and language impaired children, our results show that there is a need to use both qualitative and quantitative measures. Due to the small samples currently available, a larger study in the future is required.

Note

(1) LARSP SLO was adapted by: Martina Ozbič, Ana Praprotnik, Jerneja Novšak Brce, Damjana Kogovšek and Darija Skubic. Additional morphological page: Darija Skubic, Martina Ozbič.

References

Allen, S.E.M. and Dench, C. (2015) Calculating mean length of utterance for eastern Canadian Inuktitut. *First Language* 35 (4–5), 377–406.

Arapović, D. (1996) Naracija u djece s posebnim jezičnim teškoćama. Doctoral thesis. Zagreb: Faculty of Defectology.

Bates, E. and Goodman, J.C. (2001) On the inseparability of grammar and the lexicon: Evidence from acquisition. In M. Tomasello and E. Bates (eds) *Language Development: The Essential Readings* (pp. 134–162). Oxford: Blackwell.

Brown, R. (1973) *A First Language: The Early Stages*. Cambridge, MA: Harvard University Press.

Caselli, M.C., Casadio, P. and Bates, E. (2001) Lexical development in English and Italian. In M. Tomasello and E. Bates (eds) *Language Development: The Essential Readings* (pp. 76–110). Oxford: Blackwell.

Crystal, D. (1992) *Profiling Linguistic Disability*. London: Whurr Publisher.

Eisenberg, S.L., McGovern Fersko, T. and Lundgren, C. (2001) The use of MLU for identifying language impairment in preschool children: A review. *American Journal of Speech-Language Pathology* 10 (4), 323–342.

Fekonja Peklaj, U. (2002) Otrokov govor v kontekstu predšolskega kurikuluma. *Sodobna pedagogika* 53 (3), 94–111.

Fekonja, U., Kranjc, S. and Marjanovič Umek, L. (2005) Otrokov govorni razvoj v povezavi z njegovim spolom in izobrazbo staršev. *Psihološka obzorja* 14 (1), 53–79.

Fekonja, U., Kranjc, S. and Marjanovič Umek, L. (2003) Pripovedovanje zgodbe kot možni pristop za ugotavljanje otrokovega govornega razvoja. *Jezik in slovstvo* 48 (5), 51–63.

Fekonja, U., Kranjc, S. and Marjanovič Umek, L. (2004) Pripovedovanje zgodbe kot pristop za ugotavljanje otrokovega govornega razvoja. *Psihološka obzorja* 13 (1), 43–64.

Girolametto, L. (1997) Development of a parent report measure for profiling the conversational skills of preschool children. *American Journal of Speech-Language Pathology* 6 (4), 25–33.

Gnamuš, O. (1976) Družbeno pogojeni zaostanki v jezkovnem razvoju. *Jezik in slovstvo* 21 (5), 145–153.

Grobler, M. (2002) Otroci s specifično govorno-jezikovno motnjo. In N. Končnik-Goršič and M. Kavkler (eds) *Specifične učne težave otrok in mladostnikov: prepoznavanje, razumevanje, pomoč* (pp. 121–154). Ljubljana: Svetovalni center za otroke, mladostnike in starše.

Grobler, M. and Arapović, D. (2007) Microlinguistic analysis of narrative produced by 10-years old children with specific language impairment. *Journal of Special Education and Rehabilitation* 8 (1–2), 15–24.

Greenberg, M.L. (2006) *A Short Reference Grammar of Standard Slovenian*. Retrieved from: http://www.seelrc.org:8080/grammar/pdf/stand_alone_Slovenian.pdf or www.fran.si/slovnice-in-pravopisi/pdf/2006Greenberg.pdf

Herrity, P. (2000) *Slovenian: A Comprehensive Grammar*. New York: Routledge.

Kalin Golob, M., Gliha Komac, N., Logar, N. and Goršek Mencin, N. (2007) *O slovenskem jeziku* [On Slovenian]. First edition. Ljubljana: European Parliament Information Office for Slovenia: Ministry of Culture of the Republic of Slovenia: Government Office for European Affairs of the Republic of Slovenia.

Karmiloff, K. and Karmiloff-Smith, A. (2001) *The Developing Child. Pathways to Language: From Fetus to Adolescent*. Cambridge, MA, US: Harvard University Press.

Khan, K.S., Gugiu, M.R., Justice, L.M., Bowles, R.P., Skibbe, L.E. and Piasta, S.B. (2016) Age-related progressions in story structure in young children's narratives. *Journal of Speech, Language, and Hearing Research* 59 (6), 1395–1408.

Koltaj, P. and Žagar, I.Ž. (2007) Transkribiranje otroške argumentacije. *Šolsko polje: revija za raziskave vzgoje in izobraževanja* 18 (1–2), 171–184.

Kovačič, J. (2012) *Pripovedovanje zgodbe petletnega otroka z lažjo govorno jezikovno motnjo*. Diplomsko delo. Ljubljana: Pedagoška fakulteta UL.

Kranjc, S. (1992) Otroški govor. *Jezik in slovstvo* 38 (1–2), 19–28.

Kranjc, S. (1993) Otroški govor v zgodnjem obdobju svojega razvoja. *Anthropos* 25 (3–4), 125–137.

Kranjc, S. (1995/1996) Slovnična zmožnost otrok na besedotvorni ravni. *Jezik in slovstvo* 41 (6), 309–326.

Kranjc, S. (1997) Govorjeni diskurz. *Jezik in slovstvo* 42 (7), 307–320.

Kranjc, S. (1999) Skladnja in otroški govor. *Jezik in slovstvo* 44 (6), 197–212.

Kranjc, S. (2004) Besedni red, usvajanje prvega in učenje drugega/tujega jezika. *Jezik in slovstvo* 49 (3–4), 145–157.

Kranjc, S. (2003) Izražanje prostora v govorjenih besedilih otrok. *Slavistična revija* 51(posebna), 181–190.

Kranjc, S., Marjanovič Umek, L. and Fekonja Peklaj, U. (2003) Pripovedovanje zgodbe kot možni pristop za ugotavljanje otrokovega govornega razvoja. *Jezik in slovstvo* 48 (5), 51–63.

Kranjc, S., Marjanovič Umek, L. and Fekonja Peklaj, U. (2006) Govorni razvoj v zgodnjem otroštvu: razvojne spremembe med 3. in 4. letom otrokove starosti = Language development in early childhood: Developmental changes between the ages of three and four. *Slavistična revija* 54 (4), 351–367, 727–744.

Leonard, L.B. (2014) Specific language impairment across languages. *Child Development Perspectives* 8 (1), 1–5.

Marjanovič Umek, L., Kranjc, S. and Fekonja, U. (2005) Early versus late entry to preschool: The effect on the child's language development. *European Early Childhood Education Research Journal* 13 (2), 111–131.

Marjanovič Umek, L. and Zupančič, M. (eds) (2013) *Razvojna psihologija: izbrane teme*. Ljubljana: Znanstvena založba Filozofske fakultete.

Marjanovič Umek, L. and Fekonja Peklaj, U. (2012) Early literacy development: The role of storytelling, joint reading, and symbolic play. In M.L. Falese (ed.) *Encyclopedia of Education Research (Education in a Competitive and Globalizing World)* (pp. 13–39). New York: Nova Science Publishers.

Marjanovič Umek, L., Fekonja U. and Kranjc, S. (2004) Pripovedovanje zgodbe kot pristop za ugotavljanje otrokovega govornega razvoja. *Psihološka obzorja* 13 (1), 43–64.

Marjanovič Umek, L., Kranjc, S., Fekonja Peklaj, U. and Bajc, K. (2006) *Otroški govor: razvoj in učenje*. Domžale: Izolit.

Marjanovič Umek, L. (1990) *Mišljenje in govor predšolskega otroka*. 1. natis. Ljubljana: Državna založba Slovenije.

Nippold, M.A. (2014) *Language Sampling with Adolescents: Implications for Intervention*. (2nd edn). San Diego, CA: Plural.

O'Neill, D.K. (2007) The Language Use Inventory: A parent-report measure of pragmatic language development for 18–47-month-old children. *Journal of Speech, Language and Hearing Research* 50 (1), 214–228.

Omahna, M. (2011) *Uporaba Testa zgodba o avtobusu pri ocenjevanju pragmatične zmožnosti otrok*. Diplomsko delo. Ljubljana: Pedagoška fakulteta UL.

Owens, R.E. (1996) *Language Development: An Introduction*. Boston: Allyn & Bacon.

Papalia, D.E., Wendkos Olds, S. and Duskin Feldman, R. (2001) *Human Development*. New York: McGraw Hill.

Praprotnik, A. (2017) *Uporaba profila SLO-LARSP za analizo slovnične zmožnosti triletnih otrok*. Magistrsko delo. Ljubljana: Pedagoška fakulteta.

Sevšek, T. (2016) *Pripovedovanje zgodbe 6-9 let starih otrok s specifičnimi govorno-jezikovnimi motnjami* (Magistrsko delo). Ljubljana: Pedagoška fakulteta.

Siegler, R.S. (1998) *Children's Thinking*. New Jersey: Prentice Hall.

Tomasello, M. and Bates. E. (2001) General introduction. In M. Tomasello and E. Bates (eds) *Language Development: The Essential Readings* (pp. 1–11). Oxford: Blackwell.

Toporišič, J. (1992) *Enciklopedija slovenskega jezika [Encyclopaedia of Slovenian Language]*. Ljubljana: Cankarjeva založba.

Toporišič, J. (2000) *Slovenska slovnica [Grammar of Slovenian Language]*. Maribor: Obzorja.

Wetherby, A.M. and Prizant, B.M. (2001) *Communication and Symbolic Behaviour Scales–Infant/Toddler Checklist*. Baltimore: Paul H. Brookes Publishing Co.

Žagar, F. (1961) Razvoj izražanja osnovnošolskih učencev. *Jezik in slovstvo* 7 (3), 82–87.

Žagar, F. (1993) *Klemenov govorni razvoj v drugem letu njegove starosti*. Available also at: CHILDES, http://childes.talkbank.org/data-cmdi/childes/Slavic/Slovenian/Zagar/

6 LARSP-PE: A Developmental Language Profile for European Portuguese-speaking Children

Ana Castro, Carolina Marques and Catarina Dôro

Introduction

In this chapter, we present a brief description of a linguistic procedure for assessing the language of European Portuguese-speaking children (LARSP-PE) that may be implemented in clinical and educational settings, as a support for the assessment, screening and intervention with children with language impairment. The procedure was developed by a research group at the Setúbal Polytechnic Institute and Universidade Nova de Lisboa, following the lines of *LARSP, Language Assessment, Remediation and Screening Procedure,* originally proposed for English in Crystal *et al.* (1976). In this study, acquisition data from European Portuguese-speaking children were considered. The Portuguese varieties spoken in Brazil, Angola, Cape Verde, Guinea-Bissau, Mozambique, São Tomé e Príncipe and East Timor differ to some extend in the phonetic, lexical, morphological and syntactic domains. Therefore, the developmental scale for European Portuguese morphosyntactic development presented as a result of this study does not necessarily reflect properties of other varieties of Portuguese in this domain, such as nominal and verbal inflections, personal pronouns, determiners and possessives, null subjects, and word order in general, and the use of it as a reference for speakers of other Portuguese varieties is not entirely reliable.

Adapted (unpublished) versions of LARSP have been used by speech and language therapists in Portugal for many years, and procedures for language sample analysis along the lines of LARSP were introduced and disseminated in the training and practice of these practitioners by the persistent endeavours of Eileen Sua Kay, one of the pioneers in the field of child language disorders in Portugal. The developmental scale considered in those practices, however, was a translation, and had never been validated for European Portuguese, a fact doubtless related to the unavailability of relevant corpora. The analysis of spontaneous production data, although recognized by practitioners as highly valuable for the richness of the information it provides, is complex and time-consuming. Moreover, the absence of clear guidelines and procedures for implementing it, associated with the availability of more standardized tests and instruments for the assessment of language, meant that speech and language therapists gradually dropped the analysis of spontaneous speech samples in their practice.

Language acquisition studies in Portugal of the different dimensions of language development, both for typical and atypical populations, were largely undertaken in the last twenty years. Work developed by several teams at Universidade de Lisboa and Universidade Nova de Lisboa made available a variety of data that could finally support an adaptation of the LARSP profile into European Portuguese. The study here presented profited from the work of many researchers that shared their corpora for subsequent studies. We acknowledge, in particular, Sónia Frota and the team of Laboratório de Fonética da Universidade de Lisboa *(LumaLiDa – Linguistic Diary of Luma)*, Susana Correia, Teresa Costa and Maria João Freitas (*CCF Corpus*) and Maria Lobo, Eileen Sua Kay, Raquel Campos and Rita Campos (*RRC Corpus*).

The procedure here presented (*LARSP-PE*) provides a grid summarizing the morphosyntactic characteristics of spontaneous speech for children from 9 months to 4 years and 6 months, divided into seven stages. It can be used as a complement to the assessment of language in the morphosyntactic domain for pre-schoolers, since it provides detailed information about the language of the child through a systematic analysis of the spontaneous speech, and allows the delineation of its linguistic profile (Crystal, 1992; Crystal & Fletcher, 1979). In the next sections, we present a brief description of the main syntactic and morphological features of European Portuguese, the design of the study for the validation of LARSP-PE, and the description of the characteristics of the child profiles in the seven stages of development.

Main Syntactic and Morphological Features of European Portuguese

European Portuguese is a Romance language spoken by around 10 million people living in Portugal (mainland, and Azores and Madeira autonomous regions), as well as by a number of Portuguese emigrant communities across Europe, USA, Canada and other countries (Segura, 2013; Simons & Fennig, 2018).

Word order

At the level of the sentence, the unmarked word order in European Portuguese is SVO (Subject Verb Object), both in simple (1) and complex sentences (2).

(1) O rapaz leu um livro.
The boy read-PAST a book
'The boy read a book.'
(2) A professora disse que o rapaz leu um livro.
The teacher say-PAST that the boy read-PAST a book
'The teacher said that the boy read a book.'

However, structures of the type VSO and VOS are possible, according to the discursive status of subjects and objects: when both the subject and the object convey new information (informational focus) (3), when the object is a topic (4), or when only the subject conveys new information (5). In European Portuguese, a topic is likely to occupy the leftmost position in the sentence, and new information (informational focus) the rightmost position (Duarte, 2000, 2013).

(3) **A:** Quem é que leu o quê?
Who *é que* read-PAST the what
'Who read what?'
B: Leu o rapaz o livro e a rapariga a revista...
Read-PAST the boy the book and the girl the magazine
'The boy read the book and the girl the magazine...'
(4) Esse livro, leu-o o rapaz.
That book read-PAST-it the boy
'That book, the boy read it.'
(5) **A:** Quem é que leu a revista?
Who *é que* read-PAST the magazine
'Who read the magazine?'
B: Leu a revista a rapariga.
Read-PAST the magazine the girl
'The girl read the magazine.'

In object *wh*- and relative clauses, the order is marked as well (OSV), since the interrogative and the relative pronouns occupy the leftmost position.

(6) O rapaz que a professora viu é louro.
The boy that the teacher saw-PAST is blond
'The boy that the teacher saw is blond.'
(7) Quem é que a professora viu?
Who *é que* the teacher saw-PAST
'Who did the teacher saw?'

Complements and modifiers occur to the right of the head (8).

(8) O livro da Maria é muito interessante.
The book of-the Maria is very interesting
'Mary's book is very interesting.'

Null subjects, null objects and ellipsis

European Portuguese is a null subject language: the subject can be phonetically omitted when it expresses an argument of the main verb (9), or when it is an expletive (non-argumental or quasi-argumental), as with meteorological verbs (10)[1] (Lobo, 2013).

(9) Hoje [-] vou à praia.
Today [-] go-1SG-PRESENT to-the beach
'Today I will go to the beach.'
(10) Hoje [-] vai chover.
Today [-] go-3SG-PRESENT rain-INFINITIVE
'Today it will rain.'

It is the rich verbal inflection that allows the recovery of grammatical information about person, which is crucial for semantic and referential interpretation – (9) and (11).

(11) Hoje [-] vamos à praia.
Today [-] go-1PL-PRESENT to-the beach
'Today we will go to the beach.'

With argumental subjects, an expressed subject, such as a personal pronoun, is possible – (12) is an alternative to (9). Non-argumental or quasi-argumental subjects, on the contrary, cannot be phonetically expressed in standard varieties of EP (13).

(12) Hoje eu vou à praia.
Today I go-1SG-PRESENT to-the beach
'Today I will go to the beach.'
(13) *Hoje ele vai chover.
Today he go-3SG-PRESENT rain-INFINITIVE
'Today it will rain.'

Argumental subjects cannot be null in all contexts, since the distribution of null and expressed subjects is constrained by grammatical person (1st and 2nd person subjects are more easily null than those of 3rd person), by information structure (subject focus is typically expressed), and by the type of sentence (main or dependent) (Lobo, 2013). Ellipsis, i.e. the omission of syntactic constituents that can nevertheless be semantically interpreted, is possible in European Portuguese in different forms, such as partial ellipsis of the predicate (14), ellipsis of a sentential complement (15), verb ellipsis (16), ellipsis in questions and answers (17–19), and nominal ellipsis (20) (Matos, 2013).

(14) Hoje eu vou à praia e tu também vais.
Today I go-1SG-PRESENT to-the beach and you also go-2SG-PRESENT
'Today I will go to the beach and you also will.'

(15) A professora disse que o rapaz leu um livro mas o colega negou
The teacher say-PAST that the boy read-PAST a book but the colleague denied
'The teacher said that the boy read a book but his colleague denied it.'

(16) O rapaz leu o livro e a rapariga a revista.
The boy read-PAST the book and the girl the magazine
'The boy read the book and the girl the magazine.'

(17) **A:** Leste o livro?
Read-2SG-PAST the book
'Did you read the book?'
B: Sim.
Yes
'Yes, I did.'

(18) **A:** Quando leste o livro?
When read-2SG-PAST the book
'When did you read the book?'
B: Ontem.
Yesterday
'Yesterday.'

(19) **A:** Leio muitos livros.
Read-1SG-PRESENT many books
'I read many books.'
B: E revistas?
And magazines
'What about magazines?'

(20) Leio muitos livros em português mas poucos em francês.
Read-1SG-PRESENT many books in Portuguese but few in French
'I read many books in Portuguese but few in French.'

European Portuguese also allows a null object, possible both in oral and written modalities in less formal registers, that is different from general partial predicate ellipsis (Duarte & Costa, 2013).

(21) **A:** Viste o meu casaco preto?
See-2SG-PAST the my coat black
'Did you see my black coat?'
B: A tua mãe arrumou [-] no roupeiro.
The your mother store-PAST [-] in-the closet
'Your mother stored it in the closet .'

Noun phrases

Noun phrases in argument position are typically introduced by a determiner – a definite or an indefinite article (22) or a demonstrative (23) (Castro, 2009; Miguel & Raposo, 2013; Raposo & Miguel, 2013).

(22) O rapaz comeu uma maçã.
The boy eat-PAST an apple
'The boy ate an apple.'

(23) Este rapaz comeu essa maçã.
This boy eat-PAST that apple
'This boy ate that apple.'

Bare nominals, i.e. noun phrases not introduced by a determiner, can be singular or plural in EP and may assume a generic interpretation (24–25) or an existential indefinite interpretation (26).

(24) Adoro *sapatos.*
Love-1SG-PRESENT shoes.
'I love shoes.'

(25) O meu tio pesca *sardinha.*
The my uncle fish-3SG-PRESENT sardine.
'My uncle fishes sardines.'

(26) No ano passado só li *livros do Saramago.*
In-the year passed only read-1SG-PERFECT books of-the Saramago
'Last year I only read Saramago's books.'

Possessives are introduced by a definite or an indefinite article, occurring prenominally with a definite interpretation (27), and post-nominally with an indefinite interpretation (28). Proper names (29) and universal quantifiers (30) are also introduced by a definite article (Castro, 2006, 2009; Raposo & Miguel, 2013).

(27) A minha irmã vive em Lisboa.
The my sister live-3SG-PRESENT in Lisboa
'My sister lives in Lisbon.'

(28) Uma tia minha vive nos Açores.
A aunt my live-3SG-PRESENT in-the-PL Azores
'One of my aunts lives in Azores.'

(29) A Maria é a minha melhor amiga.
The Maria is the my best friend
'Maria is my best friend.'

(30) Todas as minhas amigas vivem na minha rua.
All-PL the-PL my-PL friend-PL live-3PL-PRESENT in-the my street
'All my friends live in the same street as I do.'

Adjectives and complements tend to appear in a post-nominal position – (21) and (26).

Inflection on nouns and verbs

Nominal inflection includes variation in gender (masculine and feminine) and number (singular and plural) in all the categories (determiners, quantifiers, pronouns, nouns and adjectives) and all show overt agreement within the noun phrase. The set of morphemes is shown in Tables 6.1 and 6.2.

Table 6.1 Nominal number inflection

NUMBER suffixes (nominal)	
plural	-s
singular	ø

Table 6.2 Nominal gender inflection for adjectives

GENDER suffixes (adjectives)	
masculine	-o
feminine	-a
invariant	-e

In the classes of nouns ending in a vowel, the plural suffix *-s* is added and there is no morphophonological change (31); nouns ending in consonants involve morphophonological singular-plural alternation, which can be considered regular since it is always predictable (32–33) (Castro, 2010).

(31) a. casa
house-SG
'house'
b. casas
house-PL
'houses'
(32) a. flor
flower-SG
'flower'
b. flores
flower-PL
'flowers'
(33) a. anel
ring-SG
'ring'
b. anéis
ring-PL
'rings'

In the case of nouns ending in *–ão*, however, three possible plural endings may occur, being a case of irregular (unpredictable) plural forms (34–36).

(34) a. mão
hand-SG
'hand'
b. mãos
hand-PL
'hands'

(35) a. leão
lion-SG
'lion'
b. leões
lion-PL
'lions'

(36) a. pão
bread-SG
'bread'
b. pães
bread-PL
'breads'

A characteristic of European Portuguese is that some prepositions – *a* ('to'), *de* ('of'), *em* ('in'), and *por* ('by') – undergo morphophonological contraction with determiners in most cases, as can be seen in the case of definite articles (Miguel & Raposo, 2013) – Table 6.3.

Table 6.3 Patterns of contraction of prepositions and determiners

PREPOSITION	DETERMINERS			
	MSG	MPL	FSG	FPL
	o	*os*	*a*	*as*
a	*ao*	*aos*	*à*	*às*
de	*do*	*dos*	*da*	*das*
em	*no*	*nos*	*na*	*nas*
por	*pelo*	*pelos*	*pela*	*pelas*

Verbal forms inflect for person, tense, mood, and aspect. Person shows, in general, six different inflections (37). Tense, mood and aspect inflection is mainly syncretic. The unmarked verbal form is 3rd person indicative present, since person, tense, mood and aspect show no overt inflection (37c).

(37) a. eu cant-o
I sing-1SG-PRESENT
'I sing'
b. tu canta-s
you sing-2SG-PRESENT
'you sing'

c. ele canta-ø
he sing-3SG-PRESENT
'he sings'
d. nós canta-mos
we sing-1PL-PRESENT
'we sing'
e. vós canta-is
you sing-2PL-PRESENT
'you sing'
f. eles canta-m
they sing-3PL-PRESENT
'they sing'

The indicative perfect displays irregular forms in many European Portuguese verbs, due to an alternation of the roots for perfective and imperfective.

(38) a. nós *faze*-mos
we know-1PL-PRESENT
'we make'
b. nós *fize*-mos
we make-1PL-PERFECT
'we made'

Verbal inflection paradigms are thus subject to many irregularities that require explicit learning.

Design of the Study

In this section, we present the method followed in the LARSP-PE study, which aimed at drawing a profile of morphosyntactic development for Portuguese pre-schoolers from 9 months to 4 years and 6 months, divided into seven stages.

The corpus

For this study, spontaneous speech samples of Portuguese children were selected from the *RRC corpus* (Campos, 2014a, 2014b), the *CCF corpus* (Correia *et al.*, 2010), and the *LumaLiDaAudy corpus* (Frota *et al.*, 2012), considering as inclusion criteria: (a) being from typically developing European Portuguese children aged from 9 months (0;9) to 4 years and 11 months (4;11); (b) the existence of at least two spontaneous speech samples of male and/or female children, distributed among the seven stages (age groups); (c) the duration of each sample being not less than 30 minutes; (d) the sample being collected in the context of adult–child interaction in play activities; and (e) being transcribed by utterance in CHILDES (Child Language Data Exchange System) or other format convertible to CHAT (Codes of the Human Analyses of Transcripts) to allow the use of CLAN (Computorized Language Analysis Program) software for some of the analyses (Ball *et al.*, 2012; Crystal *et al.*, 1989; MacWhinney, 2000; Pulido *et al.*, 2011). The full sample used is described in Table 6.4.

Table 6.4 Sample characterization

Stage	Child	Corpus	Gender	Age	MLU	Type Token Ratio	Analysable utterances	Total of Analysable utterances
I	IF	CCF	F	0;11.13	0.164	0.333	35	
I	AF	LumaLidaAudy	F	1;2.0	0.887	0.180	74	123
I	JM	CCF	M	1;5.26	0.696	0.253	14	
II	JM	CCF	M	1;6.06	0.469	0.240	61	
II	JF	CCF	F	1;10.22	0.626	0.450	91	368
II	IF	CCF	F	1;10.29	1.635	0.254	216	
III	JM	CCF	M	2;0.6	0.847	0.384	149	305
III	IF	CCF	F	2;5.24	2.389	0.337	156	
IV	JF	CCF	F	2;6.23	1.781	0.362	256	401
IV	IF	CCF	F	2;11.21	2.845	0.340	145	
V	JF	CCF	F	3;0.26	2.246	0.498	183	329
V	2A	RRC	F	3;5.01	4.065	0.297	146	
VI	8A	RRC	F	3;7.07	2.957	0.248	85	203
VI	15A	RRC	M	4,4.18	2.638	0.284	118	
VII	13A	RRC	M	4;11.16	4.839	0.291	122	266
VII	16A	RRC	M	4;7.14	4.233	0.327	144	

The sample integrates a total of 1995 analysable utterances, distributed by two or three files by stage/age group (I to VII), in which each sample corresponds to a distinct child in each stage, in a total of 16 files. Mean Length of Utterance (MLU) and Type Token Ratio (TTR) values were calculated using CLAN (MacWhinney, 2010; Pulido *et al.*, 2011).

Assigning structures to stages of syntactic development

The construction of the morphosyntactic development scale used both a qualitative and a quantitative approach. It involved an analysis, following the original LARSP procedures, with the morphosyntactic categories relevant to European Portuguese language development defined *a priori*. Subsequently, the frequency of occurrence of those morphosyntactic structures and categories in each stage at the levels of word, phrase, and clause was calculated. For these analyses, all the utterances were integrated into a database in which each utterance was coded and classified under a category at the three levels. The utterances were analysed by at least two coders and were subject to judgement agreement.

To decide which categories are acquired or under acquisition in each stage, in order to be included (or not) in the developmental scale, the criterion was their use on at least two occasions by 70% of all the children of an age group/stage. Therefore, it is considered that: (1) a structure is acquired (represented in bold in the chart) at a certain stage if, in 100 utterances, it occurs at least twice and in two children; (2) a structure is emerging (represented in grey in the chart), if a single child produces the same structure twice in 100 utterances or four times in every 100 to 200 utterances (Klee & Gavin, 2010).

Acquisition patterns in European Portuguese

The acquisition of the morphosyntactic patterns of language begins to show up when the child produces a combination of more than one word. Until 1 year and 6 months, the speech is predominantly telegraphic and holophrastic, which makes it difficult to detect morphosyntactic knowledge in production. However, it is assumed that words may assume the function of subject, verb, direct object, or indirect object (Brown, 1973; Costa & Santos, 2003; Gonçalves *et al.*, 2011; Lust, 2006). At this stage of development, nouns and verbs are the most frequent word categories produced, with adverbs and adjectives being infrequent, except for *sim* ('yes'), *não* ('no'), or *lindo* ('gorgeous') (Costa & Santos, 2003).

Between 1 year and 6 months and 2 years, the child develops the ability to combine the first words into phrases, and increases the use of noun phrases, verbs, some adjectives and some adverbs. These first productions of more than one word express already some basic properties of the language being acquired, such as the unmarked word order SVO in simple declarative sentences, complements and modifiers to the right of nouns and verbs, null subjects and *wh*-words in the leftmost position of the sentence (Corrêa & Augusto, 2017; Costa & Santos, 2003; Gonçalves *et al.*, 2011; Lobo & Soares-Jesel, 2017; Santos & Lopes, 2017).

Between 2 and 3 years, words with a grammatical function arise, such as articles, prepositions (to introduce complements or modifiers) and conjunctions (to introduce subordinate or coordinated sentences). The utterances, with two to three words, reveal the syntactic structure by the combination of lexical and functional elements. In this period, nominal inflection in gender and number emerges, with plural marking appearing mainly in nouns. Some overgeneralizations, such as the plural formation of *cão* ('dog') performed as *cãos*, instead of *cães* ('dogs'), show up (Castro, 2010; Corrêa & Augusto, 2017; Corrêa *et al.*, 2010; Ramalho, 2010). In verbal forms, the use of 'bare' forms such as the 3rd singular person is predominant, along with the imperative, as well as such overgeneralizations as *fazi*, on analogy with *comi* ('ate') instead of *fiz* ('did') (Castro, 2010; Gonçalves, 2004; Loureiro, 2000).

Over 3 years old, syntactic skills permit the production of longer simple and complex clauses, although the omission of some syntactic elements, such as clitics, conjunctions and relative and interrogative pronouns, is still observed; in parallel, overgeneralizations of the verbal and nominal morphological patterns still occur (Corrêa & Augusto, 2017; Costa & Grolla, 2017). Relatives and other subordinate clauses arise at this stage, as well as interrogative sentences with *é que* (Costa & Santos, 2003).

From 4 to 6 years of age, the length and complexity of utterances increase, and the speech is characterized by the use of adverbs, adjectives, and irregular nominal and verbal inflected forms (which reveal mastery of morphological rules and their exceptions). Passives are produced with increasing levels of mastery, as well as subject and object relatives and interrogatives and completives (Corrêa *et al.*, 2017; Lobo & Soares-Jesel, 2017; Santos, 2017; Soares, 2006). The production of all types of sentences demonstrates proficiency of morphosyntactic rules, which will be consolidated until reaching the level of adult mastery.

Table 6.5 presents a summary of information about morphosyntactic development.

Table 6.5 Morphosyntactic acquisition patterns by stage for pre-schoolers

1,0 -1,6	1;6 -2;0	2;0 -3;0	2;11 -3;2	4;0 -6;0
First rules of organization of words in sentences Telegraphic and holophastic speech Subject, verb, direct and indirect complements	Combination of words into sentences Nominal and verbal groups	Words with grammatical function, (articles, prepositions, conjunctions) Nominal and verbal inflection Overgeneralizations (in inflection)	Simple and complex interrogative sentences *é que* Clitics, personal and possessive pronouns Overgeneralizations and errors	Increased complexity Adverbs, adjectives, irregular plurals and verbal forms All types of complex sentences, including passives

Design and Description of the Adapted LARSP-PE Profile Chart

General design of LARSP-PE

The LARSP-PE chart, as shown in Figure 6.1, includes four sections, as in the original LARSP chart. Section A serves to identify the child and its analysable or problematic statements; sections B, C and D provide the analysis of the evaluator's interaction and stimulus patterns, as well as the child's responses (Ball *et al.*, 2012; Crystal *et al.*, 1976; Fletcher *et al.*, 2016).

Nome:	D.A.: _/_/___ D.N.: _/_/___ Idade: __A__M__D	Tipo de discurso:

A	**Não analisáveis** Ininteligível Ruído Simbólico Agramatical						**Problemático** Incompleto Ambíguo Estereótipos				
B	**Respostas**		Normais - Major					Normais	Anormais		
		Repetições	1	2	3+	Reduz.	Comple.	Minor	Estrut.	Ø	Prob.
	Questões										
	Outros										
C	**Espontâneo**										
D	**Reações**	Geral	Estrutural			Ø		Outros	Problemas		

		ORAÇÃO			SINTAGMA	PALAVRA
Faixa etária I (0;9-1;6)	***Minor***	Respostas		Vocativos	Outros Problemas	
	Major	**Ordens**	**Int.**	**Declarativas**	**Outros** **Problemas**	
		V	–	**V** **S/O** **O** Neg OI Mod	**N** **V** Cop Neg Adv	
	Conj.					
Faixa etária II (1;6-2;0)		VX	–	SV AX **Neg** SC **PS** SVC Obl VC **Outros**	**DN** **Cop** **Neg** PronO **Adj** PronP Num **Outros**	**2sg** Inf **Ind** PronD PronInd PronPoss
Faixa etária III (2;0-2;6)		V XY	Q	(S)VO **Mod** (S)VC **Outros** (S)VA	Prep N **Adv** PrepPronP Neg V Prep DN AuxO **Outros**	1sg Pretperf 1pl ir+Vinf PronP *PrepD Imper
Faixa etária IV (2;6-3;0)		**(S)V**	QV	**SV** **VO** **SVO** **VC** **(S)VO** **Obl** **(S)VC** **Outros**	**PronO** **Cop X** **Prep N** **Neg V** **Prep DN** AuxM Prep X DPronO **Outros**	**fem** **pl** **Pretperf** **PronD** **Inf** ***PrepD**
Faixa etária V (3;0-3;6)	e	...	**QVS**	**Coord.** **1 (+1)** **(S)VC** **Outros** **(S)VA**	**PronP** **Int** **Outros**	**PretImp** **PronP** **3pl**

	(+)			Agramaticalidades/Erros (-)					
Faixa etária VI (3;6-4;6)	**FN**	**FV**	**Oração**	**Conjunção**	**Oração**	**Sintagma**		**Palavra**	
						N	**V**	**N**	**V**
	Coord **Subord** **PrepQ** **PrepPronO**	**SVX** **Com-plexas**		e de coordenação de subordinação	Elemento: Ø ⇆ ordem concordância	D Prep PronP Ø D Ø Prep D ⇆ Prep ⇆	Ø AuxM Ø AuxO Cop	Irregular Regular	Irregular Regular
	Outros:					Ambiguos:			
Faixa etária VII (+4;6)	*Discurso*					*Compreensão sintática:*			
	Conjunção Completiva **PronCl** Outras estruturas:					*Estilo:*			
	Total de enunciados:			Número de frases por turno:		MLU:			

NOTA: Considera-se: 1) **adquirido** se, em 100 enunciados, uma estrutura ocorre pelo menos 2 vezes e em duas crianças e, 2) em aquisição, se uma criança produz 2 vezes a mesma estrutura em 100 enunciados (ou 4 em 100-200 enunciados).

Figure 6.1 LARSP-PE profile chart

The morphosyntactic development LARSP-PE chart is organized into two dimensions, one horizontal and one vertical. The horizontal dimension includes the detailed characterization of the morphosyntactic structures for each stage of language development in EP, considering clause (*oração*) and phrase (*sintagma*) levels. At the clause level, the type of sentence is identified: imperative (*ordens* 'commands'), interrogative (*int.* 'questions') and declarative (*declarativas* 'statements'), followed by their syntactic functions and internal structure. At phrase level, each syntactic constituent is described according to five types: noun, prepositional, adverbial, adjectival and verbal. Finally, at word level (*palavra*), there are six structures to consider: nominal and verbal inflections, type of verbs, pronouns, contractions, prefixes and suffixes. As previously mentioned, in this chart, the structures acquired at each stage are given in bold, while the structures undergoing acquisition are given in grey.

Vertically in the chart, the scale of morphosyntactic development is presented via seven acquisition stages, which correspond to different age-range groups.

Detailed description of LARSP-PE chart

The results are shown broken down by stage of language development, and include the structures considered to be acquired (in bold) and under acquisition (in grey).

Stage I (0;9-1;6)

In the LARSP-PE chart (see Figure 6.2), we can confirm that, until 1 year and 6 months, children's utterances are holophrases, distributed by statements ('declarativas') and commands ('ordens') with the presence of the verb. At this age range, utterances include mainly lexical words (nouns and verbs), negation (*não* 'no'), or modifiers. At phrase level, structures such as nouns (*mamã* 'mommy') and verbs (*dá* 'gives') are acquired. Some adverbs occur (*aqui* 'here'), as well as copulative verbs (*está* 'is').

As for inflectional morphology, the forms produced do not enable us to draw conclusions about the presence of verbal inflections; they are 'bare' forms, with no overt inflection. Plural nominal inflections do not seem to be present yet either. It is known, however, that, at this early stage, children still reveal phonological immaturity affecting the production of phonemes in syllable coda (post-vowel syllable position), e.g. –*s*, which is precisely the realization of some person morphemes in verbs and of plural markers in nouns. Thus, it is not clear whether the child is producing words inflected as the imperative or 3rd person singular (*dá* 'give'), or the

<table>
<tr><td></td><td colspan="4">ORAÇÃO</td><td>SINTAGMA</td><td>PALAVRA</td></tr>
<tr><td rowspan="3">Faixa etária I (0;9-1;6)</td><td>Minor</td><td colspan="3">Respostas Vocativos</td><td colspan="2">Outros Problemas</td></tr>
<tr><td rowspan="2">Major</td><td>Ordens</td><td>Int.</td><td>Declarativas</td><td>Outros Problemas</td><td rowspan="2"></td></tr>
<tr><td>V</td><td>–</td><td>V S/O O
Neg OI Mod</td><td>N V Cop
Neg Adv</td></tr>
</table>

Figure 6.2 LARSP-PE: Stage I

2nd person present indicative (*dás* 'you give') with *-s* omission. The same applies to the plural form in nouns. Nevertheless, the samples analysed were collected during symbolic play, which does make the use of the imperative plausible.

Stage II (1;6-2;0)

At stage II (see Figure 6.3), structures with two words emerge, as well as commands with two constituents (VX); verbs are present with other elements (X), as in *põe aqui* ('put here'). Statements also appear with more than one word, such as subject + verb structures (*Inês partiu* 'Inês left'), predicative or modifier (*Inês grande* 'big Inês'), subject + verb + object (*boneca tem cocó* 'doll has poop'), (temporal) adverbs (*agora partimos* 'now (we) leave'), oblique complement (*para a cama* 'to the bed'), negation (*não* 'no') and the predicative of subject (*preta* 'black').

At the phrase level, definite articles in the structure determiner + noun (*o colo* 'the lap'), negation (*não* 'no'), adjectives (*mau* 'bad'), and copulative verbs (*é* 'is') seem to be acquired. Number quantification structures (*dois* 'two'), personal pronouns (*eu* 'I'), and other pronouns such as *isto* ('this') are under acquisition. At the word level, the forms of the 2nd person singular imperative (*dá* 'give') and the indicative mode are acquired. Forms under acquisition are infinitives (*abrir* 'to open'), indefinite pronouns (*outro* 'other'), demonstrative pronouns (*esta* 'this'), and prepositioned possessive pronouns, such as *dela* ('her'). At this stage, some complex structures arise with functional elements such as determiners heading noun phrases, subject–verb or verb-complement structures and pronouns. Some adjectives seem to be already present as well as different pronominals, confirming the patterns of acquisition stated in the literature (Corrêa & Augusto, 2017; Costa & Santos, 2003; Gonçalves *et al.*, 2011).

	ORAÇÃO						SINTAGMA		PALAVRA	
Faixa etária II (1;6-2;0)		VX		SV	AX	**Neg**	**DN**	**Cop**	**2sg**	Inf
			–	SC		**PS**	**Neg**	PronO	**Ind**	PronD
				SVC		Obl	**Adj**	PronP	PronInd	
				VC		**Outros**	Num	**Outros**	PronPoss	

Figure 6.3 LARSP-PE: Stage II

Stage III (2;0-2;6)

Between 2 years and 2 years and 6 months (see Figure 6.4), at clause level, we observe the presence of three constituents in the utterance, and the consistent presence of modifiers and adverbs. Commands consist of a verb combined with other elements (*espera lá* 'wait there!'), and interrogatives emerge (*e este?* 'and this one?'). In statements, null subjects are already produced frequently. At phrase level, personal pronouns (*eu* 'I'), prepositional phrases consisting of preposition and noun (*de neve* 'of snow'), preposition, article and noun (*para a Julieta* 'for the Juliet'), and preposition and personal pronoun (*para mim* 'for me') are already present. Verbal negation also shows up (*não sei* 'don't know'). With respect to morphological development during this stage, the past tense forms begin to appear (*tirou* 'took'), as well as the 1st person singular present tense (*eu quero* 'I want'), and the 1st person plural (*nós temos* 'we have'). This stage is still characterized by the presence of the auxiliary verb *ir* ('to go') combined with main verbs in the infinitive (*vou buscar* 'I am going to get'), expressing future events. According to Gonçalves *et al.* (2011), auxiliary verbs and infinitive inflection marking emerge later in development; nonetheless, these structures seem to be under acquisition at this stage.

	ORAÇÃO					SINTAGMA		PALAVRA	
Faixa etária III (2;0-2;6)		V XY	Q	(S)VO	**Mod**	Prep N	**Adv**	1sg	Pretperf
				(S)VC	**Outros**	PrepPronP	Neg V	1pl	ir+Vinf
				(S)VA		Prep DN	AuxO	PronP	*PrepD
							Outros	Imper	

Figure 6.4 LARSP-PE: Stage III

Stage IV (2;6-3;0)

At stage IV, shown in Figure 6.5, age ranging from 2 years and 6 months to 3 years, at the clause level, commands are acquired and include null subjects (*filma!* 'film!'); simple *wh*-questions are under acquisition (*quem é?* 'who is he/ she?'). Both lexical and null subjects are observed in statements, as well as direct and oblique objects, and predications of the subject (*eles sobem* 'they go up'; *porque eu queria ir ver os animais* 'because I wanted to go see animals'; *limpar o banco* 'clean the chair'; *tem um livro novo* 'he/ she has a new book'; *é o porco* 'it is the pig'). At phrase level, demonstrative pronouns surface as acquired structures (*esta* 'this'; *com isto* 'with this'), as well as noun ellipsis (*o da Polergarzinha* 'the of the Littlefinger'). Prepositional phrases combined with elements such as adverbs (*para aqui* 'to here') and other pronouns (*a outra* 'the other one') are being acquired. Also, modal auxiliary verbs begin to show up (*pode ir* 'he/ she/ it can go'), as do copulas (*é um cavalo* 'is a horse') and verbal negation (*não tem* 'he/ she/ it has not'). At word level, data support the acquisition of feminine and plural markers (*branca* 'white', *grandes* 'large'), past perfect inflection (*caímos* 'we fall'), infinitives (*beber* 'to drink'), demonstrative pronouns (*este* 'this'), and the contraction of the preposition with a determinant (*desta* 'of this').

	ORAÇÃO					SINTAGMA		PALAVRA	
Faixa etária IV (2;6-3;0)		**(S)V**	QV	**SV**	**VO**	**PronO**	**Cop X**	**fem**	**pl**
				SVO	**VC**	**Prep N**	**Neg V**	**Pretperf**	**PronD**
				(S)VO	**Obl**	**Prep DN**	AuxM	**Inf**	***PrepD**
				(S)VC	**Outros**	Prep X	DPronO		
							Outros		

Figure 6.5 LARSP-PE: Stage IV

Stage V (3;0-3;6)

Between 3 years and 3 years and 6 months (Figure 6.6), partial interrogative sentences are acquired (*o que é isto?* 'what is this?'), as well as predicative structures with adverbs (*estão aqui* 'they are here'). At phrase level, intensity adverbs also appear (*muito* 'a lot'). At word level, the consistent use of personal strong pronouns (*ele* 'he'), verbal inflection in the imperfect (*queria* 'he/ she/ it wanted'), and 3rd person plural present tense (*estão* 'they are') may be seen. The production of clitic pronouns and subordination processes, expected up to three years and six months, is not observed at this stage (Costa & Santos, 2003; Gonçalves *et al.*, 2011).

	ORAÇÃO					SINTAGMA	PALAVRA
Faixa etária V (3;0-3;6)	e	–	QVS	Coord. (S)VC (S)VA	1 (+1) Outros	PronP Int Outros	PretImp PronP 3pl

Figure 6.6 LARSP-PE: Stage V

Stage VI (3;6-4;6)

At stage VI, shown in Figure 6.7, coordination and subordination structures are acquired, illustrating more complex structures at clause level. At phrase level, we observe the acquisition of constructions involving prepositions combined with interrogative pronouns (*para quê?* 'for what?') and other pronouns (*com nada* 'with nothing'). At this age, when children reach an improved mastery of an increasing number of complex mophosyntactic structures, it is worth analysing errors arising from the overgeneralized use of morphosyntactic rules in the verbal and nominal domains, a parameter considered in the original LARSP chart (Ball *et al.*, 2012; Crystal *et al.*, 1976, 1989). Furthermore, according to the LARSP procedure, grammatical structures should be classified according to the processes of subordination and coordination that are already systematic at this stage, as well as to the absence (Ø) or change in the order (⇆) of any morphosyntactic structures present in the sentences produced. The absence or change in the order of structures is also applicable at phrase level, considering words as pronouns, prepositions, determiners, main verbs and auxiliary verbs.

<table>
<tr><td rowspan="5">Faixa etária VI (3;6-4;6)</td><td colspan="3">(+)</td><td colspan="7">Agramaticalidades/Erros (-)</td></tr>
<tr><td>FN</td><td>FV</td><td>Oração</td><td>Conjunção</td><td>Oração</td><td colspan="3">Sintagma</td><td colspan="2">Palavra</td></tr>
<tr><td rowspan="2">Coord
Subord
PrepQ
PrepPronO</td><td rowspan="2">SVX
Com-
plexas</td><td rowspan="2"></td><td rowspan="2">e
de coordenação
de subordinação</td><td rowspan="2">Elemento:
Ø
⇆ ordem
concordância</td><td>N</td><td>V</td><td></td><td>N</td><td>V</td></tr>
<tr><td>D Prep PronP
Ø D Ø Prep
D ⇆ Prep ⇆</td><td>Ø AuxM
Ø AuxO
Cop</td><td></td><td>Irregular
Regular</td><td>Irregular
Regular</td></tr>
<tr><td colspan="5">Outros:</td><td colspan="5">Ambíguos:</td></tr>
</table>

Figure 6.7 LARSP-PE: Stage VI

Stage VII (+4;6)

After 4 years and 6 months, the length and complexity of the children's utterances increase, resulting from the full mastery of the processes of subordination and the use of clitic pronouns, which are already acquired (see Figure 6.8). At this stage the variety of structures produced is considerable, so the chart includes as open 'questions' three parameters: *other structures* ('outras estruturas'), including any complex structures which were not included in previous stages; *syntactic comprehension*: ('compreensão sintática'), where aspects of syntactic comprehension can be reported; and *style*: ('estilo'), which assumes the report of any syntactic and morphological preferences that characterize the speech of the child under analysis.

Faixa etária VII (+4;6)	*Discurso*		*Compreensão sintática:*
	Conjunção Completiva	**PronCl**	
	Outras estruturas:		*Estilo:*

Figure 6.8 LARSP-PE: Stage VII

In general, LARSP-PE confirms the data reported in the literature regarding the acquisition of syntactic and morphological patterns in European Portuguese of children from 9 months to above 4 years and 6 months. The nature of the data (only spontaneous production) may explain why some specific structures, identified by some studies via experimental data, are not so salient in this study. Furthermore, minor divergences with respect to the timing of acquisition and the emergence of some structures may be due to the natural variability that affects individuals in language development processes.

Conclusions

A procedure such as LARSP-PE enables us to describe the characteristics of language development of European Portuguese-speaking children in the domains of syntax and morphology, as well as the systematization of those characteristics in a morphosyntactic developmental profile, comprising seven stages, from 9 months to 4 years and 6 months.

This tool can be used in the context of screening, assessment and intervention in language, as a complementary support for the establishing of a linguistic profile. The morphosyntactic development scale is divided into seven age groups, including clause, phrase and word levels. It makes available an outline of the specific morphosyntactic development patterns for European Portuguese, in which the morphosyntactic structures show increasing complexity through the stages. The chart allows the assessment of the strengths and weaknesses of children's grammatical repertoire, contributing to a better knowledge of their linguistic profile; it also allows the planning and monitoring of intervention in cases where this is needed. LARSP-PE helps clinicians and educators establish the pattern of morphosyntactic development in language-impaired children in clinical or educational settings, as well as providing a more directed therapeutic intervention.

Note

(1) [-] represents the null subject.

References

Ball, M., Crystal, D. and Fletcher, P. (2012) *Assessing Grammar: The Languages of LARSP*. Bristol: Multilingual Matters.

Brown, R. (1973) *A First Language; The Early Stages*. Cambridge, MA: Harvard University Press.

Campos, A.R. (2014a) A Extensão Média de Enunciado como indicador de desenvolvimento linguístico no português europeu. Master dissertation, Instituto Politécnico de Setúbal and Universidade Nova de Lisboa. https://comum.rcaap.pt/handle/10400.26/7743

Campos, R.J.P.M. de. (2014b).*Rácio Type-Token e D como indicadores de desenvolvimento linguístico no português europeu*. Master dissertation, Instituto Politécnico de Setúbal and Universidade Nova de Lisboa. https://comum.rcaap.pt/handle/10400.26/7742

Castro, A. (2006) On Possessives in Portuguese. PhD dissertation, Universidade Nova de Lisboa and Université Paris 8.

Castro, A. (2009) Possessivos e artigo definido expletivo em PE e PB. *Revista Veredas* 10, 1–2. https://veredas.ufjf.emnuvens.com.br/veredas/article/view/374

Castro, A. (2010) Aquisição de morfologia de plural em português europeu: Sobre a produtividade das regras. In *XXV Encontro Nacional da Associação Portuguesa de Linguística* (pp. 277–289). Lisboa: APL.

Corrêa, L.M.S. and Augusto, M.R.A. (2017) Primeiros passos na aquisição da sintaxe: o sintagma nominal. In M.J. Freitas and A.L. Santos (eds) *Aquisição de língua materna e não materna: Questões gerais e dados do português* (pp. 121–54). Berlin: Language Science Press. https://doi.org/10.5281/zenodo.889427

Corrêa, L.M.S., Augusto, M.R.A. and Castro, A. (2010) The role of D in the ascription of gender to novel animate nouns in early language acquisition: Evidence from Brazilian and European Portuguese. In J. Costa, A. Castro, M. Lobo and F. Pratas (eds) *Language Acquisition and Development; Proceedings of GALA 2009*. Newcastle-upon-Tyne: Cambridge Scholars Publishing.

Corrêa, L.M.S., Augusto, M.R.A. and Lima-Júnior, J.C. (2017) Passivas. In M.J. Freitas and A.L. Santos (eds) *Aquisição de língua materna e não materna: Questões gerais e dados do português* (pp. 201–224). Berlin: Language Science Press. https://doi.org/10.5281/zenodo.889433

Correia, S., Costa, T. da and Freitas, M.J. (2010) *Corpus of European Portuguese Phonological Development*. https://doi.org/10.21415/T53034

Costa, J. and Grolla, E. (2017) Pronomes, clíticos e objetos nulos: dados de produção e compreensão. In M.J. Freitas and A.L. Santos (eds) *Aquisição de língua materna e não materna: Questões gerais e dados do português* (pp. 177–199). Berlin: Language Science Press.

Costa, J. and Santos, A.L. (2003) *A Falar Como os Bebés*. Lisbon: Editorial Caminho.

Crystal, D. (1992) *Profiling Linguistic Disability*. London: Whurr Publishers Ltd.

Crystal, D., Fletcher, P. and Garman, M. (1976) *The Grammatical Analysis of Language Disability*. London: Edward Arnold.

Crystal, D. and Fletcher, P. (1979) Profile analysis of language disability. In C.J. Fillmore, D. Kempler and W.S-Y. Wang (eds) *Individual Differences in Language Ability and Language Behaviour* (pp. 167–88). New York: Academic Press.

Crystal, D., Fletcher, P. and Garman, M. (1989) *Grammatical Analysis of Language Disability* (2nd edn). London: Cole and Whurr.

Duarte, I. (2000) *Língua Portuguesa; Instrumentos de Análise*. Lisboa: Universidade Aberta.

Duarte, I. (2013) Construções de Topicalização. In E.B.P. Raposo, M.F.B. do Nascimento, M.A.C. da Mota, L. Segura and A. Mendes (eds) *Gramática do Português* (Vol. I, pp. 401–426). Lisboa: Fundação Calouste Gulbenkian.

Duarte, I. and Costa, J. (2013) Objeto nulo. In E.B.P. Raposo, M.F.B. do Nascimento, M.A.C. da Mota, L. Segura and A. Mendes (eds) *Gramática do Português* (Vol. II, pp. 2339–2348). Lisboa: Fundação Calouste Gulbenkian.

Fletcher, P., Ball, M. and Crystal, D. (2016) *Profiling Grammar – More Languages of LARSP*. Bristol: Multilingual Matters.

Frota, S., Vigário, M., Matos, N., Cruz, M. and Jordão, R. (2012) LumaLiDaAudy.

Gonçalves, F., Guerreiro, P. and Freitas, M.J. (2011) *O conhecimento da língua: percursos de desenvolvimento*. Lisboa: DGIDC/Ministério da Educação.

Gonçalves, F.M.R. (2004) *Riqueza Morfológica e Aquisição da Sintaxe em Português Europeu e Brasileiro*. PhD dissertation, Universidade de Évora.

Klee, T. and Gavin, W.J. (2010) Reference data for the LARSP profile chart for 2- and 3-year-old children. https://ir.canterbury.ac.nz/handle/10092/4101

Lobo, M. (2013) Sujeito nulo: Sintaxe e Interpretação. In E.B.P. Raposo, M.F.B. do Nascimento, M.A.C. da Mota, L. Segura and A. Mendes (eds) *Gramática do Português* (Vol. II, pp. 2309–2335). Lisboa: Fundação Calouste Gulbenkian.

Lobo, M. and Soares-Jesel, C. (2017) Interrogativas, relativas e clivadas. In M.J. Freitas and A.L. Santos (eds) *A aquisição de língua materna e não materna; Questões gerais e dados do português* (pp. 225–248). Berlin: Language Science Press. https://doi.org/10.5281/zenodo.889435

Loureiro, J. (2000) Aquisição de ordem de palavras e de flexão verbal no Português Europeu : produção vs compreensão João Loureiro. Master dissertation, Universidade Nova de Lisboa.

Lust, B.C. (2006) *Child Language; Acquisition and Growth*. Cambridge: Cambridge University Press.

MacWhinney, B. (2010) The CHILDES Project: Tools for analyzing talk (3rd ed.). Mahwah, NJ, NJ: Lawrence Erlbaum Associates. http://talkbank.org/manuals/CHAT.pdf

Matos, G. (2013) Elipse. In E.B.P. Raposo, M.F.B. do Nascimento, M.A.C. da Mota, L. Segura and A. Mendes (eds) *Gramática do Português* (Vol. II, pp. 2351–2386). Lisboa: Fundação Calouste Gulbenkian.

Miguel, M. and Raposo, E.B.P. (2013) Determinantes. In E.B.P. Raposo, M.F.B. do Nascimento, M.A.C. da Mota, L. Segura and A. Mendes (eds) *Gramática do Português* (Vol. I, pp. 819–879). Lisboa: Fundação Calouste Gulbenkian.

Pulido, M.T., Simões, M., Moreira, M. and Branco, T. (2011) Manual de Transcrição do Programa CLAN. Centro de Linguística da Universidade Nova de Lisboa.

Ramalho, A.M. (2010) *Aquisição do plural nos nomes terminados em ditongo nasal*. Master dissertation, Universidade de Évora.

Raposo, E.B.P. and Miguel, M. (2013) Introdução ao Sintagma Nominal. In E.B.P. Raposo, M.F.B. do Nascimento, M.A.C. da Mota, L. Segura and A. Mendes (eds) *Gramática do Português* (Vol. I, pp. 703–734). Lisboa: Fundação Calouste Gulbenkian.

Santos, A.L. (2017) Alguns aspetos da aquisição de orações subordinadas completivas. In M.J. Freitas and A.L. Santos (eds) *A aquisição de língua materna e não materna; Questões gerais e dados do Português* (pp. 249–273). Berlin: Language Science Press. https://doi.org/10.5281/zenodo.889437
Santos, A.L. and Lopes, R.E.V. (2017) Primeiros passos na aquisição da sintaxe: Direcionalidade, movimento do verbo e flexão. In M.J. Freitas and A.L. Santos (eds) *A aquisição de língua materna e não materna; Questões gerais e dados do português* (pp. 155–175). Berlin: Language Science Press. https://doi.org/10.5281/zenodo.889429
Segura, L. (2013). Geografia da Língua Portuguesa. In E.B.P. Raposo, M.F.B. do Nascimento, M.A.C. da Mota, L. Segura and A. Mendes (eds) *Gramática do Português* (Vol. I, pp. 71–81). Lisboa: Fundação Calouste Gulbenkian.
Simons, G. and Fennig, C.D. (eds) (2018) *Ethnologue: Languages of the World*. https://www.ethnologue.com/
Soares, C. (2006) La syntaxe de la périphérie gauche en portugais européen et son acquisition. PhD dissertation, Université Paris 8.

Appendix

Glossary of abbreviations

⇆	change of order
(S)V	Null Subject + Verb
(S)VA	Null Subject + Verb + Adverb
(S)VC	Null Subject + Verb + Complement
(S)VO	Null Subject + Verb + Object
*PrepD	contraction of the preposition with a determiner
1 pl	first person plural
1 sg	first person singular
2 sg	second person singular
3 pl	third person plural
Adj	adjective
Adv	adverb
AuxM	modal auxiliary verbs
AuxO	other auxiliary verbs
AX	Adverb + Other element
C	The morphosyntactic categories represented by C include the oblique complement structures, complements the subject's modifier and predicative
CCF corpus	Correia *et al.* (2009) corpus
Coord.	coordination structures
Cop	Copulative Verb
Cop X	Copulative Verb + Other element

D	Determiner
DN	Determiner + Noun
D pronO	Determiner + Other Pronouns
Fem	Feminine
Imper	Imperative
Ind	Indicative mode
Inf	Infinitives
Int	intensity adverbs
Ir + Vinf	verb *ir* (to go) + main verb in the infinitive
LARSP	Language Assessment, Remediation and Screening Procedure
LumaLiDaAudy corpus	Frota, Vigário, Matos, Cruz, & Jordão, (2012) *corpus*
MLU	Mean Length of Utterance
Mod	Modifier
N	Noun
Neg	Negation (Adverb)
Neg V	Verbal negation
Num	Number quantification structures
Ø	Absence
O	Object
Obl	Oblique complement
OI	Indirect Object
OSV	Object + Subject + Verb
PE	stands for 'European Portuguese'
Pl	plural markers
Prep DN	Preposition + Determiner + Noun
Prep N	Preposition + Noun
Prep X	Prepositional phrases + Other element
PrepPronP	Preposition + Personal pronoun
PrepQ	Preposition + Interrogative pronoun
PretImp	Verbal inflection in the imperfect
PretPerf	Past perfect
PronD	Demonstrative pronouns
PronInd	Indefinite pronouns

PronO	Other Pronouns
PronP	Personal pronouns
PronP	Personal pronouns
PronPoss	Possessive pronouns
PS	Predicative of subject
Q	Interrogative type/interrogative pronouns
QV	*Wh*-question + Verb
QVS	parcial interrogative sentences
RRC corpus	Campos (2014[a]) and Campos, (2014b)
S	Subject
SC	Subject + Complement
Subor	Subordination structures
SV	Subject Verb
SVC	Subject + Verb + Complement
SVO	Subject + Verb + Object
V	Verb
V XY	Verb + Other element + any element other than X
VC	Verb + Complement
VO	Verb + Object
VOS	Verb + Object + Subject
VSO	Verb + Subject + Object
VX	Verb + Other element
X	Other element
Y	any element other than X

7 CS-LARSP: Colombian Spanish Morphosyntactic Development Profile

Maryluz Camargo-Mendoza, Ana Isabel Codesido-García and Elena Garayzábal-Heinze[1]

Introduction

In this chapter, the Colombian Spanish Morphosyntactic Development Profile (hereafter CS-LARSP), based on a cross-sectional corpus of Spanish-speaking children from Colombia, is introduced. The profile itself derives from the doctoral thesis submitted by the first author (Camargo, 2013; Camargo & Garayzábal, 2015). The chapter begins with a brief overview of Spanish grammar, explains how the CS-LARSP was designed and then describes the profile itself and the structures to be expected at each stage.

Spanish Grammar

According to Greenberg's Universals (Greenberg, 1963), the Spanish language is an SVO language although with a flexible syntagmatic order. For example, we can say:

(a) Mañana iremos de paseo (*Tomorrow we will go for a walk*)
(b) Iremos mañana de paseo (*We will go tomorrow for a walk*)
(c) De paseo iremos mañana (**For a walk we will go tomorrow*)
(d) Mañana de paseo iremos (**Tomorrow for a walk we will go*)
* (c) and (d) are not ungrammatical, but they are not frequently employed.

Spanish is a pro-drop language, which implies that the pronominal subject can be omitted, as there is a high presence of verbal inflections identifying the sentence subject (Codesido *et al.*, 2012). Regarding morphology, nouns, adjectives, determiners and pronouns are considered as variable elements due to the fact that they can be inflected in both number (singular/plural) and gender (masculine/feminine). Verbs are also considered variable elements because of the verb conjugation (1st -ar; 2nd -er; 3rd -ir), verb tenses (present, past, future), verb mood (indicative, subjunctive, imperative), verb person (1st, 2nd, 3rd), verb number (singular/plural) and verb voice (active/passive).

In Spanish, some inflected forms are considered canonical (non-marked forms), whereas other inflected elements are formed by adding morphemes to the standard inflected form. The Spanish canonical inflections are the following: gender (masculine), number (singular) and verb tense (present).

(e) Number Inflection: La muñeca bonita/Las muñecas bonitas (*The pretty doll/The pretty dolls*)
(f) Gender: La mano/El niño (*The hand/The boy*)
(g) Conjugation: amar/beber/reír (*to love/to drink/to laugh*)
(h) Verb Tense: (Yo) canto, cantaba, cantaré (*(I) sing/I was singing/I will sing*)
(i) Mood: /(Que tú) cantes / Canta (tú) (*That you sing/Sing (as an imperative)*)
(j) Person: (Yo) canto, (Tú) cantas, (Él, Ella) canta, (Nosotros/as) cantamos, (Vosotros/as) cantáis, (*Ellos/as) cantan ((I)) sing, ((You)) sing, ((He/She)) sings, ((We/You/They)) sing*)
(k) Voice: Cervantes escribió *Don Quijote de la Mancha/Don Quijote de la Mancha* fue escrito por Cervantes (*Cervantes wrote Don Quijote de la Mancha / Don Quijote de la Mancha was written by Cervantes*).

Besides these variable Spanish categories, there are also invariant categories such as adverbs, conjunctions, prepositions and interjections. Regarding sentences, two important issues must be emphasized in relation to negative and interrogative sentences. Negative sentences are marked with a '*no*' preceding the verb:

(l) No quiero ir al colegio (*I don't want to go to school*)

Regarding interrogative sentences, they can be formulated by using an affirmative structure SVO and adding an interrogative intonation (m), by changing order (n) or by using interrogative particles at the beginning of the sentence (e.g. *qué* 'what', *cómo* 'how', *cuándo* 'when', etc.) (o):

(m) ¿María está resfriada? –SVO (*Mary has a cold?*)
(n) ¿Está María resfriada? –VSO (*Has Mary a cold?*)
(o) ¿Qué le pasa a María? – Wh-question VO (*What is wrong with Mary?*)

Spanish Profiles

In Spanish there are some linguistic development profiles already developed. The most popular among them deal with phonetics and phonology, and are the following: *Análisis del Retraso del*

Habla[2] *–A-RE-HA–* (Aguilar & Serra, 2003), *Evaluación Fonológica del Habla Infantil*[3] *–EFHI–* (Bosch, 2004), and *Análisis del Retraso del Lenguaje*[4] *–A-RE-L–* (Pérez & Serra, 1998). This last profile is quite general; it does not deal with phonetics or phonology but with Spanish morphosyntax, rather superficially. The Spanish phonological development profile (*EFHI*), is basically complete. The morphosyntactic profile named PERSL (*Procedimiento de Evaluación, Rehabilitación y Screening Lingüístico – A procedure for assessment, remediation and linguistic screening*), is the first LARSP-based profile. The authors refer to it as a 'preliminary' version (Codesido *et al.*, 2012: 279). The CS-LARSP is intended to systematize in a detailed manner the characteristics of Colombian Spanish and to this end we made use of a large homogeneous sample of speakers from Bogotá, the capital city of Colombia.

There is a wide variety of spoken Spanish. In general, there is a difference between the Spanish spoken in Spain and the Spanish spoken in the Americas. Each Spanish-speaking country shows, therefore, specific linguistic characteristics at every level. This new version of LARSP for Spanish focuses, in particular, on data directly related to the acquisition of Spanish from Bogotá's interior Andean region of Colombia. CS-LARSP for stage I offers data directly obtained from 19 children. CS-LARSP stages II–VI are based on a 50 children-sample (as shown in Table 7.1), and CS-LARSP stage VII was based on a sample of 36 children from Bogotá. Finally, we can note that CS-LARSP is based on monolingual children from Bogotá and it uses data from a total of 105 children.

CS-LARSP Design

Sample and participants

The corpora used to devise the CS-LARSP were based on the information collected from 105 children, 54 girls and 51 boys, aged from 10 months to 6 years and 7 months (see Table 7.1). These children were monolingual Spanish speakers. Among them, 63% were attending a kindergarten or preschool educational institutions, while the other 37% stayed at home being taken care of by their mothers. Regarding those going to preschool (66 children), 10.6% were aged between 2 and 3 years old and 89.4 % were older than 3. Most of the participants belonged to the low socioeconomic class (28.5%), to lower- middle class (41%) and middle class (24%),[5] see Table 7.2; they were all either the second born child (37.1%), or the only child (35.2%).

When collecting the linguistic data, we went directly to the homes and also to the preschool institutions. In both places, a prenatal questionnaire was given to parents or caretakers. The questionnaire dealt with the child's prenatal and perinatal background and asked about possible language disabilities. Parents and caretakers signed an informed consent

Table 7.1 Participants classified according to their age

Age	0;10-1;05	1;06-2;00	2;01-2;06	2;07-3;00	3:01-3;06	3;07-4;06	4:07-6:07
Girls	9	6	4	4	4	5	23
Boys	10	4	5	6	6	6	13
Subtotal	19	10	9	10	10	11	36
					Total	105	

Notice: age is provided according to year; month.

Table 7.2 Participants classified according to social classes (percentage)

1 Class	2 Class	3 Class	4 Class	5 Class	6 Class	No answer
3,7	28,5	41	24	0,9	0	1,9

form so that the children could be audio and video recorded. Any children having a complex clinical background were excluded from the study. All participants took a whispered voice test. Before data collection, two or three visits took place in order to let the children get to know the researchers as well as the recording camera.

Material

Two types of material were used during the recordings, depending on whether the recording took place at home or at the educational institution. With those children being recorded at home, their own toys were used. Those recorded in the institutions would play with the game 'Play-Doh Dr. Drill'N Fill' (© 2008 Hasbro).[6] This game contained a patient's head (which could be opened), a dental high-speed handpiece, a tooth brush, a clip, a dental saliva ejector, a model brace and three play-doh blocks. The book *A boy, a dog and a frog* by Mercer Mayer (1967)[7] was used with all the participants. This book consisted of 30 pages with drawings without text, and it tells the story of a boy who goes for a walk in the woods with his dog, meets a frog and tries to catch it; after several attempts, he gives up and goes back home. The frog feels lonely and follows both the child and the dog. When arriving home, the frog finds them taking a bath and joins them.

Recording procedures and contexts

All participants were video-recorded. A Sony DCR-SX44 video recorder and a Panasonic RR-US361 sound recorder were used. The children at home were recorded in four communication contexts between them and their parent(s) or caretaker(s): bath time, dressing-up time, playing time and book-reading time (of *A boy, a dog and a frog*). During these first two moments (bath-time and dressing-up time), caretakers were asked to proceed with their everyday routines and child–caretaker interactions. At playing time, they were asked to offer the child his/her favourite toys. Regarding reading time, they were asked to proceed as they would usually do when reading other books. All parents had previously read stories to their children. Reading time was included in the collecting procedure because it is considered a social activity in which both adults and children exchange information regarding a story (Muñoz & Anwandter, 2011). Further, this book in particular, with no text in it, was selected in order to promote communication: parents could freely decide what to talk about during the communicative interaction (Cornell & Broda, 1995; Muñoz & Anwandter, 2011).

Regarding the educational institution's recordings, two activities were used. In the first activity children would play at being dentists with a peer of a similar age. During the activity itself, both children had to discover what the game was about and then play. Once that game was over, the second activity would take place: every child had to narrate the 'frog story' through the drawings in the book. Children were encouraged to respond by the experimenter, who would say, for example, 'They say you are the best story-teller of all pupils!'. Children would go over the book narrating what they saw in each of the drawings in the book.

As mentioned above, we focused on obtaining a speech language corpus largely obtained through spontaneous and everyday activities. The Frog Story – a semi-structured activity – was included, though, for two reasons: first, this activity is nothing new for children going to educational institutions, being something common in this context and part of their everyday activities; secondly, it has been shown that, when children tell stories, more words per sentence are produced and the syntax tends to be more complex (Coloma *et al.*, 2007). Of course, we were aware of the fact that shared reading was not going to help 10-month-old children produce more complex sentences and it would end up being another communicative interaction activity.

Transcription and analysis

All recordings were orthographically transcribed and the grammatical analyses were annotated according to the SALT software conventions – *Systematic Analysis of Language Transcripts* – 2012 version (Miller & Iglesias, 2012).

First, a decision-making process took place in order to decide how to split the corpus. Following SALT criteria, the corpus was split into Communicative Units (CUs), defined as 'clauses which cannot be divided, otherwise their essential meaning would get lost' (Miller & Iglesias, 2012).

Once the corpus had been segmented, each CU was annotated according to LARSP methodology into three levels: clauses, phrases (also known as clusters) and words. A more detailed description can be found in Camargo

(2013) and Camargo and Garayzábal (2015). After having all CUs annotated according to the three levels of analysis, a database was built, and a percentage of each structure's occurrence was calculated using *Software R*, (R Core Team, 2012). Finally, once the percentage occurrence was calculated, the morphosyntactic profile began to be drawn up. The structures annotated would cover seven stages, according to the 50% criterion: a structure would be first included in a stage if it appeared in, at least, 50% of the corpora. This criterion was previously used by Maillart, Parisse and Tommerdahl (2012) for F(rench)-LARSP and by Dijkstra and Schlichting (2012) for their Frisian adaptation. A 30% criterion was also employed, as implemented by Maillart *et al.* (2012), in order to define some of the structures.

Final Profile

All in all, 11,212 complete, intelligible clauses were analysed. The resultant morphosyntactic profile can be seen in Figure 7.1. All structures have been classified, as already mentioned before, according to three levels of analysis: clause, phrase and word (conventions in Table 7.3).

Stage I (10 months–1;5 years)

Stage I is characterized by one-element statements, classified according to minor and major clauses. Minor clauses include *answers* (yes, no, mh), *vocatives* (mummy, aunt, etc.), and *exclamations* (ah!, ay!), defined as *others*. Major statements include imperative verb commands, *Vimp^* (go, look), nouns, *N* (water, baby) and *others* such as adjectives, adverbs, etc. Statements accomplishing the 50% criteria are vocatives and nouns; those accomplishing the 30% criteria comprise answers and, even though imperative verbs reached only a 21%, these were included in the table in order to highlight their presence among children's first words; the symbol ^ was assigned to indicate that their presence will increase in the following stages.

Structures implying questions do not appear in the stage due to the low percentage of utterances including Question pronouns or Wh-words. In fact, for children at this age questions are stated through question-like intonation applied to isolated words (i.e. ¿este? (*this?*).

Stage II (1;06–2;00 years)

Stage II includes structures which mainly combine two elements. In this stage, the chart was divided into three sections: 1. Clause: subdivided into commands, questions and statements; 2. Phrase and 3. Morpheme.

Clause

Commands during this stage are basically expressed by combining the verb *mirar (look)* together with another particle. We can also see some

CS-LARSP

Nombre	**Edad**	**Fecha de Muestra**
A Inanalizable 1. Inintelegible 2. Sonido simbólico 3. Alterada		**Problemático** 1. Incompleto 2. Ambiguo 3. Estereotipado

B Respuestas		Repetitions	**Respuesta Normal**							**Respuesta Anómala**		Problemas
			Mayor						Menor			
Tipo de Estímulo	Total		**Elíptica** 1	2	3+	**Reducida**	**Completa**			Estructural	Ø	
Preguntas												
Otros												
C Espontáneo			General				Estructural	Ø		Otros	Problemas	
D Reacciones												

Etapa I (10m- 1;5)	Menor	Respuestas	Vocativos	Otros	Problemas	
	Mayor	**Orden** Vimp^	**Pregunta**	**Aserción** N	Otros (Adj, A)	Problemas

	Conec.	**Claúsula**			**Sintagma**	**Palabra**
Etapa II (1;6- 2;0)		MiraX Vimp(X)	Q^	V SV NegX AX VO/se^ S/VC^ otros	DN Pron Cop cN^ PrN^ NN^ otros	Gen Dimin Ger Ind-Pres3s Ind-Pps3s Imp2s
Etapa III (2;1- 2;6)		MiraX(Y)	QX^	SVO/se SVC NegXY SVA^ AVO/se^ otros	PrDN^ XcX 1aux^	Inf Ind-Pres1s
Etapa_V (2;7-3;■)	*y*	MiraXY(Z) VimpX(Y) Subord	(pr)QVX	VOdOi SVO/seA SVO/seC^ NegXYZ Coord1 Subor1 otros	(D)NPrDN	Pl Ind-Pres2s Ind-Pres1p Ind-Pps1s Ind-Pps3p Ind-Pretim3s Enclit *Aum**
Etapa V (3;1- 3;6)	enton. luego desp. *c* *s*	VimpXY(Z) Coord/Yuxta	QVXY Tag	A/SOiVOd SOiVOdA/C* AAXY SVCA^ Yuxta Coord2+ Cierre:YA 2neg* otros	DNAdj IntenX	Part Ind-Pres3p *Ind-Pps2s** *Ind-Pps1p** *Sub-Pres2s** *Ind-Fut3s** *Ind-Fut3p**

	Imprecisiones			**Cláusula**	**Sintagma**	**Palabra**
	(-) **Oración**	(-) **Sintagma verbal**	(-) **Morfema**			
Etapa VI (3,7-4,6)	Concord. V Ø	aux/V Ø *Nominal*	**V** Irre. Reg.	XYZAA/C+ Subord2+ Compar Q!	PrDNAdj* v_V *2 aux**	Imp1p *Ind-Pretim1s** *Ind-Pretim2s** *Sub-Pres1s** *Sub-Pres3s** *Sub-Pres3p** *Sub-Pretim1s** *Sub-Pretim3s** *Superl**
Etapa VII (4,7-6,7)		D DØ Pr PrØ Pron. PronØ	**N**	2Oi 2Od Estilo Directo cierre: colorín/fin *> 5;06 Ser Intensivo*	*CoordSN** *Aposic**	Ind-Pretim3p *Ind-PretPC3s** *Ind-PretPlus3s** *Ind-PretPlus3p** *Ind-PretPC1s** *Ind-PretPC2s** *Ind-Pret PC3p** *Ind-Con3s** *Ind-Con3p** *Ind-Fut1s** *Ind-Fut2s** *Ind-Fut1p** *Imp3p**

Número total de oraciones	LME en palabras	LME en morfemas

Figure 7.1 CS-LARSP Chart

Table 7.3 CS-LARSP Conventions

( )	Optional Element	Ger.	Gerund
^	completes the 50% threshold in previous stages	Imp.	Imperative
1aux	Auxiliary Verb	Ind.	Indicative
1p	1st person, plural	Inf.	Infinitive
1s	1st person, singular	Inten.	Intensifier
2 aux.	2 Auxiliary Verbs	Irre.	Inappropriate irregular Verb Conjugation
2 Od	Two Direct Objects	Mira	*'mirar' (to look) verb*: *mire* (you look), *mira* (he/she looks)
2 Oi	Two Indirect Objects	N	Noun
2neg	Double Negative	Neg.	Negative
2p	2nd person, plural	O	Object
2s	2nd person, singular	Od	Direct Object
3p	3rd person, plural	Oi	Indirect Object
3s	3rd person, singular	Part.	Participle
A	Adverb	Pl	Plural
Adj	Adjective	Pps	*Pretérito perfecto simple* (Simple past)
Aposic	Apposition	Pr	Preposition
Aum	Augmentative	Pr Ø	Preposition Omitted
aux/V Ø	Main verb or Periphrasis' auxiliary verb omitted	Pres.	Present
C	Complement	Pretim.	*Pretérito imperfecto* (Imperfect)
c	Conjunction	PretPC	*Pretérito perfecto compuesto* (present perfect)
c	Coordinative Conjunction	PretPlus	*Pretérito pluscuamperfecto* (pluperfect)
cierre:ya	Narration ends using *'ya' (already)*	Pron.	Pronoun
Compar.	Comparative Clauses	Pron Ø	Pronoun Omitted
Concord.	Agreement Difficulties	Q	Interrogative Words
Cond	Conditional	Q!	Wh-Exclamations
Conec.	Connective Words	Reg.	inappropriate regular Verb Conjugation
Coord1	One Coordinate Structure	S	Subject
Coord2+	More than two Coordinate structures	*s*	Subordinate Conjunction
CoordFN	Nominal Phrase Coordinated	se	*Reflexive 'se'*
Cop	Copular Verb	Sub	Subjunctive
*cursiva**	50% or 30% Threshold Unaccomplished	Subor2+	More than two Subordinate Clauses

(Continued)

Table 7.3 (*Continued*)

D	Determiner	Subord.	Subordinate Clause
D Ø	Determiner Omitted	Superl.	Superlatives
desp.	Afterwards	Tag	Tag/Affirmative questions
Dimin.	Diminutive	V	Verb
Enclit.	Enclitic	Vimp	Imperative Verb
enton.	'Entonces' (then)	V Ø	Verb Omitted
Estilo directo	Direct Style Subordination	v_V	Auxiliary and Main Verb Separated
Fut.	Future	X, Y o Z	Any other Element
Gen.	Genre Agreement	*y*	'*y*' (and) Conjunction
AVO/se	AVO o AVse	Yuxta	Juxtaposition

(-): here grammatical ambiguities/inaccuracies can be included.

other isolated imperatives, as in stage I, followed by another particle. As can be seen on the chart, when an element is included in brackets – ( ) – it means that the element is optional at this stage. The symbol X, (later Y, Z) indicates the presence of any other element. This way, commands appear as two different structures, the two-element combination and one which may include a second element or not:

-MiraX: i.e. *mira doce, mire casa* (*look twelve, look home*)
-Vimp(X): Vimp i.e. *toma* (*take*)
Vimp + interjection i.e. *venga pues* (*come on then*)
Vimp + O i.e. *vea sapo* (*see toad*)

As in stage I, the main way to express questions is through one or two elements with question intonation. WH-forms such as *qué* (what) and *por qué* (why) are present, though they are limited. Even though the WH-structure does not reach either the 50% or the 30% criteria, it has been included at this stage for two reasons: firstly because it was already occasionally present in the previous stage; secondly while it will not reach the 50% criterion until stage IV, where some more complex question structures are also present, we can already see it being used at this stage. This means that the acquisition process is dynamic. The transitional stages are very interesting and indicate how the child's language develops and point out as well what could be relevant in order to distinguish a divergent from a delayed development.

Statements combining mainly two elements:

-V: i.e. *cható* (saltó, *jumped*)
-SV: i.e. *la niña bañal* (la niña se va a bañar, *the girl is getting a bath*)
-NegX: SNeg→ *el vaso no* (*the glass no*);
SV→ *no peo* (no puedo, I *can not*),
NegVcop→ *no está* (*not here is*)

-AX: AVcop→ *aquí etá* (aquí está, *here it is*),
AV→ *así sató* (así saltó, *like this it jumped*)
-VO/se^: VO→ *la dañó, bañé mi manos* (*broke it, washed my hands*);
seV→ *se baña, se abrió* (*he/she bathes, it opened*)
-S/VC^: SC→ *lopa ninda* (*la ropa está linda, the clothes are pretty*),
VC→ *cayó a agua* (el niño cayó al agua, *the child fell into the water*).

The two former structures including the ^ symbol, represent the combination of only two elements. The symbol / included in between indicates the presence of either the first or the second element: for example, S/VC would include the Subject plus a Complement or a Verb plus a Complement. For this stage, a 30% criterion was applied, as 50% is only reached at stage III, a stage which shows three-element structures clearly fixed.

Phrase

The isolated nouns found in stage I start appearing next to determiners, conjunctions, prepositions and other nouns. Some personal, possessive and demonstrative pronouns start to appear as well, together with the copula verb *ser/estar* (to be):

-DN: i.e. un niño, mi mano, la foto (*a boy, my hand, the picture*)
-NN*: i.e. loción papi (la loción del papi, *the lotion of daddy*)
-cN*: i.e. y sapo, y rana (*and toad, and frog*)
-PrN*: i.e. pala Ateque (para Guateque, *to Guateque*)
-Pron: i.e. yo, mío, éste (*I, mine, this one*)
-Cop: i.e. aquí <u>está</u>, no <u>está</u> (*here it is, it is not*)

The convention of marking some forms with * highlights that these do not reach the 50% criterion or that they appear here but will disappear in later stages.

Morpheme

In this stage, different types of word inflections were recorded – all of them reaching the 50% criterion. Among them, we observed the following: gender agreement (firstly between determiner and noun), gerunds, diminutives, indicative verb inflections in present, past and imperative:

-Gen: <u>la</u> fich<u>a</u>, <u>el</u> nen<u>é</u> (*the token, the baby boy*)
-Dimin: cas<u>ita</u>, mam<u>ita</u> (*home-tiny or sweet home, mother-tiny or mammy*)
-Ger: tá mañ<u>ando</u> (se está bañando, *-he/she- is taking –a- bath*), abaj<u>ando</u> (trabajando, *working*)
-Ind/Pres3s: ota ez se ca<u>e</u> (otra vez se cae -el niño-, *and again –the child- falls*)
-Ind/Pps3s: así salt<u>ó</u> (*and so –he/she- jumped*)
-Imp2s: ñáñate (báñate, *take a bath*), mire, mira (*look*)

Stage III (2;01–2;06 years)

Clause

In this stage only one symbol appears regarding commands: MiraX(Y). Compared to the previous stage, here a third particle may appear (Y).

MiraX: Mira el sapo (*look the toad*)

or

MiraXY i.e. mire eso un pollo (*look that a chicken*)

Questions in stage III are indicated by the following symbol QX^, included following a 30% criterion, i.e. ¿qué cosas?, ¿qué color? (*which things?, which colour?*)

Statements are three-element structures:

-SVO/se: SVO→ yo veo a(l) niño (*I see -the- child*);
VSO→ cayó balde niño (*fell bucket child*);
SOV→ El camino la dañó (the road him/her damaged);
seVS→ se cayó el niño (*-himself- felt the boy*)
-SVC: SVcopC→ este es mío (*this is mine*);
VcopCS→ está sucio este, está fría el agua (*-it- is dirty this -one-, -it- is cold the water*)
-NegXY: ANegV→ ya no puedo (*-I- cannot any longer*);
NegVcopS→ no está el balde (*there is no bucket*);
ONegV→ una foto no tengo (*a picture I –do-not have*)
-SVA^: SVA→ la ficha dañó otra vez (*the counter broke again*);
VSA→ cepilla el niño así (*brush the child this way*);
SVcopA→ ese es así (*that one is this way*)
-AVO/se^: AOV→ sí la baña (*indeed she washes her*);
OAV→ éste sí quiero (*this one I do want*);
AVO→ dónde están los zapatos (*where are the shoes*);
seVA→ se fue allá (*she left there*)
-Otros: AOA→ sí agua acá (*yes water here*);
AVVoc→ ya voy tío (*already coming brother*);
cOV→ porque lo regañaron (*because he was scolded*)

Phrase

At the phrase level there are three symbols representing word combinations for both noun phrases and verb phrases. Regarding verb phrases, auxiliary verbs are now present when expressing verb periphrasis. Noun phrases are preceded by prepositions and some nouns or verbs start being coordinated through a conjunction, mainly *y* (*and*):

-PrDN^: en la poceta, para la(s) niñas (*in the WC, for -the- girls*)
-XcX: niño y sapo, correr y correr (*child and toad, run and run*)
-1aux^: (el niño) se <u>va a bañar</u> (*-the child- <u>is going to take</u> a bath*); (la rana) <u>está mirando</u> no más (*-the frog- <u>is</u> just <u>looking</u>*)

Morpheme

Here we observe the same inflections as those from the former stage though at a higher frequency. We note the presence of one of the non-finite verb forms, the infinitive, as well as the presence of the first person singular indicative:

Inf: no vas hacer chichí, se va a bañar *(-you-are not go-ing- -to- pee, she is take-ing- a bath)*
Ind/Pres1s: yo veo (al) niño, quiero esto (*I see ((the)) child, -I- want this*)

Stage IV (2;07–3;00 years)

Clause

Stage IV is characterized by two phenomena: one, the increase of elements in this clause level; two, the first occurrence of coordinate and subordinate clauses.

The number of elements making up commands increases: some contain three, others four, elements. We also observed some subordinate commands, mostly including the verb mira (*look*):

MiraXY(Z): MiraXY→ míra*lo* (en) la sala (*look –at- it ((in)) the room*);
MiraXYZ→ míre*la* allá en el lago (*look –at- her there in the lake*)
VimpX(Y): VimpX→ coja esta (*get this –one-*);
VimpXY→ déje*lo* ahí (*leave it there*); Paula coge una (*Paula gets one*)
Subord: Mire+O→ mire ese es (*look that's –it-*); mira yo quiero esto (*look I want this*)
Vimp+O→ come este (que) está rico (*eat this one ((that)) is yummy*)

In earlier stages we indicated the fact that questions stated by using question pronouns or adverbs were not the most common. In fact, it is only at the present stage that Q and QX questions reach the 50% threshold. Nevertheless, consistent three-element questions predominate and, besides the question form, a verb is now included (prQVX); we also observe questions followed by prepositions: ¿en dónde va esto? ¿para qué ponemos eso? (*Where does this go? Why are we putting this on?*)

At this stage, statements include from three to four elements. Coordinate and subordinate structures are present as well. The occurrence of two direct and indirect objects is observed:

-VOdOi: OiOdV→ me lo compro, te lo cuento (*-I- (me) buy it, -I- it to you tell*);
OiVOd→ me presta la planchita (*me borrow -you- the ironing machine*)
-SVO/seA: AseVS→ así se cepilla uno (*this is how you brush yourself*);
ASVO→ una vez un niño estaba mirando la rana (*once a boy was watching the frog*)

-SVO/seC: SOVC→ yo las pongo grandes (*I wear them big*);
SseVC→ la mascota se paró con cinco patas (*the pet stood on five legs*)
-NegXYZ: El niño no coge el sapo, yo no me oriné (*the boy does not hold the toad, I did not pee*)
-Coord1: una rana se subió acá y el perro estaba (en) el agua (*a frog went up there and the dog was ((in)) the water*)
-Subord1: Adverbial→ lo regañaron porque se fueron (*they scolded him because they left*)
Noun→ yo quiero estarme con este (*I want to be with this one*)

Phrase

At this stage noun phrases or clusters become more complex and follow the following pattern: DNPrDN, i.e.: *un cepillo de dienes, un charco de lodo, un reguero de agua (a toothbrush, a mud pond, a water trickle).* Occasionally, they are introduced by prepositions, especially when they work as adverbial phrases, i.e. *en la casa del niño* (*at the child's home*).

Morpheme

Verb inflections in the indicative mood display a greater variety. Number agreement between determiner and noun and between some nouns and adjectives starts to take place here. As well, some pronouns located at stage II start being present as enclitic pronouns next to an imperative verb. These enclitic pronouns also appear next to non-finite verb forms – gerunds or infinitives:

-Pl: las manos; los dientes; las cosas (*the -s plural- hands; the -s plural- things*)
-Ind/Pres2s: ves?; tú te llamas Jimenéz-Torrez (-*You- see? Your name is Jimenéz-Torrez*)
-Ind/Pres1p: no le contamos nada; la espichamos (*we do not tell him anything; we smash it*)
-Ind/Pps1s: ya lo perdoné; yo pinté el perro (*already him I forgave; I draw the dog*)
-Ind/Pps3p: y corrieron así; se pusieron el balde (*and they run -simple past- this way; they put -simple past- bucket on*)
Ind/Pretim3s: una rana estaba (en) la punta (d) el agua (a frog was ((at)) the border ((of)) the water)
-Enclit: míra*la*; míra*lo*; dá*melo*; pegándo*le*; quitar*le* (*look-at-her; look-at-him/it; give it to me; get it*)
-Aum*: grandote, bocota, cabezota (*very big, enormous mouth, very big head*)

The presence of augmentatives was scarce: among the corpora collected, only five of them appeared and each only once. This has been included in this stage and marked by the symbol * to highlight that it is the first time that it has been used and also to indicate that in future stages it will not occur, neither will it reach the 50% criteria.

Stage V (3;0–3;06 years)

Clause

At this stage we observed three- to four-element commands as well as some coordinate and juxtapositional commands:

-VimpXY(Z): VimpXY→ deja eso ahí (*leave that there*);
-VimpXYZ→ mételo bien Paula (*put it properly inside, Paula*)
-Coord: Coord→ échalo y echa esto también así (*throw it and throw this as well this way*)
-Yuxta→ oye, mira; toma, dale (*listen, look; take -this-, go on*)

Questions become more elaborated and question tags emerge:

-QVXY: ¿Por qué se dañó esto? ¿Por qué no funciona esto? ¿Qué le pasó (a) eso? ¿Profe por qué viniste aquí? (*Why did this get broken? Why doesn't this work? What happened ((to)) that? Teacher, why did you come here?*)
-Tag: y yo con esta, ¿sí?; es el turno de David, ¿cierto?; y no puede hablar, ¿ves? (*and me, I use this one, don't I?; it's David's turn, right?; and he/she/it cannot talk, see?*)

Statements reach four to five elements. We also observed two or more coordinate and clausal juxtapositions:

-A/SOiVOd: AOiVOd→ ahora me toca mi turno (*now it is my turn*);
SOiVOd→ yo te cepillo los dientes; yo te lo presto (*I -will- brush your teeth; I -will- lend it to you*)
SOiVOdA/C: SOiVOdA→ Esa canción me la enseñó mi mamá ya; (*that song, my mother taught it to me already*)
SOiVOdC→ yo le cepillo los dientes con un cepillo (*I brush his*[8] *teeth with a brush*)
-AAXY: <u>ahora</u> lo colocamos <u>aquí</u>; <u>aquí</u> <u>sí</u> va su cabeza (*now we –will- place it here;*)
-SVCA^: AVcopSC→ acá está el sapo por mentiroso (*there it is the toad the liar*); SVcopAC→ el perro estaba acá con el niño (*the dog was here with the child*)
-Yuxta: pero hay un problema, yo iba a consentirte (*but there is a problem, I was going to spoil you*)
-Coord2+: entonces el niño se quitó el balde de la cabeza <u>y</u> lo botó <u>y</u> al perro lo mataron los policías (*then, the boy took the bucket of his head and he threw it away and the dog was killed by the police*)
-2neg*: tú <u>no</u> vas a hacer <u>nada</u> (*you are not going to do anything*)
-Cierre:Ya/otro: YA→y el sapo perdonó al perro... ya; Otro→y se acabó el cuento (*ALREADY→the toad forgave the dog...already; Another →and the story is finished*)

At this stage, the option Cierre: Ya/Otro (*Ending: Already/Another*) was included to indicate the particular way in which stories end. In former stages, this was not noticeable in the corpus. Double Negatives, even if the occurrence was not that high, were included in this stage because it is here where they reached the highest frequency.

Phrase

Noun phrases accompanied by adjectives as well as intensifiers can be found at this stage:

-DNAd: una rana brava; la camiseta sucia; las muelas rojas (*an angry frog; a dirty t-shirt; red teeth*)
-IntenX: muy duro; muy malo; muy bien (*very hard; very bad; very well*)

Morpheme

New verb inflections are detected here, but only two accomplished the 50% criterion. The rest of them appear for the first time in this stage and will only reappear occasionally in following stages:

-Part: quedó trabado; no lo ha cepillado (*he got stuck; -He/she- has not brushed it*)
-Ind/Pres3p: faltan algunos; los niños deben hacer esto (-there are- *some missing; children must do this*)
-Ind/Pps2s*: ¿por qué me mandaste aquí?; ¿por qué viniste aquí? (*Why did you send me here?, why did you come here?*)
-Ind/Pps1p*: le pusimos esto, no lo sacamos (*we put him/her this; -we- did not take it out*)
-Sub/Pres2s*: no lo vayas a abrir; no dejes el largo (*don't go and open it; don't leave the long one*)
-Ind/Fut3s*: ¿será que se murió?; ¿dónde estará? (*maybe he/she died?; Were will -it/she/he- be?*)
-Ind/Fut2p*: ¿no serán para ponerlos? (*don't you think these should be worn?*)

The 'connective words' column includes five symbols representing the most frequently occurring connective words within the corpus: enton. (entonces or *then*), luego (*later*), desp. (después, *afterwards*), as well as *c* and *s* to refer to either coordinate or subordinate connective words.

Stage VI (3;07–4;06 years)

In stages VI and VII, there are no new structures worth listing regarding commands or questions. Therefore, no symbols have been included in the corresponding columns. Instead, the most common 'inaccuracies' were included there, marked as (-). Statement, Phrase and Words do include new structures.

Clause

Stage VI's statements comprise four symbols representing five or more elements, subordinate sentences which appear several times, comparatives and exclamations using *¡qué!* (*what!*).

- XYZAC/A +: SAseVC→ Esto siempre se deja quieto (*This must always be kept still*)
SANegVcopC→ El gris todavía no está listo (*the grey one is not ready yet*)
AASOiVAOd→ Ahí sí tú le pones así los dientes (*there you do put out this way the teeth*)
AAseVA→ ya casi se acaba ahí (*-it is- almost finished there*)
AASVOA→ allá sí estaba el sapo haciendo la boca así (*there sure was the toad doing like this with its mouth*)
SAOiOdVA→ yo solo se la estoy dando así (*I am just giving it to him/her this way*)
-Subord2: vé que no quiere compartir; toca cuando se los hagamos porque o si no se rompe (*-you- see how he/she does not want to share; it's his/her turn whenever we do it because otherwise it'll break*)
-Compar: la tuya no te quedó tan bien como la mía (*yours is not as nice as mine*)
-Q!: ¡pero qué chévere este juego!; ¡pero qué molestia! (*How fun is this game!; what a discomfort!*)

Phrase

Prepositional noun phrases are now followed by adjectives. Regarding verb phrases, main and auxiliary verbs are now separated within the same clause and two auxiliary verbs are used in the same clause:

-PrDNAdj*: con la cara brava; de la otra coca; en la otra cabeza (*with an angry face; from the other recipient; in the other head*)
-v_V: acá está el niño jugando; se estaba ahí secando; tenemos que primero armarlo (*here the boy is playing; it was getting dry there; we have to build it first*)
-2aux*: va tocar imaginar; no he podido destapar (*we'll have to imagine; I could not uncover it*)

Morpheme

At this stage, the only stable inflected verb is the imperative, first person plural. Some other inflections related to the subjunctive mood are detected. Some superlatives are also found here:

-Imp1p: abrámoslo; arreglemos; miremos (*let's open it; let's fix it; let's look*)
-Ind/Pretim1s*: quería gritarle (*I wanted to scream at him*)

-Ind/Pretim2s*: que tú estabas (*you were there*)
-Sub/Pres1s*: espera que yo le haga la lengua (wait until I've done his/her tongue)
- Sub/Pres3s*: espere que (él) abra la boca (*I hope ((he)) opens the mouth*)
-Sub/Pres3p*: tenemos que (esperar) que crezcan los dientes (*we have to ((wait)) until the teeth grow*)
-Sub/Pretim1s*: quisiera jugar hartas veces (*I'd like to play a thousand times*)
-Sub/Pretim3s*: quería que se montara su mamá (*-he/she- wanted her mummy to get on*)
-Superl*: todísima; durísimo (*all of it; real hard*)

Stage VII (4;07-on)

Clause

In this last stage, double objects appear in the same clause, direct-style subordinate clauses appear when narrations take place, and specific structures appear to end stories. As well, after 5;06 years old a special use of the verb 'ser' (to be) emerges and this phenomenon is called '*ser intensivo*' (*intensive to be*[9]):

-2Oi: al niño se le cayó el vaso; van a pegarle a la rana; dígale a la señora (*the child dropped the glass; they are going to hit the frog; tell it to the woman*)
-2Od: el cepillo yo lo cogía; este pedacito lo metemos acá (*the brush I took it, this little piece we'll put it in here*)
- Estilo directo: y el niño *dijo, regresa*; y él no puedo saltar porque él *dijo, ayúdame* con el perro (*and the boy said, come back; and he said I cannot jump because he said, help me with the dog*)
-Cierre: Colorín/fin: colorín colorado este cuento se (ha) acabado (*and they lived happily ever after*)
Fin de la historia (*End of story*)
Fin (*The End*)
-Ser Intensivo: y atrapó *fue* al perrito; la que va *es* gris; mi mamá tiene *es* otro de estos juegos (*and he caught went the doggy; now goes is the grey one; my mummy has is one of these games*)

Phrase

Among the last developments observed regarding noun phrases, we find complex coordinate clauses and appositions:

-Aposic: se estaban bañando los dos, el perro y el niñito (*they both were taking a bath, the dog and the little child*)
Y acá cogió al perrito, su mascotica (*and here he grabbed the dog, his little pet*)

Morpheme

The following were recorded:

-Ind/Pretim3p: el niño y el perro estaban caminando; el niño y el sapo se bañaban (*the boy and the dog were walking; the boy and the toad were having a bath*

-Ind/PretPC3s*: este cuento se ha terminado; acá ninguno ha crecido (*this story is over; here nobody grew up*)

-Ind/PretPlus3s*: y se había bañado con el perro; un niño había llegado (*and he had taken a bath with the dog; a boy had arrived*)

-Ind/PretPlus3p*: y no había agua después cuando se habían bañado (*and there was no water left when they had taken a bath*)

-Ind/PretPC1s*: no le he arreglado los dientes; yo ya los he lavado (*I have not fixed the teeth; I have already washed them*)

-Ind/PretPC2s*: usted no ha ido a odontología (*you have not been to the dentist*)

-Ind/PretPC3p*: a mí sí me han hecho cosas; y los otros no han crecido (*they have done things to me; and the others have not grown*)

-Ind/Con3s*: ¿(eso) sería así? (*would ((that)) be that way?*)

-Ind/Con3p*: ¿qué le echarían? (*what would they give them?*)

-Ind/Fut1s*: y con gris pondré la estrella (*and I will paint the star wit grey*)

-Ind/Fut2s*: verá que es rosada (*you will see that it is pink*)

-Ind/Fut1p*: oye pronto te cazaremos (*listen we will soon catch you*)

-Imp3p*: oigan (*listen*)

Error column in stages VI and VII

As mentioned before, stage VI and stage VII are divided into three columns in order to highlight and identify the elements which children have trouble with and where they commit some kind of mistake in clauses, phrases or words. In the following examples, the symbol (*) is included to denote omissions and those comprising non-adult forms contain only the symbol *:

Regarding clauses, we still observe some agreement and number mistakes as well as some verb omissions:

-Concord: número: hacerle la(s*) líneas; ¿este* serán los dientes? (*draw a (s*-the-) lines; is this* might be the teeth?*)

-Gen: este* es la blanca (this* is the white one)

-VØ: eso (es*) para que se cepille (*that ((is*)) to brush your teeth*)

With respect to phrases and verb periphrasis, some auxiliaries or main verbs are omitted. Omissions also affect determiners, prepositions and pronouns:

-aux/V Ø: aux: por acá (hay que*) meterle las muelas (*around here ((we have to*)) put it the teeth*)

-V: toca (hacerlo*) con esto (*it's turn ((to do it*)) with this*)

-D: y después los* ninito estaba muy bravo (*and then the-plural-* boy was very upset*)
-DØ: y acá estaba feliz él porque estaba feliz (el*) sapo (*and here he/she/it was happy because he was happy (the*) toad*)
-Pr: el color de* que tú quieras (*the color that which* you prefer*)
-PrØ: el niño tenía atrapado (a*) el perro (*the boy had caught ((the*)) dog*)
-Pron.: echarlos* los dientes (*grow them* the teeth*)
-PronØ: el perro (se*) estaba rascando (*the dog was scratching ((himself*))*)

In relation to words, some mistakes with regular and irregular verb conjugations as well as some mistakes with some nouns, have been observed:

-Irre: así no caberá*; se había ponido* esta carie (*this way it is not going to fitted*; he had putted* this caries*)
-Reg: la rana se metió al baño a metiersese* (*the frog got into the bath to get itselfself**)
-N: vamos a sacar una carie* (let's grab a caries*)

Finally, the CS-LARSP shows exactly the same sections as those on the original English LARSP regarding the first part of the table, sections A, B, C and D. Other authors have confirmed how these sections can be maintained when creating new LARSP-based profiles, since the information compiled there does not focus on specific characteristics of a certain language (Ball, 1988; Hickey, 1990; Jin *et al.*, 2012; Samadi & Perkins, 1998).

Conclusions

The CS-LARSP morphosyntactic profile described in this chapter has been based on a cross-sectional corpus of 105 Spanish-speaking children from Colombia aged from 10 months to 6 years and 7 months. This is the second profile designed for the Spanish language based on LARSP methodology, and the first one for Spanish spoken in Colombia, though the CS-LARSP was based on a larger sample compared to the PERSL sample.

The present CS-LARSP description highlights key transitional differences between stages II and III, which outlines the dynamic nature of the language acquisition process. These transitional stages may well be useful in identifying a potential pathological development. At the same time, this CS-LARSP version has allowed us to clearly observe the presence of the '*ser intensivo' (intensive to be)* in children's speech. This specific mark has only been observed in Colombian Spanish-speaking adults (Albor, 1986; Montes, 2005) and in Caracas-Venezuela (Sedano, 1990), and there are no other studies reporting such a feature. For future studies we suggest the analysis not only of a wider cross-sectional sample, but also longitudinal samples in order to show a more reliable Spanish morphosyntactic development profile.

Notes

(1) Translated by Ainhoa Robles Baena.
(2) *Speech Delay Analysis.*
(3) *Phonological Evaluation of Children's Speech.*
(4) *Analysing Delayed Language Development.*
(5) According to the Rule 142 of 1994 from the Republic of Colombia, socioeconomic status is classified as follows: 1) poor-poor, 2) poor, 3) poor-middle, 4) middle, 5) middle-upper class and 6) upper class.
(6) In Spanish *El Dentista Bromista.*
(7) In Spanish *Un niño, un perro y una rana.*
(8) Translator note: the Spanish structure is in fact the following '*I brush him the teeth*'.
(9) In the 'intense to be' sentences the verb *to be* appears after a second verb, i.e.: 'He/She caught *went* to the dog' versus 'He/She caught the dog'. Such sentences have sometimes been considered as mistakes in child speech but, in fact, this phenomenon has been attested also in adults in Bogotá (Montes, 2005) and is also used all over Colombia (Albor, 1986), as well as Caracas, Venezuela (Sedano, 1990).

References

Aguilar, E. and Serra, M. (2003) *AREHA: Análisis del retraso del habla.* Barcelona: Edicions Universitat de Barcelona.

Albor, H. (1986) Uso e interpretación de 'ser' en construcciones galicadas y en 'Él necesita es descansa'. *Thesaurus*, Tomo XLI (pp. 173–186). Bogotá: Instituto Caro y Cuervo.

Ball, M. (1988) LARSP to LLARSP: The design of a grammatical profile for Welsh. *Clinical Linguistics & Phonetics* 2 (1), 55–73.

Bosch, L. (2004) *Evaluación fonológica del habla infantil.* Barcelona: Masson.

Camargo, M. (2013) S-LARSP: Perfil de desarrollo morfosintáctico del español. Tesis doctoral no publicada. Universidad Autónoma de Madrid.

Camargo, M. and Garayzábal, E. (2015) Perfil de desarrollo morfosintáctico del español de Colombia: S-LARSP. *Revista de Logopedia, Foniatría y Audiología* 35 (1), 62–76.

Codesido, A., Coloma, C., Garayzábal, E., Marrero, V., Mendoza, E. and Pávez, M. (2012) Spanish acquisition and the development of PERSL. In M. Ball, D. Crystal and P. Fletcher (eds) *Assessing Grammar: The Languages of LARSP* (pp. 245–281). Bristol: Multilingual Matters.

Coloma, C., Peñaloza, C. and Fernández, R. (2007) Producción de oraciones complejas en niños de 8 y 10 años. *Revista de Lingüística Teórica y Aplicada* 45 (1), 33–44.

Cornell, E. and Broda, L. (1995) Age-related differences in the organization of parent–infant interactions during picture-book reading. *Early Childhood Research Quarterly* 10, 317–337.

Dijkstra, J. and Schlichting, L. (2012) Frisian TARSP. Based on the methodology of Dutch TARSP. In M. Ball, D. Crystal and P. Fletcher (eds) *Assessing Grammar: The Languages of LARSP* (pp. 189–207). Bristol: Multilingual Matters.

Greenberg, J. (1963) *Universals of Language.* Cambridge, MA: MIT Press.

Hasbro (© 2008). *El Dentista Bromista.*

Hickey, T. (1990) ILARSP: A grammatical profile of Irish. *Clinical Linguistics & Phonetics* 4 (4), 363–376.

Jin, L., Oh, B. and Razak, R. (2012) C-LARSP: Developing a Chinese grammatical profile. In M. Ball, D. Crystal and P. Fletcher (eds) *Assessing Grammar: The Languages of LARSP* (pp. 208–229). Bristol: Multilingual Matters.

Maillart, C., Parisse, C. and Tommerdahl, J. (2012) F-LARSP 1.0: An adaptation of the LARSP language profile for French. *Clinical Linguistics y Phonetics* 26 (2), 188–198.

Mayer, M. (1967) *A Boy, a Dog and a Frog*. New York: Dial Books.
Miller, J. and Iglesias, A. (2012) *Systematic Analysis of Language Transcripts* (SALT), Version 2012 [Computer Software], SALT Software, LLC.
Montes, J. (2005) Anotaciones lingüísticas y correcciones idiomáticas. Bogotá: Aequus Editor.
Muñoz, B. and Anwandter, A. (2011) *Manual de lectura temprana compartida: ¿Por qué es importante y cómo leer con niños y niñas de 0 a 7 años?*. Gobierno de Chile: Consejo Nacional de la Cultura y las Artes.
Pérez, E. and Serra, M. (1998) *A-RE-L. Análisis del retraso del lenguaje*. Barcelona: Ariel Practicum.
R Core Team (2012) *A Language and Environment for Statistical Computing*. R Foundation for Statistical Computing, Viena.
República de Colombia. Ley 142 de 1994, del 11 de julio. Diario Oficial 41.433 del 11 de julio de 1994 (Rule 142 of 1994, July 11th from the Republic of Colombia. Official Journal 41.433, July 11th 1994).
Samadi, H. and Perkins, M. (1998) P-LARSP: A developmental language profile for Persian. *Clinical Linguistics & Phonetics* 12 (2), 83–103.
Sedano, M. (1990) Hendidas y otras construcciones con ser en el habla de Caracas. Caracas: Universidad Central de Venezuela.

8 Towards a Micro-profile of Bangla Verb Inflection

Asifa Sultana, Stephanie Stokes, Thomas Klee and Paul Fletcher

Introduction

Bangla or Bengali, an Indo-Aryan language, has branched out from Sanskrit (600–650 BC) through Prakrit, an intermediate language. Bangla is widely spoken in Bangladesh, in the Indian states of PashchimBanga, Assam and Tripura, and among the Bengali migrant population in countries such as the USA, UK, Australia and Canada, and many Middle-Eastern countries. There are over 107 million first language speakers of Bangla in Bangladesh (Bangladesh Bureau of Statistics, 2011) and 83 million speakers in different states of India (Encyclopaedia Britannica, 2016). With a total of 250 million first and second language speakers, Bangla is considered the 6th largest among the languages of the world (Comrie, 2005; Klaiman, 2008). Modern Bangla, in the 19th and 20th century, had two varieties which were used in specific contexts: the *shadhu bhasha* was used in official documents and in literature, and the *chalita bhasha* was used in informal, everyday conversation. Although the former variety is obsolete now, situations of diglossia are still observed in the Bangla-speaking regions. The account of the acquisition of verb inflection that we outline below draws on children's spontaneous language samples and elicitation data collected from a major Bangla-speaking region – Dhaka, Bangladesh. There are two varieties of the language in use in Dhaka. The Standard variety is the norm in spoken and written formal contexts, while the Colloquial one is primarily a spoken variety in informal situations. Although there are some differences in the specific grammatical markers used in these language varieties, the same conjugation principles are maintained in both.

Grammatical Sketch of Bangla

The canonical word order in Bangla is Subject–Object–Verb. However, a considerable amount of flexibility is permitted within the word order.

These three examples of a transitive simple sentence show the same three words in SVO, OVS and OSV order:

(1a)	Bimal	Anil-ke	mar-l-o.
	Bimal	Anil.acc	hit.pst.3p
	Bimal hit Anil.		
(1b)	Anil-ke	mar-l-o	Bimal.
	Anil.acc	hit.pst.3p	Bimal
	Bimal hit Anil.		
(1c)	Anil-ke	Bimal	mar-l-o.
	Anil.acc	Bimal	hit.pst.3p
	Bimal hit Anil.		

The arguments in each of the sentences in (1a)–(1c) are in the same relationship with the verb, and all the sentences are grammatical, conveying the same meaning in Bangla regardless of their order in the sentence. However, word order in Bangla is manipulated to achieve specific pragmatic purposes.

Bangla is a null-subject language, i.e. the projection of the subject in a sentence is not always obligatory. As a language with rich inflectional morphology, Bangla often allows for adequate information to be derived from the inflected verbs which is why an obligatory projection of the subject is not always required. For example,

(2a)	bhat	kha-chch^h-i.	
	rice	eat.pres.prog.1p	
	(I am) eating rice.		
(2b)	Eta	bol-l-e	keno?
	this	say.pst.2p	why
	Why did (you) say this?		
(2c)	Ekhon	ki	kor-ch^h-e?
	now	what	do.prog.3p
	What is (he) doing now?		

The sentences in (2a)–(2c) demonstrate the null-subjecthood allowed in Bangla with 1st, 2nd and 3rd person subjects. Each of these sentences is grammatical in Bangla without overtly realising the subject.

In Bangla, the equivalents of the English utterances with 'be' copulas do not require a verb. Therefore, a sentence in English such as 'This is a book' has the following representation in Bangla:

(3)	Eta	ekta	boi.
	This	a	book
	This (is) a book.		

Verb Morphology

Bangla verb morphology exhibits agglutinative features: the grammatical markers are attached to the stem in a linear, incremental fashion where one marker performs only one grammatical role. In a fusional language such as English, the inflection –ed denotes both temporal and aspectual information. However, there is a one-to-one relationship between morphemes and their functions in Bangla. For example, the inflected verb form 'hashch^{h}ilam' (hash-ch^{h}i-l-am) (was laughing) carries four elements: stem (hash-), progressive aspect marker (-ch^{h}i-), past tense marker (-l-), and 1st person marker (-am). Agglutination, a typical feature of the Dravidian languages, is considered a Dravidian influence on Bangla (Mazumdar, 1920), and the presence of the properties we see in the Bangla verb inflectional paradigm is likely to be a reflection of that.

Bangla verbs are marked for aspect, tense, and person (Campbell, 1995). The verbal form does not signal number- and gender-related information. All verbal inflections are suffixes that attach to the stem depending on the grammatical information that needs to be expressed. The stems rarely occur in bare forms. Tense and aspect markers are overtly realized when required, while the person marker is almost always obligatory. Table 8.1 summarizes the situation for three verb forms, present simple, present progressive and past progressive, with two verbs, one with vowel-final stem. Any differences between the inflections of the two verbs are morphophonological, arising from the nature of the stem-final segment.

Aspect

Two types of aspectual information are realized on Bangla verbs: progressive and perfective. The progressive aspect marker is used to indicate an ongoing action regardless of the time when the action takes place. The progressive aspect marker is overtly realized in present and the past progressive forms. However, the past marker in (4b) entails a phonological modification of the progressive marker via an epenthetic vowel:

(4a)	ami	golpo	bol-ch^{h}-i.
	I	(a) story	tell.prog.1p
	I am telling a story.		
(4b)	ami	golpo	bol-ch^{h}i-l-am.
	I	(a) story	tell.prog.past.1p
	I was telling a story.		

The perfective aspect marker, on the other hand, is used in contexts denoting the completion of an action. The marker is realized on present and past perfect verb forms. Again in (5b) an epenthetic vowel precedes the past inflection:

(5a)	ami	golpo	bol-ech^{h}-i.
	I	(a) story	tell.perf.1p
	I have told a story.		

Table 8.1 Verb morphological paradigm in Bangla (the general form is verb stem–aspect marker–tense marker–person marker)

	Verb form	Verb stem 1: /por-/	Verb stem 2: /k^ha-/
Present	Simple/ 1st person Verb root - Ø- Ø- i	Ami boi pori I book(s) read	Ami k^hai I eat
	Simple/ 2nd person Verb root - Ø- Ø- o	Tumi boi poro You book(s) read	Tumi k^hao You eat
	Simple/ 3rd person Verb root - Ø- Ø- e	She boi pore (S)he book(s) reads	She k^hae (S)he eats
	Progressive/ 1st person Verb root - ch^h- Ø- i	Ami boi porch^hi I (a) book am reading	Ami k^hachch^hi I am eating
	Progressive/ 2nd person Verb root - ch^h- Ø- o	Tumi boi porch^ho You (a) book are reading	Tumi k^hachch^ho You are eating
	Progressive/ 3rd person Verb root - ch^h- Ø- e	She boi porch^he (S)he (a) book is reading	She k^hachch^he (S)he is eating
	Perfect/ 1st person Verb root - ech^h- Ø- i	Ami boi porech^hi I (a) book have read	Ami k^heyech^hi I have eaten
	Perfect/ 2nd person Verb root - ech^h- Ø- o	Tumi boi porech^ho You (a) book have read	Tumi k^heyech^ho You have eaten
	Perfect/ 3rd person Verb root - ech^h- Ø- e	She boi porech^he (S)he (a) book has read	She k^heyech^he (S)he has eaten
Past	Simple/ 1st person Verb root - Ø- l- am	Ami boi porlam I (a) book read	Ami k^helam I ate
	Simple/ 2nd person Verb root - Ø- l- e	Tumi boi porle You (a) book read	Tumi k^hele You ate
	Simple/ 3rd person Verb root - Ø- l- o	She boi porlo (S)he (a) book read	She k^helo (S)he ate
	Progressive/ 1st person Verb root - ch^hi- l- am	Ami boi porch^hilam I (a) book was reading	Ami k^hachch^hilam I was eating
	Progressive/ 2nd person Verb root - ch^hi- l- e	Tumi boi porch^hile You (a) book were reading	Tumi k^hachch^hile You were eating
	Progressive/ 3rd person Verb root - ch^hi- l- o	She boi porch^hilo (S)he (a) book was reading	She k^hachch^hilo (S)he was eating
	Perfect/ 1st person Verb root - ech^hi- l- am	Ami boi porech^hilam I (a) book had read	Ami k^heyech^hilam I had eaten
	Perfect/ 2nd person Verb root - ech^hi- l- e	Tumi boi porech^hile You (a) book had read	Tumi k^heyech^hile You had eaten
	Perfect/ 3rd person Verb root - ech^hi- l- o	She boi porech^hilo (S)he (a) book had read	She k^heyech^hilo (S)he had eaten
Future	Simple/ 1st person Verb root - Ø- b- o	Ami boi porbo I book(s) will read	Ami k^habo I will eat
	Simple/ 2nd person Verb root - Ø- b- e	Tumi boi porbe You book(s) will read	Tumi k^habe You will eat
	Simple/ 3rd person Verb root - Ø- b- e	She boi porbe (S)he book(s) will read	She k^habe (S)he will eat

(5b)	ami	golpo	bol-ech^{h}i-l-am.
	I	(a) story	tell.perf.past.1p
	I had told a story.		

In non-progressive and non-perfective aspect situations (e.g. present simple), the aspect markers are considered to have a null form, and only the person marker is attached to the stem.

(6)	She	protidin	boi	por-e.
	He/She	everyday	book(s)	read.3p
	He/She reads books every day.			

Tense

Distinct markers are used to express tense-related information in Bangla independently of aspectual information. Overt marking is used to denote future time (7a), and past time (7b). There is, however, no overt marker for present tense, and these forms simply have a person suffix attached to the verb stem (7c):

(7a)	She	boi	por-l-o.
	He/She	(a) book	read.past.3p
	He/She reads a book.		
(7b)	She	boi	por-b-e.
	He/She	(a) book	read.fut.3p
	He/She will read a book.		
(7c)	She	boi	por-e
	He/She	(a) book	reads
	He/She reads a book		

Person

Three different person markers are used to denote 1st, 2nd and 3rd person agents. As noted earlier, person markers are the only obligatory inflections required with a verb stem.

(8a)	Ami	protidin	boi	por-i.
	I	everyday	book(s)	read.1p
	I read books everyday.			
(8b)	Tumi	protidin	boi	por-o.
	You	everyday	book(s)	read.2p
	You read books everyday.			
(8c)	She	protidin	boi	por-e.
	He/She	everyday	book(s)	read.3p
	He/She reads books every day.			

The Bangla verb morphological paradigm is relatively transparent with a one-to-one relationship between the grammatical forms and functions. The resulting transparency has significant implications for language acquisition. Children learning an agglutinative language appear to master the morphological details of the ambient language earlier than children learning a fusional language with complex morphological coding (Chakraborty & Leonard, 2012; Xanthos *et al.*, 2011).

We now turn to an examination of findings emerging from Bangla child language research that reveal the developmental course of verb inflection in Bangla.

Verb Morphology in Typically Developing Children

Studies on Bangla child language development are scarce. There are three recent studies on Bangla verb form acquisition. Working with a group of 37 typically developing children between 1;6 to 4 years, Chakraborty and Leonard (2012) examined children's use of first, second and third person present and past progressive forms. From the accuracy and error rates calculated from their elicitation tasks, the authors concluded that second person forms were late to emerge both in the present and the past forms. Children were found to replace the second person endings by first or third person forms. Given that mean scores were high (present progressive 86%, past progressive 79%) the authors concluded that, aside from person error, those tense and aspect combinations did not offer significant challenges for children. However, these findings may not accurately reflect verb inflection performance generally in this age range. Chakraborty and Leonard's conclusions were based on data from only half the original sample, as it turned out that 18 of the children could not reach criterion on the elicitation tasks they attempted. Sultana (2016), again using elicitation, found that verb forms requiring the tense marker without aspect marker, i.e. the past simple, were rarely used by children, and confirmed that forms taking only the aspect marker in absence of a tense marker, e.g. present perfect, were frequent (Sultana, 2016).

In the context of this limited previous research, we present here further data from two sources – spontaneous speech samples, and a more extensive elicitation study with a much larger sample (Sultana *et al.*, 2016). Via these two studies we can provide a clearer picture of verb form development in Bangla. We begin with an analysis of the spontaneous speech samples.

Verb forms in spontaneous speech

Data

The data come from a cross-sectional study involving spontaneous speech samples from three groups of typically developing children: the

Table 8.2 Participant profile

	Age (months)	Utterances	M:F
Group 1 [n = 6]	M = 25.67; SD = 1.51	M = 166.67; SD = 61.21	2:4
Group 2 [n = 6]	M = 34.83; SD = 2.64	M = 230.5; SD = 41.07	1:5
Group 3 [n = 6]	M = 48; SD = 1.55	M = 181.17; SD = 94.76	6:0

first of mean age 25.67 months (so close to two years of age); the second of mean age 34.83 months, so close to three years; and finally a group whose mean age was four years (Table 8.2). There were six children in each group, and they formed a subset of the subjects in the Sultana *et al.* (2016) elicitation study described later in the chapter. The children were recruited from daycare centres and pre-schools in Dhaka, Bangladesh. The identification of the children as typically developing was based on parents responding in the negative to questions like 'Do you have any concern about your child's speech, language or hearing' and 'Has anyone in your family had a speech or language delay or disorder'. Children were also required to be monolingual speakers of Bangla. Four of the six daycare centres operated as part of four companies and they catered for children of employees from all levels of the company. Therefore, although the group recruited for the study was not deliberately representative of the Bangla-speaking population, it was a diverse group, with children belonging to low to high socioeconomic backgrounds.

Analysis

The spontaneous language samples of children were transcribed and coded using Systematic Analysis of Language Transcripts (SALT) (Miller *et al.*, 2012) by the first author. A list of the verb-form codes used is presented in Appendix 1. Minor utterances were identified in the samples, and excluded from the analysis to generate scores based on major utterances (for the minor-major utterance distinction see Crystal *et al.*, 1989: 44). The production of the inflected verb forms were then calculated for 100 major utterances. A productivity criterion was applied: only forms with at least two instances (tokens) were considered to be productive and entered in the analysis. This criterion is consistent with previous LARSP analyses of English data (e.g. Klee & Gavin, 2010). Frequencies of inflections meeting the criterion, per 100 major utterance, are presented in Table 8.3. We also present the percentage of children using a particular inflection in Table 8.4. (Tables 8.3 and 8.4 use the SALT codes to identify verb inflections – these are listed and glossed in Appendix 1). We utilized this information as follows: if 4/6 children in a group (66.67%) provide the inflection (i.e. met the frequency criterion) it is regarded as emerging; if all the children used the form, then it is considered to be acquired.

Table 8.3 Production of the verb forms calculated for 100 major utterances[1]

Verb forms	Two-year olds	Three-year olds	Four-year olds
	Mean (SD)	Mean (SD)	Mean (SD)
PS1P	2.47 (3.18)	5.58 (3.26)	4.13 (2.06)
PS2P	0 (0)	0.27 (0.65)	0.55 (1.34)
PS3P	9.51 (12.21)	7.28 (3.33)	17.59 (5.98)
PSP1P	0.63 (1.54)	0 (0)	0.58 (1.42)
PSP2P	54 (0.85)	0 (0)	0 (0)
PSP3P	4.78 (5.30)	0.36 (0.87)	0.36 (0.87)
PP1P	0 (0)	2.29 (2.88)	0.23 (0.57)
PP2P	0 (0)	0 (0)	0 (0)
PP3P	0.92 (1.56)	4.25 (2.94)	4.18 (4.68)
PPF1P	1.68 (2.07)	2.39 (2.24)	2.94 (2.33)
PPF2P	2.61 (5.58)	1.96 (2.24)	0.18 (0.43)
PPF3P	4.78 (7.38)	6.09 (1.49)	8.52 (3.68)
PTS1P	0 (0)	0 (0)	0 (0)
PTS2P	0 (0)	0 (0)	0.24 (0.58)
PTS3P	0 (0)	0.76 (1.35)	4.80 (4.68)
PTP1P	0 (0)	0 (0)	0 (0)
PTP2P	0 (0)	0 (0)	0 (0)
PTP3P	0 (0)	0 (0)	0.24 (0.058)
PTPF1P	0 (0)	0 (0)	0 (0)
PTPF2P	0 (0)	0 (0)	0 (0)
PTPF3P	0 (0)	0 (0)	0 (0)
F1P	5.87 (5.41)	5.77 (3.26)	2.65 (2.41)
F2P	0.86 (2.11)	1.62 (1.98)	1.65 (1.51)
F3P	8.34 (6.72)	11.45(4.76)	10.62 (4.70)
IMP2P	14.20 (10.98)	13.37 (6.38)	6.98 (3.61)

Findings

Two-year olds

Of the inflected verb forms, PS3P (Present Simple third person), PSP3P (Present Simple for Present Progressive third person), PPF3P (Present Perfect third person), F1P (Future first person) and F3P (Future third person), constituted the majority of verb forms in these children's utterances.

Aspect

Use of the perfective aspect marker was observed at this stage. The marker was used to refer to immediate actions. For example, *Khorgosh*

Table 8.4 Percentage of children in each group producing the verb inflections

Verb forms	Two-year olds	Three-year olds	Four-year olds
PS1P	50%	83.33%	100%
PS2P	0%	16.67%	16.67%
PS3P	83.33%	100%	100%
PSP1P	16.67%	0%	16.67%
PSP2P	33.33%	0%	0%
PSP3P	66.67%	16.67%	16.67%
PP1P	0%	66.67%	16.67%
PP2P	0%	0%	0%
PP3P	16.67%	100%	66.67%
PPF1P	50%	66.67%	100%
PPF2P	33.33%	66.67%	16.67%
PPF3P	50%	100%	100%
PTS1P	0%	0%	0%
PTS2P	0%	0%	16.67%
PTS3P	0%	33.33%	100%
PTP1P	0%	0%	0%
PTP2P	0%	0%	0%
PTP3P	0%	0%	16.67%
PTPF1P	0%	0%	0%
PTPF2P	0%	0%	0%
PTPF3P	0%	0%	0%
F1P	83.33%	100%	66.67%
F2P	16.67%	50%	66.67%
F3P	100%	100%	100%
IMP2P	83.33%	100%	100%

rakhsi [(I) have put the rabbit], *Oshudh dise* [(The doctor) has given medicine]. However, the perfective aspect marker was observed only in present tense context; the past perfect forms did not emerge at this stage.

The use of overtly realized progressive marker was minimal at this stage. Note that colloquial Bangla used in Dhaka permits the use of Present Simple form to refer to the Present Progressive.

Children at this stage were found to use the Present Simple forms, i.e. PSP1P, PSP2P, PSP3P, that were functional equivalents of their Present Progressive counterparts. For example,

(9) ki kor-o
what do-2P
What are (you) doing?

(10) Ora twinkle twinkle dekhe
they twinkle twinkle watch-3P
(They) are watching twinkle twinkle

The use of Present Simple for Present Progressive was significantly lower among the older groups of children. None of the aspect inflections reached emerging status in Table 8.4.

Tense

Bangla present tense markers have a null representation while there is overt marking of past and the future tenses on verbs. Children at this stage did not produce any past tense marker; there were no instances of the Past Simple, Past Progressive or Past Perfect forms. The perfective actions were all expressed using the Present Perfect forms. Note that, unlike English, Bangla Past Simple forms have very restricted application; they are observed in specific contexts as narratives while most of the perfective actions are indicated through the Present Perfect forms (cf. Sultana, 2015). This is likely to have delayed the emergence of the Past Simple forms in children's speech. The future tense marker appears to be one of the most dominant markers at this stage. While children's use of future tense markers were restricted to Future Simple forms, these, in first, second and third person combinations, constituted a significant portion of children's utterances. Table 8.4 indicates in particular an emerging status for the 1stperson future inflection.

Person

With a few exceptions, person markers are the only obligatory forms in Bangla. This is likely to have contributed to children's early use of these markers in their speech. Across all inflected verb forms, the use of third person marker (*Bhat khabe* [(She) will eat rice]) outnumbered those of the first (*Eta ami bhangbo* [I will break this]) and the second person markers (*Woofwoofke diba* [(You) will give to woofwoof]) (Table 8.3). Children also exhibited preferences towards the third person forms over the first person forms. In line with the previous studies conducted cross linguistically, the second-person forms appeared in fewer numbers compared to both first and third person forms (cf. Chakraborty & Leonard, 2012 for Bangla; Bassano *et al.*, 2001, for German and French). There were inflected verb forms (Present Progressive) that appeared only in third-person forms while the first and the second person counterparts remained absent (Table 8.3). Note that by the criterion established for Table 8.4, Present Simple third person, Future first person and Future 3rd person inflections are acquired by two-year olds. One reason for the low frequencies for second person variants in the data may be the ubiquity of a form not yet mentioned, the imperative. Two-year olds, in common with their older counterparts, used this form more frequently (at 14.2 instances per 100 major utterances) than any other inflection, and five of the six children in the group supplied it. The extensive use of this form in the early stages of acquisition is consistent with the fact that the imperative form in Bangla is structurally simple. The Bangla imperative form consists of the verb stem and only the person marker. For example,

(11) Mom jala-o
Candle light-2P
Light (the) candle

Three-year olds

A further year of language experience marks a significant development in children's use of overtly inflected verb forms (Table 8.3). Whereas for two-year olds we can see from Table 8.4 that only three inflections can be regarded as mastered, nine of the ten inflections (excluding the PSP forms) are in this category for three-year olds.

Aspect

While the use of the perfective aspect marker increased in children at this age, it still remained exclusive to present tense contexts. No instances of children's use of Past Perfect forms were observed in this group of children. This stage marked the emergence of the overt Present Progressive marker. This development is in line with the notable decline in the use of Present Simple for Present Progressive. However, children at stage II exhibited no instances of the progressive aspect marker in the past or future contexts. From Table 8.4 we can designate first person Present Progressive as emerging, and third person Present Progressive as acquired. For Present Perfect, first and second persons are emerging, while all children in the sample provided the third person form.

Tense

The past tense marker began to appear at this age. Children at this stage exhibited a few instances of the past tense marker in the Simple Past context (*Ki korlo?* [What did (he) do?]). However, the marker was still absent in Past Perfect contexts. The use of the future tense marker continued to be a dominant inflection produced by children at this stage.

Person

The possible pattern of emergence, i.e. third > first > second person marker, observed among two-year-old children was consistent with the order observed in their three-year-old peers. In all contexts, the production of the third person marker surpassed the production of the first and second person markers respectively (e.g. Present Simple, Present Progressive, Future Simple). Also, whenever a new form emerged, it appeared in the third person context (e.g. Past Simple).

Four-year olds

Children's increasing use of the inflected verb forms is clear in the four-year-old children. It is evident looking across the groups that, as they get older, children use inflections more frequently, and use a greater variety of verb forms, some that could be argued to be cognitively more challenging to process.

Aspect

While the Present Perfect form continued to occur frequently at this stage, productive use of the Past Perfect form was still absent in children's language. The emergence of the progressive aspect marker in the present context coupled with the decline in the Present Simple for Present Progressive observed with three-year olds continued with this older group. Children's development with regard to the use of aspect markers was manifested in the emergence of the Past Progressive forms, which can now be deemed acquired for first and third person. Children began to use the Progressive aspect marker in past contexts; for example, *Ki korchhilo?* [What was (he) doing?].

Tense

Children at this stage exhibited a significant increase in the use of the Past Simple form, with all six children in the group using the inflection. However even at this age Bangla-speaking children are still resistant to extending the past tense marker to Progressive and Perfect aspect forms. Out of the six inflections involved, there is only one that appears in the data, a third person Past Progressive, used by a single child in this group. The future tense marker, used in all three person–marker combinations, remains a dominant inflection for four-year olds.

Person

The relationship among the three person markers remained the same, i.e. the third person marker had the highest frequency, followed by the first and the second person markers. Second person forms emerged for many verbs at this stage. For example, children were found to use the second person form in a variety of morphological contexts (*Tumi shunte pele* [You got to hear it], *Dekhechho?* [Have (you) seen?], *Cup e kore pani khabe?* [Will (you) drink water from (a) cup?]).

Verb Forms via Elicitation

An advantage of an elicitation procedure is that it can provide information on error forms as well as forms that the child has mastered, and so provides a more rounded picture than spontaneous speech data. Sultana *et al.* (2016) explored verb inflections in 70 Bangla-speaking children between the ages of 1;11 and 4;3. The focus of the study was on three inflections, the Present Simple, the Present Progressive and the Past Progressive. For the present simple, responses were elicited in structured conversations, while for the two progressive forms, responses were elicited via pictures. Only third person forms were tested. Across the sample as a whole, the Present Simple form was used with the highest accuracy (mean = 88%), followed by the Present Progressive (mean = 67%) and the Past Progressive forms (mean = 44%). Children's performance across the three tasks differed significantly. The errors made by the children were also analysed, to determine if there were consistent error patterns for target forms. In attempts at the present progressive, the most common error was present simple. And for past progressive targets the tendency was for children to use the present progressive. When correct responses and errors were analysed together using a cluster analysis, three groups of children emerged, based on their performance on percent correct and percent error measures (Sultana *et al.*, 2016). The first group used the present simple for both present progressive and past progressive. The second group used the present progressive when past progressive was required. The third group made very few errors. It seems reasonable to conclude that there is a developmental sequence starting with the emergence of the present simple followed by present and past progressive forms respectively. The order of acquisition can be explained in relation to the structural and cognitive complexities of the forms. As we have seen in discussing the spontaneous speech data, Present Progressive forms are more complex than Present Simple forms, in requiring an aspect morpheme in addition to a person marker. And Past Progressive requires aspect, tense and person morphemes.

Verb Forms in Children with Language Impairment

There is no history of studies of language impairment in Bangladesh, and no infrastructure exits for the identification of or intervention with children with specific language impairment (SLI) or developmental language disorder. There is no identified SLI population in Bangladesh. Participants in the small group of nine children recruited for a pilot study did not go through any formal assessments such as taking standardized tests before involvement in this study. However, they were all attending a special school and as confirmation of their language difficulties, reports of the assessments done by the school or by other clinical experts were collected for each child. The inclusion of these children was largely based on these reports. All children were below age ten (age range 47–112 months). The study was aimed at identifying the challenges to morphological development in Bangla-speaking children with language impairment, but we should make clear that the participants were a mixed group with distinct cognitive difficulties that included autism, Down's syndrome, intellectual disorder and developmental delay. Hence any conclusions must be tentative.

This group was presented with the same elicitation procedures as the typically developing (TD) children reported in Sultana *et al.* (2016). Mean percent correct scores in response to the elicitation probes were as follows: Present Simple, 53.29%; Present Progressive, 27.78%; Past Progressive, 8.89%. At much lower levels of accuracy, these values mirror the trend in the TD children. There was considerable individual variation however: for example, scores on the Present Progressive ranged from 0 to 60%. Scrutiny of errors made by the children with LI also showed considerable similarity to those of TD children. When the target form was not available in the repertoire, children with language impairment tended to choose what the typically developing children also chose as a possible substitute. For example, the Present Simple form did not have any other dominant verb conjugation as substitute except for infrequent uses of the Present Perfect form. Performance was also similar to the typically developing children on the Present and the Past Progressive tasks. In the Present Progressive task, a dominant non-target form was the Present Simple form as it was for the typically-developing group. Finally, similarity was also observed in the errors between the groups on the Past Progressive task. The dominant errors were the Present Simple and the Present Progressive forms.

The Micro-Profile

The term 'micro-profile' in the title of this chapter harks back to some early efforts to drill down into the structure of English, at some specific points in the original LARSP profile where it was felt that more detail would be of clinical utility. So Garman (1979) provided an exhaustive account of what was at that time known about development at the one-word stage. And Fletcher (1979) brought together the then current information on verb auxiliary and inflection development in English. The intention of these elaborations of specific areas of the original profile was to enable clinicians to sharpen their assessments in specific areas of the profile chart, and to furnish them with better guidance for remediation. The level of structural detail built into a grammatical profile is always a matter of judgement for its architects, and different languages pose different problems. For English, the paucity of inflection does not present any hard choices. But the complexity of Bangla verb inflection reflected in Table 8.1 will entail decisions about what information about verb inflection to include in a comprehensive profile for Bangla analogous to the English LARSP, and what to leave out. For the moment we are postponing that judgement and providing a *micro-profile* of verb inflection development from 2 years to 4 years, based on the spontaneous speech and elicitation data we have summarized. The micro-profile appears as Appendix 2, and uses the SALT codes of Appendix 1 to identify verb forms.

The organization of the micro-profile makes clear that the agglutinative character of verb forms in the language is directly reflected in the developmental sequence in Bangla-speaking children. The only firm acquisition at two years of age is the person-only Imperative form. By three years, the person-only third person Present Simple form is mastered, as is the first person Future, which requires tense and person markers. Children at three years are also developing aspect + person forms for both Present Progressive and Present Perfect. By four years we see the consolidation of future forms, and the emergence of the first form that involves three verb morphemes, the Past Progressive. Significant as the structural character of the language is in influencing acquisition, it is important to stress that there are other factors that play a part. As noted above, Past Simple tense is restricted to particular contexts, and present perfect is more usually applied to completed past events. So frequency presumably plays a role in the relatively late appearance of past tense, which, despite its relatively simple structure, is not mastered until four years. We should also remember that the inferences we draw from the language samples derive from just six children in each group, and further work will be required to consolidate the picture presented in the micro-profile, and to understand the remainder of the developmental course beyond 48 months, as children move towards mastery of the full range of forms described in Table 8.1.

Note

(1) A fuller version of Table 3, including confidence intervals for each variable, can be obtained from the first author at bdliza@gmail.com

References

Bangladesh Bureau of Statistics (2011) Population and Housing Census 2011: Socio-economic and demographic report. Retrieved from http://www.sid.gov.bd/wpcontent/uploads/2014/01/Socio_Economic.pdf

Bassano, D., Maillochon, I., Klampfer, S. and Dressler, W. (2001) The acquisition of verb morphology in French and Austrian-German: II. Data Analysis. *Enfance* 53, 117–148.

Campbell, G.L. (1995) Bengali. In G.L. Campbell (ed.) *Concise Compendium of the World's Languages*. London & New York: Routledge.

Chakraborty, R. and Leonard, L.B. (2012) A brief research report on acquisition of verb inflections in Bengali-speaking children. *Journal of Advanced Linguistic Studies* 1 (1-2), 41–53.

Comrie, B. (2005) Language. *Microsoft Encarta Online Encyclopedia*, 2005. Microsoft Corporation.

Crystal, D., Fletcher, P. and Garman, M. (1989) *The Grammatical Analysis of Language Disability* (2nd edn). London: Cole & Whurr. Available from University of Canterbury Research Repository, http://hdl.handle.net/10092/5483

Fletcher, P. (1979) Micro-profile of the stage III verb phrase. In D. Crystal (ed.) *Working with LARSP* (pp. 132–140). London: Edward Arnold. Available from University of Canterbury Research Repository, http://hdl.handle.net/10092/5482

Garman, M. (1979) Micro-profile of Stage 1. In D. Crystal (ed.) *Working with LARSP* (pp. 119–131). London: Edward Arnold. Available from University of Canterbury Research Repository, http://hdl.handle.net/10092/5482

Indo-Aryan languages (2016) In *Encyclopædia Britannica*. Retrieved 22nd March 2016 from http://www.britannica.com/EBchecked/topic/286348/Indo-Aryan-languages
Klaiman, M.H. (2008) Bengali. In B. Comrie (ed.) *The World's Major Languages* (pp. 417–436). London: Routledge.
Klee, T. and Gavin, W.J. (2010) *LARSP Reference Data for 2- and 3-year-old Children*. Christchurch, NZ: University of Canterbury Research Repository, http://hdl.handle.net/10092/4980
Mazumdar, B.C. (1920) *The History of the Bengali Language*. Asian Educational Services.
Miller, J.F., Gillon, G. and Westerveld, M. (2012) Systematic Analysis of Language Transcripts (SALT), New Zealand Instructional Version 2012 [Computer software]. Middleton, WI: SALT Software, LLC.
Sultana, A. (2015) Morphosyntactic Development of Typically- and Atypically-developing Bangla-speaking Children (Unpublished doctoral dissertation). University of Canterbury, Christchurch, New Zealand.
Sultana, A., Stokes, S. Klee, T. and Fletcher, P. (2016) Morphosyntactic development of Bangla-speaking preschool children. *First Language* 36, 637–657.
Sultana, A. (2016) Morphological development of Bangla-speaking children: A pilot study. *The EFL Journal* 7 (1), 73–92.
Xanthos, A., Laaha, S., Gillis, S., Stephany, U., Aksu-Koc, A., Christofidou, A. ... and Dressler, W. U. (2011) On the role of morphological richness in the early development of noun and verb inflection. *First Language* 31 (4), 461–479. doi:10.1177/0142723711409976

Appendix 1

SALT Codes for Bangla

[ps1p]	Present simple 1st person
[ps2p]	Present simple 2nd person
[ps3p]	Present simple 3rd person
[psp1p]	Present simple for progressive 1st person
[psp2p]	Present simple for progressive 2nd person
[psp3p]	Present simple for progressive 3rd person
[pp1p]	Present progressive 1st person
[pp2p]	Present progressive 2nd person
[pp3p]	Present progressive 3rd person
[ppf1p]	Present perfect 1st person
[ppf2p]	Present perfect 2nd person
[ppf3p]	Present perfect 3rd person
[pts1p]	Past simple 1st person
[pts2p]	Past simple 2nd person
[pts3p]	Past simple 3rd person
[ptp1p]	Past progressive 1st person
[ptp2p]	Past progressive 2nd person
[ptp3p]	Past progressive 3rd person
[ptpf1p]	Past perfect 1st person

[ptpf2p]	Past perfect 2nd person
[ptpf3p]	Past perfect 3rd person
[f1p]	Future 1st person
[f2p]	Future 2nd person
[f3p]	Future 3rd person
[imp2p]	Imperative 2nd person

Appendix 2

Micro-profile for Bangla verb inflections, two–four years of age*

	Person	Tense+Person	Aspect+Person	Aspect+Tense+Person
Two Years	IMP2P PS3P(E)	F1P(E)		
Three Years	PS1P(E) PS3P	F1P	PP1P(E) PPF1P(E) PPF2P(E) PPF3P	
Four Years	PS1P	F2P(E) PTS3P F3P	PP3P(E)	PTP3P(E)

*(E) indicates that the form is 'emerging' at this point, as evidenced by the percentage of children using it in the spontaneous speech sample (Table 8.4) or the elicitation procedure in Sultana et al. (2016).

9 Adapting LARSP to Turkish: TR-LARSP Part II

Özlem Cangökçe Yaşar and Seyhun Topbaş

Introduction

This chapter outlines the second part of the study for the adaptation of LARSP to Turkish (TR-LARSP); for the first part see Topbaş *et al.* (2012). In our study we analysed 70 children (30 female, 40 male) aged between 9 and 67 months who were all monolingual and born to Turkish-speaking families. The children were grouped into age categories according to the LARSP age criteria. Accordingly, these stages were included: stage I: 09–18 months; stage II: 19–24 months, stage III: 25–30 months; stage IV: 31–36 months; stage V: 37–42 months; stage VI: 43–54 months and stage VII: 55 months and above (Cangökçe-Yaşar & Topbaş, 2018).

The data of this study are composed of speech samples obtained from the children. Speech samples were collected in one session via video recording, lasting approximately 1.5 hours for each child. For the children aged between 9 and 24 months we used spontaneous speech recordings with baby–mother–researcher interaction. The therapist and the mother used toys and materials that the child liked or became excited about in his/her own environment. With the older children we used picture compositions from the phonological subtest of the SST (Sesletim ve Sesbilgisi Testi-Articulation and Phonology Test, Topbaş, 2004).

In our first part of the study (Topbaş *et al.*, 2012) we analysed 20 children (8 females, 12 males). In that study we could only present the first five stages of TR-LARSP due to the age profile of the data. With an extended sample we have now completed the missing stages of the profile and make some minor changes in general. However, the overall results support first part of the study.

Because of the agglutinative structure of Turkish, there is a wide range of suffixes that we must consider including in the TR-LARSP chart. Further, there were some processes like reduplication and scrambling that we wanted to mention in the developmental period. Therefore, we have added inflections in a new column at the right-hand side of the chart.

Other structures and grammatical structures that we wanted to mention are under the 'word type/other' column.

Types of Utterance

In the adaptation of TR-LARSP, 4500 utterances were analysed. After the analysis process 83 morphosyntactical structures were identified in children's speech. These structures were categorically grouped under 16 headings to allow a statistical analysis. Only the morphosyntactical structures that were used by more than 50% of the children were analysed. While drawing up this list, Göksel and Kerslake (2005) was followed. These structures are shown below.

1. Existential sentences
2. Copular sentences
3. Embedded sentences
4. Bound sentences
5. 2-element sentences
6. 3-element sentences
7. 3+ element sentences
8. Conjunctions
9. Question sentences
10. Determiners
11. Noun phrases
12. Adverbial clauses
13. Complex structures
14. Case suffixes
15. Possessive suffixes
16. Postposition

Morphosyntactical structures that were seen in more than 50% of the children

1. Negation suffix: -mA
2. Comment suffix: Ø
3. Aspect: -(y)E
4. Aspect /Aorist: -Ir
5. Future: -AcAk
6. Past: -dI
7. Aspect/Evidential: -mIş
8. Aspect: -Iyor

Stage I

Stage I is based on data from nine children. Our analysis was based on 450 utterances from this group. The structures that were seen in all of the stage I

Table 9.1 Stage I

Minor	Responses 40	Vocatives 72	Other 39	Problem 13		
Major	*Comm*	*Quest*	*Statement*	*Inflection*		
	C	Q	(S)V	-DI[1]	ACC	1S
			V_{neg}	Ø	LOC	3S
				DAT	mA_{neg}	

ACC: accusative, LOC: Locative, DAT: Dative, V_{neg}: Verb with negative marker, S: Singular.

children were root and inflected verbs, question words, and nouns. In terms of Minor sentences, there were 40 responses, 72 vocatives, 39 other and 13 problem structures. For Major sentences, there were 51 comments, 10 questions, 106 statements and 100 morphological inflections were analysed.

In our 2012 study we divided stage I into two sub-categories named stage 1A and stage 1B. But after analysing the data noted above, we combined these two categories. To make this combination, we applied a 30% 'must be seen' criterion to the structures. In other words, if a structure was not seen in 30% of the children's speech, we did not add the structure to the chart.

Inflections are analysed under two sub categories, *verbal inflections* and *nominal inflections*. These inflections and the whole structures of stage I can be seen in Table 9.1.

The uninflected verbs were labelled as comments as they are in bare forms. These verbs also represent the imperative mood as in *aç-* ('open'), *git-* ('go') and *gel-* ('come'). So, they are categorized as statements and put under the statement column.

In Table 9.2 there are examples of noun and verb categories. Near the end of the stage *–DI* and negative marker *–mA* is attached to the verbs. The use of progressive *–Iyor* is described in our earlier study and was included in that study's stage 1B. However, the use of the suffix is under 30% so we did not add it to stage I of the current description.

Question word *ne?* is seen with the locative case suffix *-dE* to ask the place of someone or something *ne:dE* ('where').

Table 9.2 Stage I: Categories

Command	Quest	Noun	Verb
aç- 'open' al- 'take'	ne:-dE where-LOC-3S	muz 'banana' ayı 'bear'	git-me go-NEG
gel- 'come'		fil 'elephant' bebe 'baby'	dü:tü fall-PAST

At the statement level, children use single word statements. Indeed, all the children tend to communicate with single word utterances. As we mentioned before, by the end of stage I, two-element structures can be seen; however, the majority of the children do not use these structures. It was difficult to determine the age ranges, as there seems to be an overlap between stage I and stage II. Thus, we used the 30% criterion to set a border between these two stages. Two-element structures did not pass the 30% criterion in stage I and the emergence of these structures is assigned to stage II.

Stage II

Data for stage II comes from eight children. In this period, sentences contain two-element structures. The use of nominal and verbal markers with multi-member suffixes increases. The latest version of stage II can be seen in Table 9.3.

Table 9.3 Stage II

Command	Q	Statement	Phrase	Word type/other	Inflections	
BakX *look*	Q	SV_{EX}	NP (Adj N)	Pronoun	Poss	Voice
VX	XQ	SV	NP (N N)	Det_{dem}	*-Iyor*	GEN
XV		SV_{EXneg}			*-AcAK*	
		SAV				
		SV_{COP1}				

SV_{EX}: *Subject–verb existential sentence,* SV_{EXneg}: Subject–verb negative existential sentence, SV_{COP1}: Subject–verb copular type 1 sentence, Det_{dem}: Demonstrative determiner, GEN: Genitive, Poss: Possessive.

There are three structures *VX*, *XV* and *BAK+X* in the Command category. *VX* and *XV* structures are formed with the attachment of a structure before or after the verb. BAK+X is commonly seen at this stage. The verb *bak* 'look' is used differently from its basic meaning 'to look' and from other bare verbs in the command category. This verb is used to attract the attention of the communication partner. The use of command structures can be seen in Table 9.4. In question sentences, differing from stage I, *X+Q* can be seen. Question words are, *ne* 'what', *nerde*, 'where' and *kaç* 'how many/much'.

As we mentioned before at the clause level, stage II differs from our original study. All the grammatical roles of the structures are assigned correctly by the children. The forms of statements were found to be SV, SV_{cop1}, SV_{ex1} and SV_{ex1NEG}.

In stage II copular markers begin to emerge. In the example in Table 9.5, there is no suffixation at the right end of the noun *okul* 'school'. The copular marker *-dir,* forms a nominal predicate when attached to a noun: 'okulda + *dır*'. The Copular marker is usually omitted in the spoken

Table 9.4 Stage II: Commands

Command			
BAKX			
bak	**X**	**Category**	**Extra Info**
Bak **'look'**	küçücük 'very small'	Verb+Noun	-cUK (nom inf.)
E	**X**		
ver **'give'**	o-nu Verb+*Det*$_{dem}$ +*ACC* *'this'*		
X	**E**		
Anne **Mommy**	gel come	Noun+*Verb*	

Nom inf: Nominal inflection.

Table 9.5 Stage II: Statements

Statement		
S	**V**	
Gemi **boat**	git-iyo go+ASP+3S	
'Boat is going'		
Ece **Ece**	oku-du read+PAST+3S read	
'Ece read'		
Subject	**Object**	**Verb**
Ben **I**	tarak comb	al-dı-m take+PAST+1S
'I bought comb'		
Subject	**Adverbial**	**Verb**
Sen **you**	doktor-a doctor+DAT	git go
'You, go to a doctor'		
Subject	**Verb**$_{cop1}$	
Abi **brother**	okul-da *Ødır* school+LOC+*Øcop*	
'Brother probably at school'		
Subject	**Verb**$_{ex1}$	
Araba **car**	var there is	
Subject	**verb**$_{ex1NEG}$	
Ekmek **bread**	yok there is not	

Cop: Copula, Ex: Existential, NEG: Negative, ASP: Aspect.

Table 9.6 Stage III

Command	Q	Statement	Word type/other	Phrase	Inflections
VXY	XYQ QXY XQY $VQ_{ml}X$	OV_{cop2} SV_{cop2} SOV_{cop1} SAV	Değil- not dA (topic marker) çünkü (conjunction) scrambling Det_{ind} Det_{class}	Pronoun N Adv V	PL ABL *-mlş* *-(y)E* *-Ir* 2S

Det_{ind}: Indefinite determiner, Det_{class}: Classification determiner, PL: Plural, ABL: Ablative, 2S: Second person singular.

language, and the omitted suffix is showed as a null category in the example. Existential sentences used with *var* 'there is' and *yok* 'there is not' are also observed at this stage.

Stage III

Data for stage III came from 10 children. At this stage statements usually contain three elements. Stage III has an increase in sentence structure types compared with stage II. Also new grammatical processes emerged. All of the morpho-syntactical structures of stage III can be seen in Table 9.6.

At the statement level, $OV_{cop2,}$ $SV_{cop2,}$ SOV_{cop1} and SAV sentence forms are used. The details, with examples, can be found in Table 9.7.

Table 9.7 Stage III: Statements

Statements		
Subject	**Adverbial**	**Verb**
O **That**	kaydırak-tan slide+ABL	kay-ı-cam slip+FUT+1S
'I will slip from that slide'		
O **That**	makine-de machine+LOC	yıka-n-mış wash+V+EVD+3S
'It has washed in that machine'		
Object	**$Verb_{cop2}$**	
Pis **Dirty**	ol-du be-PAST	
Subject	**$Verb_{cop2}$**	
Kaza **Accident**	ol-du happen-PAST	
Subject	**Object**	**$Verb_{cop1}$**
Bu **This**	kurbağa frog	*Ødır* is

Cop_2: Copular type 2, FUT: Future, LOC: Locative, V: Voice, ASP: Aspect, EVD: Evidential.

In our research we coded the verb *ol-* as 'copula type 2- (cop_2)'. In stage III, the copular function of the verb *ol-* 'be' emerges. In this use, the verb shows whether there is a static or a dynamic meaning. The examples are two element ones because the emergence of the verb was observed in two-element compound structures. Also, copula type 1 *-Ødır* is omitted and can be seen in three-element structures with the null category.

Değil 'not' has a negating meaning and is used especially in linking type nominal sentences. It can combine with the suffixes that occur in nominal predicates, namely copular markers. In stage III, children tend to use *değil* to state negativity. Ex: *soğuk değil* 'it is not cold', but they rarely use the word for linking. Ex: *O değil bu* 'It is not that, this is it'.

When the suffix *–dA* is written separate from the preceding noun it becomes a topic marker and discourse connective. It could have several functions such as adversative and additive in the sentence. At this stage children use different forms of the topic marker *–dA*. Examples can be seen in Table 9.8.

Table 9.8 Stage III: *-dA* topic marker

Topic Marker		
O-nu	***da***	**al-a-yım**
That-ACC	***too***	**take-OPT-1S**
'I take that one *too*'		
Bu *da*		**babası**
That is		**father-POSS&2S**
'That is his father' (presenting someone else before and secondly pointing to the father)		
Beni *de* götür		
Me *too* take-AOR-3S		
'Take me *too*'		

AOR: Aorist, OPT: Optative.

The causal conjunction *çünkü* 'because' emerges at stage III. It has a causative meaning in which the later clause explains the cause of the first one. Children can use *çünkü* in different positions in the sentence. At this stage children develop scrambling. The most scrambled word order is SVO. This could be due to the possibility of flexible word order in Turkish. They also scramble *çünkü* and use the conjunction at the beginning of the sentence with no previous information. Examples of *çünkü* can be seen in Table 9.9.

The inflections that emerge in stage III are evidential *–mIş*, aspect *–Ir* and *–(y)E*. In the word type/other category determiners can be seen. At this stage children start to use the indefinite determiner *bir* 'a', and the classification determiners *böyle, öyle* 'like this/ like that'.

Table 9.9 Stage III: Conjunction

Çünkü-conjunction

Sana ver-me-z	***çünkü***	**kır-ıyo-sun**
You give-NEG-AOR	**because**	**break-ASP-2S**

'He does not give it to you because you break it'

Çünkü	**bil-m-iyor-um**
Because	**know-NEG-ASP-1S**

'Because I do not know'

Determiners

O *bir araba*
This is *a* Det$_{ind}$ car

Böyle	**oje**	**sürüyosun**
***Like that* Det$_{class}$**	**nail polish**	**apply-ASP-2S**

'You apply nail polish *like that*'

Stage IV

In stage IV, we analysed 10 children between 31–36 months of age. At this stage four-element structures can be seen. The most important point in this stage is the emergence of complex sentences with subordinate clauses.

Table 9.10 Stage IV

Statement		Word type/other	Phrase	Inflections
ASV$_{ex1}$	SAV+	*diye*	PP	*-Inlyor*
SAAV	E$_a$	*-ki*		*-mIşDI*
SOV+	E$_n$	Compounds		
SOAV	B$_{same}$	Conj *sonra*		
SAOV	B$_{dif}$	Det$_{quan}$		
ASV				

The forms of statements at this stage are found in 11 categories as mentioned in Table 9.10. The detailed information about statement types and examples can be seen in Table 9.12 (see later). With the increased use of conjunctions, clitics and compounds, children begin to make more syntactical operations and more complex sentences. These complex structures can cause problems as we mentioned in our first TR-LARSP chapter (Topbaş *et al.*, 2012).

A postpositional phrase is formed with a noun followed by a postposition. The postposition is the head of the phrase and the noun phrase is its complement. In stage III there are two postpositions that we identified in children's speech. These are *için gibi*, and *–(y)lA/ile*. Examples of the postpositions are given in Table 9.11.

Table 9.11 Stage IV: Phrase-level categories

Postpositional Phrase	***diye***
kuş koymak için **bird putting for** **'for putting bird'**	Karlar gelmesin *diye* süpürdü Snow-PL come-NEG so that sweep-PAST-S2 'She swept so that the snow wouldn't come'
çakmak-la yak-(t)ım **with the lighter flicked I** **'I flicked with the lighter'**	Hop *diye* düştüm Oops as fall-PAST-1S 'I fell as oops'
Bizim lamba-mız gibi **Our lamp-PL3 like** **'Like our lamp'**	
-ki	**Det$_{quan}$**
çanta-sı(n)da-ki kitabı **case+POSS+LOC+*ki*** **'the book in her case'**	Şeker-ler-in hepsi-ni ye-di-m Candie-PL-GEN hepsi-ACC ate-PAST-1S 'I ate all of the candies'.

diye is the converbial form of the verb *de-* 'say'. It can function as a subordinator marking noun clauses and adverbial clauses. At this stage *diye* is used at the end of sentences and specifies the cause of the action. Examples of *diye* can be seen in Table 9.11.

-ki emerges as a complex adjectival in stage III. Phrase constructions are made with locative-marked *-dA* expression or possessive-marked *-IN* expressions. Examples of *–ki* can be seen in Table 9.11.

Complex inflections attach more than one suffix to one verb. This stage is a productive stage for verbal inflections. Children can attach two verbal inflections to a verb.

At this stage, four-member inflectional suffixes occur. Children can construct verbal paradigms such as *-InIyor* and *–mIşDI*. *-In* is a reflexive voice suffix. It attaches to transitive verbs to form an intransitive verb. It has a meaning that the action is performed by the person him/herself. It is combined with the aspect marker *-Iyor*. These structures are used correctly and with the right grammatical roles by the children. They can produce appropriate sentences in the right contexts. Examples of these suffixes can be seen in Table 9.12.

At this stage children can produce bare finite noun clauses as exemplified in Table 9.12 as embedded noun statements. Also, they can produce finite noun clauses with a subordinator with *diye* and the verb *–de* 'say'. Mostly, they drop the preceding superordinate clause and finish the sentence after *diye* as in the examples in Table 9.11. But the grammatical roles and the context of the sentences are used correctly by the children.

Non-finite adverbial clause markers can be seen at this stage. In most of the examples the *–(y)IncA* converbial suffix is added to the verb. Also *–mAk için* is used as an adverbial subordinator by the children. These adverbial subordinators are termed embedded adverbial clauses and examples can be seen in Table 9.12.

Table 9.12 Stage IV: Statement level

Statements			
Adverbial	**Subject**	**Verb$_{ex}$**	
Bur-da **Here-LOC**	hayvan-lar animal-PL 'animals'	var 'is'	
Adverbial	**Subject**	**Verb**	
Ordan **There-LOC**	oje 'nail polish'	ak-ıyor pour-ASP	
Subject	**Adverbial**	**Verb+**	
Ben **'I'**	abla-m-ın okul-u-na sister-POSS school-DAT	git-ti-m go+PAST+1S 'went'	
Subject	**Adverbial**	**Adverbial**	**Verb**
Ben **'I'**	bugün 'today'	okul-a school-DAT 'to school'	git-mi-ce-m go+NEG+FUT+1S will not go
'I will not go to school today'			
Subject	**Object**	**Verb+**	
Ben **'I'**	kırmızı başlıklı kız 'little red riding hood'	oku-du-m read+PAST+1S 'read'	
Subject	**Adverbial**	**Object**	**Verb**
Biz **'we'**	öğretmenle 'with the teacher'	resim-ler 'picture-PL'	çiz-iyor-uz draw+ASP+1P 'drawing'
Subject	**Object**	**Adverbial**	**Verb**
Biz **'we'**	çiş-imiz-i pee-PL1-ACC	tuvalet-e toilet-DAT	yap-ıyor-uz do+ASP+1P
We pee to the toilet			
Embedded Statements (Adv)			
Sarı **'Yellow'**	yan-ınca light-ADV	hemen 'immediately'	hazır ol-uyor-sun ready be-ASP-2S 'you get ready'
Embedded Statements (Noun)			
Kurt **'The wolf'**	burda 'here'	ev-ine git-mek ' home-POSS go-N	istedi 'want'
Bound Statements (Same)			
Banyo-da **Bathroom-LOC**	sabun-u soap-ACC	al-mış take-EVD	yıka-n-ıyo wash-V-ASP
Bound Statements (Different)			
Ama bura-ya **but here-LOC**	bir tane-si-ni one piece-GEN-ACC	çek-ti-m take-PAST-1S	ol-ma-dı be+NEG+ PAST

(Continued)

Table 9.12 *(Continued)*

Complex Verbal Inflections	
-lnlyor	yıka-n-ıyor wash+V+ASP+3S 'He is taking a shower'
-mIşDI	yarış-mış-tı-k compete+EVD+PAST+1P 'We competed against each other'

Bound sentences are those that consist of a minimum of two predicates that refer to the same subject or a different subject. In this type of sentence there is no conjunction word or inflection to link the sentences. Word stress and, in writing, the use of a comma makes the distinction between the sentences. At this stage children can use these types of syntactic structures especially in storytelling. Prosodic characteristics of the sentences are attached correctly by the children.

Stage V

This basis for the analysis at this stage is data from 11 children. At this stage sentences contain five elements. Also, we saw three-element sentences of types that we did not see before. Another important point is that the reciprocal pronoun emerges in this stage. The morphosyntactical categories of this stage can be seen in Table 9.13.

This stage is a more complex form of stage IV. The length of the sentences in words increases. Children can construct more complicated structures and join them more easily. With the increase of word knowledge and use of more complex suffixes children can produce more complex sentences. They can use and join subordinate clauses more often. Stage V is more productive than stage IV. The number of noun phrases and adjectival phrases in this stage also increases.

As seen in Table 9.14, children's statements are getting longer in this stage. Further, they use the copular verb *dIr* more effectively and construct different forms of sentences that were not seen in the former stages.

At this stage, the types of conjunctions increase. In particular, through the second part of the stage, children could use conjunctions more often and they could join sentences correctly. Also, they use the right

Table 9.13 Stage V

Statement		Word type/other	Inflection
SAOV+	SAV_{cop1}	Conj: ki, ve, ama, ile	*-lllr*
ASV_{cop1}	OSV	Reciprocal pronoun *birbirleri*	*-llmlş*

Table 9.14 Stage V: Statements

Statements				
Subject	**Adverbial**		**Object**	**Verb+**
O 'he/she'	çay-ın tea-GEN	iç-i-ne in-POSS-DAT	şeker 'sugar'	atıyo put+ASP+3S
Adverbial	**Subject**			**Verb$_{cop1}$**
Burası **'Here'**	yata(ğ)-ın bed-GEN 'bedspread'	örtü-sü spread-POSS		*-dIr Ø*
Subject	**Adverbial**			**Verb$_{cop1}$**
Annem **'My mom'**	çok 'very'	güzel beatiful		*-dIr Ø*
Object	**Subject**		**Verb**	
Abi-yi **'Brother-ACC'**	elektrik 'electric'		çarp-mış shock-EVID+3S	

conjunction in the right context. The most commonly used conjunctions are *ile* and *ama*. The reciprocal pronoun *birbir-* is used in the context where two parties act mutually. *Birbir-* is obligatorily inflected for person by combining with the plural possessive suffixes. These forms can be further inflected for case. Examples can be seen in Table 9.15.

Table 9.15 Stage V: Conjunctions and reciprocal pronoun

Conjunctions
Ama 'but'
Ama anne-m iste-m-iyo **But my mother want-NEG-ASP** **'But my mother does not want'**
Ve 'and'
Kitap ve defter var **Book and notebook there are** **'There are book and notebook'**
ile 'with'
Bişi ile su-(y)u karıştır-ıyo-sun **Stg with water-ACC mix-ASP-2S** **'You mix something with water'**
Ki 'so'
Ben o-(n)dan kork-ma-m ki **I him-ABL afraid-NEG-1S so** **'I am not afraid of him so'**
Reciprocal pronoun
Tabanca-(y)la birbirlerini vur-uyor-lar **Gun- each other shot-ASP-PL** **'They shoot each other with a gun'**

Table 9.16 Stage V: Complex inflections

Complex Inflections		
-Illr	Kapı açılır open+V+AOR 'door opens'	
-Ilmlş	Kaza Accident 'accident has been made'	yap-ıl-mış make+V+EVID

Complex inflections that we see in this stage are *–Illr* and *–Ilmlş*. Especially with the increased control of the language, children begin to use more complex structures in telling stories or about something that happened. *–Illr* is the combination of the passive voice suffix *–Il* plus an aspect suffix. It can be attached to transitive and intransitive stems. It turns transitive verbs to intransitive ones. In this complex structure *–Il* and aspect *–Ir* , in the second example *–Il* and evidential *–mlş* are combined. The examples of complex inflections can be seen in Table 9.16.

Stage VI

This stage is based on data analysed from 11 children aged between 43–53 months of age. At this stage, statements consist of five elements. Children become more productive and construct more subordinate clauses with conjunctions. Command and question categories, however, do not have any structures specific to this stage. In the inflection category, there is an increase in the variety and usage of complex inflections. Children use verbal suffixes more productively. The new structures in stage VI can be seen in Table 9.17.

Table 9.17 Stage VI

Statement	Inflections	
E_{adv} 1	*-Irmlş*	*-IyorDI*
Discourse	*-IlDI*	*-Iyormlş*

At this stage embedded adverbial clauses expand. In the example in Table 9.18, we can see that two subordinate clauses that are formed with the adverbial clause suffix *–Ip* are included. Also in that example, the child uses two conjunctions, *çünkü* and *sonra*, in the same sentence. There is no other new form of sentence construction in this stage.

Table 9.18 Stage VI: Statements

Embedded Adverbial Clause 1						
Çünkü eve	gid-ip go-CONJ	okul	kıyafetlerimi	giy-ip wear-CONJ	sonra	gid-ice-m go-FUT-1S
'Because, I go home and wear my school clothes and after this I'll go'						

Table 9.19 Stage VI: Complex inflections

Complex Inflection	
-IyorDI	bil-m-iyor-du-m know+NEG+ASP+PAST+1S 'I did not know'
-Iyormlş	yi-yor-muş eat+ASP+EVD+3S 'he/she was eating'
-Irmlş	yap-tır-mış do+V+EVD+3S 'he/she made it done'
-IlDI	Boz-ul-du break+V+PAST+3S 'it broke'

At this stage complex inflection types are more productive. Examples of suffixes that can be seen are given in Table 9.19.

Stage VII

The last stage of TR-LARSP, stage VII represents the analysis of 11 children's data. These children were aged between 55–67 months. At this stage, statements contain multiple elements. The acquisition of the morphosyntactical structures is nearly completed. Being at the end of the acquisition period children begin to show their own choices of language use. Thus, they have a higher ability to use or manipulate their language. However, at this stage command and question categories do not show any significant developments. The children could produce question sentences in the same forms as at previous stages but with more words or phrases. In the inflection category complex structures that emerged before were used more productively by the children. The only suffix newly emerging in this stage is the possibility marker *–Abil*. The new structures that emerged in stage VII can be seen in Table 9.20.

At this stage we see that the sentence forms expand. More noun phrases and adjectival phrases are used in the sentences. The use of different types of adverbial in the sentences also increases. Pointing to a location correctly,

Table 9.20 Stage VII

Statement			Word type/Other	Inflections
SAAAV	E_n	1	Conj: ondan sonra, hem de	-Abil
ASOV				

Table 9.21 Stage VII: Statements

Statements

Subject	**Adverbial**	**Adverbial**	**Adverbial**	**Verb**
O **him/her**	bur-da here-LOC	merdiven-ler- den stair-PL-ABL 'from the stairs'	Anne-si-(y)le Anne-ACC- CONJ 'with her mom'	in-iyo come down- ASP 'come down'
'He is coming down from the stairs with her mom here'				
Adverbial	**Subject**	**Object**	**Verb**	
Bur-da **Here-LOC**	anne-si mom-ACC 'her mom'	bir şey something	Dök-üyo pour-ASP	
'Her mother pouring something here'				
Subject	**Adverbial**	**Adverbial**	**Object**	**Verb**
Dede-m **Grandfather-POSS**	bana to me	hergün everyday	balon balloon	al-ıyor buy-ASP-3S
'My grandfather buys ballon to me everyday'				

time expressions, and explaining the time of the actions can all be seen. With this emergence of the almost complete morphosyntactical structure of Turkish, children begin to attach words correctly in the right order. Examples of the statements of stage VII can be seen in Table 9.21.

Temporal conjunction *ondan sonra*, and additive conjunction *hem de* emerge in this stage. *Hem, hem de* conjunctions usually emphasise the equal status and function in an utterance of two or more persons, objects or events (Göksel & Kerslake, 2005). Sometimes it is only used for adding extra information to the sentence. At this stage children use *hem de* for adding extra information to their sentence. These conjunctions can be seen in Table 9.22.

Table 9.22 Stage VII: Conjunctions

Temporal conjunction

Ondan sonra **'after that'**					
Ondan **sonra** ***After that***	**balı(ğ)-ın** **fish-GEN**	**ağ(ı)z-ın-dan** **mouth-POSS-ABL**	**köpük-ler** **bubble-PL**	**çık-ıyo** **come out-ASP**	
'After that bubles are coming out from fish's mouth'					
Additive conjunction					
Hem de 'also'					
Başka **Other**	**toka-lar-ım** **hairclip-PL-POSS**	**da** **too**	**var** **have**	***hem de*** **also**	**yeni** **new**
'I have other hairclips *also* new too'					

Table 9.23 Stage VII: Inflection

Inflection

-Abil	Ayıcık	gel-ebil-di come+MOOD+PAST+3S
	'Little bear *able to come* (at last)'	

Name:			**Age:**	**Date:**		**Type:**	
Stage I (0,9 - 1,6)	**Minor**		*Responses*		*Vocatives*	*Other*	*Problems*
	Major	Comm	Quest	Statement	Inflections		
		V	Q	(S)V V_{NEG}	-DI DAT ACC	LOC -*mA*$_{Neg}$	1S 3S
Stage II (1,6-2,0)	Conn.	Clause			Word type/Other	Phrase	Inflections
		Bak X VX XV	XQ	SV_{EX} SV SOV $SV_{EX(NEG)}$ SV_{COP1}	Det_{dem} Pronoun	NP(Adj N) NP(N N)	Voice Poss Gen *-Iyor* *-AcAK*
Stage III (2,0 - 2,6)	*çünkü*	VXY XYV	XYQ QXY XQY $VQ_{mI}X$	OV_{COP2} SV_{COP2} SOV_{COP1} SAV	*değil* *dA-* Topic marker Det_{ind} Det_{class} scrambling	Pron N	PL ABL *-mIş* *-(y)E* *-Ir* 2S
Stage IV (2,6 - 3,0)	*sonra*	VXY+ XYV+	QXY+ $SOV+Q_{mI}$	ASV ASV_{EX} SAAV SOV+ SOAV SAOV SAV+ E_A E_N B_{same} B_{dif}	*diye* *-ki* Compounds Det_{quan}	PP NP +	*-InIyor* *-mIşDI*
Stage V (3,0 - 3,6)	*ve* *ama* *ile* *ki*			ASV_{COP1} SAOV+ SAV_{COP1} OSV Coord 1 1+ Subord 1 1+	Reciprocal pronoun *birbirleri*		*-IlIr* *-IlmIş*
Stage VI (3,6 - 4,6)	*Conn+* *Discourse*			E_{ADV} 1 1+			*-IrmIş* *-IlDI* *-IyorDI* *-IyormIş*
Stage VII (4,6 -+)	*ondan* *sonra* *hem* *hem de*			SAAAV E_N 1 1+			*-Abil*

Figure 9.1 TR-LARSP profile

At this stage the *–Abil* suffix is seen. This suffix expresses an action's possibility to happen. The example of the suffix can be seen in Table 9.23. In Figure 9.1, the whole TR-LARSP chart can be seen.

Conclusion

In this chapter we finalized our study of the adaptation of LARSP to Turkish as TR-LARSP. We found that the TR-LARSP comprehensively represented the language acquisition of the children studied.

TR-LARSP is a reference tool for speech and language therapists. Recording the developmental data and the emergence of the morpho-syntactic structures of children in one chart provides the opportunity to make a rapid assessment of the child's language. Also, speech-language therapists can easily plan a therapy program concerning the grammatical requirements for the development of the children. The TR-LARSP chart may be a good starting point for further research for developing clinically useful materials in the field of speech and language therapy for Turkish.

Note

(1) During suffixation morphophonological alternations may occur due to vowel and consonant harmony in that all grammatical suffixes harmonize with the last vowel of the lexical stem. Thus, a suffix may have different forms and the alterable sounds in suffixation are usually indicated by capital letters. For detailed information see; Topbaş *et al.* (2012).

References

Cangökçe-Yaşar, Ö. and Topbaş, S. (2018) Profiling morpho-syntactical development of cochlear implanted children with TR-LARSP. *Clinical Linguistics & Phonetics* 32 (3), 181–192.

Göksel, A. and Kerslake, C. (2005) *Turkish: A Comprehensive Grammar.* Routledge.

Topbaş, S. (2004) Türkçe Sesletim-Sesbilgisi Testi (SST) [Turkish Articulation and Phonology Test]. *Ankara, Turkey: Milli E.*

Topbaş, S., Cangökçe-Yaşar, Ö. and Ball, M.J. (2012) LARSP for Turkish (TR-LARSP). In M.J. Ball, D. Crystal and P. Fletcher (eds) *Assessing Grammar: The Languages of LARSP* (pp. 282–305). Bristol: Multilingual Matters.

10 T-LARSP: A Grammatical Profile for Tamil

R. Lalitha Raja

Introduction

The Language Assessment Remediation and Screening Procedure (LARSP) is a linguistic profile chart framed for English by David Crystal and colleagues (e.g. Crystal, 1979) with a later revised version (Crystal *et al.*, 1989; Crystal, 1992), that summarizes the significant grammatical characteristics of children's language at different stages of normal language development. By analysing the language of a child, the clinician can determine the structures used by the child and structures where the child is having problems (Donaldson, 1995). LARSP is the most widely used tool for profiling grammatical constructions that children produce in spontaneous language samples in clinical settings. The profile structure has seven stages relating to chronological age, with an interpretation covering the structural organization: sentence, clause, phrase and word types (Müller *et al.*, 1981). Although there is a high demand for assessment tools, their development in many languages is still in its formative years. The provision of a Tamil version of LARSP is particularly urgent for the Tamil-speaking community. Developing such a profile for Tamil is challenging due to the linguistic structure of Tamil which differs from European languages, its diglossic character, and the varieties of dialects. Construction of the profile is also constrained by the lack of normative data. The data for the present work aim to give the picture of child language development in five stages (0-1, 1-2, 2-3, 3-4, 4-5). Data have been drawn from 96 children residing in five different districts of Tamil Nadu and from the TV programme 'Kutty-cutties' an adult and child interactive programme.

The Structure of Tamil

Tamil is one of the major languages of the Dravidian family of languages spoken in Southern India, predominantly by people of Tamil Nadu, Puducherry, Andaman and the Nicobar Islands, and Sri Lanka.

It has been given official status in Tamil Nadu, Puducherry, and Andaman and the Nicobar Islands.

Tamil has some distinguishing morphophonemic, syntactic and stylistic features. Agglutination of suffixing morphemes, free order of words in sentences, and head-final structure of phrases are some of the features that distinguish this language from European languages. Added complexity comes from its diglossic characteristics with the presence of both high and low varieties, besides a vast number of registers and dialects.

Morphology

To describe morphology, this study adopts the Kothandaraman (1997) model of description to describe the grammatical categories of Tamil. Tamil grammatical categories can be divided into word classes and particle classes. The word classes of Tamil have 10 categories: Noun, Verb, Adjective, Adverb, Intensifier, Conjunction, Interjection, Introductory, Summoners and Responsives. The particle classes of Tamil have five categories also: suffix (case and number), postposition, verbal participles, clitics, and fillers. Word formation with verbs and nouns in the Tamil language is agglutinative.

Agglutinative features

As an agglutinative feature, Tamil morphs are added in sequence (i.e. agglutinated or concatenated), thus words and even phrases are formed by adding suffixes which can be both derivational and inflectional onto the root form of the word.

Noun

A noun is a word which is capable of taking a case suffix. The following examples illustrate the structure of a noun with various suffixes and particles.

/peɳ	kaɭ	uk	ku	ɑ:kɑ:	mɑʈʈum	t̪ɑ:n	ɑ:	ɑʈɑ:/
Nst.	Pl.	Filler	Cs	Pp.	Cl.1	Cl.2	Cl.3	Cl.4.[1]
Woman	plural	---	to	for	only	only	is it	dear

Is it only for the women, dear?

/ɑ:ɳ	kɑɭ	in	ɑ:l	mɑʈʈum	t̪ɑ:n	ɑ:	ɑʈɑ:/
Nst.	Pl.	Filler	Cs	Cl.1	Cl.2	Cl.3	Cl.4.
man	plural		because of	only	only	is it	dear

Is it only because of the men, dear?

A noun stem (Nst.) can take one or more suffixes or particles as shown above. The number suffix, filler and the clitics (Cl) can occur with both nouns and verbs, whereas the case suffix (Cs) and the postpositions (Pp.) can occur only with nouns.

Case

The case marker is a suffix that occurs with a noun and changes the syntactic function of that noun. The following are the case suffixes in Tamil. Nominative is unmarked, Accusative is /-ɑi/, Associative/Sociative is /-o:ʈu ~ -oʈu/, Instrumental is /-ɑ:l/, Causative is /-ɑ:l/, Dative is /-ku/, Genitive is /-ɑt̪u/, Locative is /-il/, and Vocative is /-ee/.

Postpositions

Postpositions are the word-like elements which perform the function of the case suffix and are classified into five groups.

1. Accusative post positions come next to the accusative case suffix /-ɑi/
2. Dative post positions come next to the dative case suffix /-ku/
3. Genitive post positions come next to the genitive case suffix – /-ɑtu/ (optional)
4. Locative post positions come next to the locative case suffix – /-il/
5. Plain post positions, with examples of their use, are

/uʈɑn/	/ennuʈɑn/	(with me)
/ku:ʈɑ/	/enku:ʈɑ/	(with me)
/uʈɑijɑ/	/kɑnnɑnuʈɑijɑ/	(of Kannan)
/ʋɑcɑm/	/enʋɑcɑm/	(with me)
/iʈɑm/	/enniʈɑm/	(on/with me)
/ʋɑɾɑi/	/pɑt̪t̪uʋɑɾɑi/	(up to ten)
/ɑ:kɑ/	/pɑt̪t̪unɑ:ḷɑ:kɑ/	(for the (past) ten days)
/ɑ:kɑ/	/ɑɾɑcɑɾɑ:kɑ/	(as king)
/t̪o:ɾum/	/vi:ʈut̪o:ɾum/	(at every house)
/ɑ:ɾɑ/	/kɑɳɳɑ:ɾɑ/	(eyeful)

Clitics

Clitics, based on the order of occurrence, are grouped into four categories.

Clitics.1 (cl.1)

The following are the clitics which come under cl.1

/mɑʈʈum/ 'only', /mɑ:t̪t̪irɑm/ 'only', /ku:ʈɑ/ 'also', /-um/ 'also', and /-ee/ 'only'[2]

Clitics.2 (cl.2)

The following are the clitics which come under cl.2

/-t̪ɑ:n/ 'only', /-ɑ:ʋɑt̪u/ 'at least', /-e:num/ 'at least', /-ɑ:kilum/ 'at least', and /-ɑ:jinum/ 'at least'

Clitics.3 (cl.3)

The following are the clitics which come under cl.3

/-ɑ:/, /-e:/, and /-o:/ are interrogative markers

'e:' and 'o:' function as interrogative markers only when they are preceded by /t̪ɑ:n/

Clitics.4 (cl.4)

The following are the clitics which come under cl.4
/ɑʈɑ:/ for Masculine non-honorific, /ɑʈi/ for Feminine non-honorific, /uŋkɑ/ for honorific.sg., and /uŋkɑ/ for honorific.pl.

Verb

Any word which is capable of taking a tense marker is a verb and conjugates for person-number-gender. In addition to this, a verb may be qualified by an adverb or adverbial, and it may be changed into an adjectival or adverbial participle.

The complex structure of the verb may consist of: Verb stem + Aspe ct + Voice + Modal + Tense + PrNrG (person, number gender):

/eɻut̪ik - kɑ:ʈʈɑ - ʋɑikkɑp - pɑ:ɾ - t̪t̪ - ɑ:n - ɑ: - ɑʈɑ:/
write and show to make try (past) 3sg.masc. Q(did he) is it that-dear
Vst - (Aux.^{ASP}) -(Aux.^{VC})-(Aux.^{M})-Tns - PrNrG - (cl. 3) (cl. 4)
'Is it that dear he tried to make (one) to write and show?'

The aspectual auxiliaries are added to the verbal participial forms (e.g. /cejt̪u/, /colli/, etc.). They are classified into 12 in Tamil (Kothandaraman, 1997). They are; Progressive /koɳʈiru/, Perfective / iɾu/, Definitive /ʋiʈu/, Trial /pɑ:ɾ/, Demonstrational /kɑ:ʈʈu/, Reflexive /koɭ/, Reciprocal /koɭ/, Accidental /po:/, Contemptive /t̪olɑi/, Preservative /ʋɑi/, Benefactive /ɑɾuɭ/, and Habitual /ʋɑ:/. /-ɑ:/ is a marker indicating questioning which is considered as a clitic in Tamil (Kothandaraman, 1997).

In Tamil, the modal auxiliaries; inceptive /po:/, attemptive /pɑ:ɾ/, probablitative /ku:ʈu/, obligatory /ʋe:ɳʈu/, future negative /mɑ:ʈʈu/, and factive negative /illɑi/ are added to the infinitive forms of the verbs.

Passivization markers /pɑʈu~pɑʈʈ-/ and causative markers /ʋɑi-/ are classified under the voice auxiliaries that follow Vst in Tamil.

Negative forms are complex in Tamil and the spoken variety has most complex structures. For example:

cejjɑ+mɑ:ʈʈ+ɑ:n
to do not 3sg.m.
he will not do -- present and future
cejjɑ+ʋillɑi 'literal/standard form' /cejɑlɑ 'spoken'
to do not past.
he did not do -- past, where person number gender marking will not be marked.

/mɑ:ʈʈ-/ is classified as a modal auxiliary and is used to denote negation for future and /illɑi/ for past.

The informal imperative is unmarked in Tamil, e.g. /col/ 'say' – with no suffix.

The desiderative suffix is /-ɑʈʈum/, and /- kkɑʈʈum/ occurs with stems.
Ex: /ʋɑɾɑʈʈum/ 'let (sub.) come', /pɑʈikkɑʈʈum/ 'let (sub.) read'

The Optative suffix is /–kɑ/ which has an alternant /–kkɑ/. Ex:. /pɑṯikkɑ/ '(I wish)
you/he/she/they etc. read', celkɑ'(I wish) you/ he/she/ they etc. go'
The potential suffix is /- ɑlɑ:m/ and its variants are /- kɑlɑ:m/ and /-kkɑlɑ:m/ e.g : /po:kɑlɑ:m/ '.....may go', /pɑṯikkɑlɑ:m/ '.....may read', /collɑlɑ:m/ '..... may say'

The structure of the prohibitive form, which may also be called a negative imperative, is Vst. + neg.s + 2.pers.Sg. The negative marker is ɑ:t and its variants are /kɑ:t̪/ and /kkɑ:t̪/, e.g : /po:kɑ:t̪e:/ 'don't go', /n̪ɑṯɑ:kkɑ:t̪e:/ 'don't walk', /sollɑ:t̪e:/ 'don't say'.

Syntax

The sentence structure of Tamil is SOV. However, it has free word order due to morphological case marking. Also, it is a pro-drop language in that pronominal subjects can be omitted.

Free word order

/ɾɑ:mɑn	kɑṯɑikku	ceṉɾɑ:n/
Rama	shop-to	went

The alternative word orders, /kɑṯɑikku ɾɑ:mɑn ceṉɾɑ:n/ and /kɑṯɑikku ceṉɾɑ:n ɾɑ:mɑn/ etc. are also grammatically accepted in Tamil.

Pro- drop feature

/ʋɑɾu+kir+ɑ:n/
V + tense + PrNrG
come + present tense + 3sg.masc
'he comes'
/ʋe:kɑmɑ:kɑ ʋɑɾukirɑ:n
quickly come + present tense + 3sg.masc.
Adv. + V + tense + PrNrG
'he comes quickly'

The example specifies that the subject is IIIrd person-singular-masculine through the PrNrG concord, though the subject is not there in the sentence. So due to the concord feature, pro-drop is allowed in Tamil.

Coordination

Coordination can be classified into two broad classes: (1) Correlative and (2) Non-correlative.

Correlatives which come under coordinating conjunctions are:

/-um/	/n̪i:jum n̪ɑ:num/	You and I
/-o:/	/n̪i:jo: n̪ɑ:no:/	You or I
/-ɑ:ʋɑṯ̪u/	/n̪i:jɑ:ʋɑṯ̪u n̪ɑ:nɑ:ʋɑṯ̪u/	You or I

Correlatives which come under subordinating conjunctions are:

/ɑ:nɑ:l --um/ as in /ɑʋɑɾ ʋɑɾuʋɑ:ɾɑ:nɑ:l n̪ɑ:num ʋɑɾuʋe:n/
if he comes I also will come
/enrɑ:l --um/ as in /ɑʋɑɾ ʋɑɾuʋɑ:ɾenrɑ:l n̪ɑ:num ʋɑɾuʋe:n/
if he comes I also will come
Non-correlatives which come under coordinating conjunctions are:
/ɑ:nɑ:l/ 'but', /ɑt̪ɑnɑ:l/ 'therefore', ɑ:kɑijɑ:l 'so', /illɑije:l/ 'if not so', / illɑ:viʈʈɑ:l/ 'if not so', /iɾun̪t̪ɑ:lum/ 'even so', /ɑ:nɑ:lum/ 'even so'
Non-correlatives which come under subordinating conjunctions are:

/-um/	/ɑʋɑɾum ʋɑɾɑʋillɑi/	he did not come, either
/-ɑ:ʋɑt̪u/	/ɑʋɑɾɑ:ʋɑt̪u ʋɑn̪t̪iɾukkɑlɑ:m/	at least he could have come

Diglossic feature

Tamil is a diglossic language; that is, there is a large disparity between the written form of the language and the spoken form. These differences are found in the usage of grammatical features, vocabulary and pronunciation. The spoken form of /ʋi:ʈʈiliɾun̪t̪u/ is /ʋi:ʈləɾn̪t̪ɨ/ 'from home'. Children's productions are only of the spoken variety and have grammatical variations according to the spoken variety of language.

Standard	*Spoken*	*meaning*
/solliɾin̪t̪ɑ:ɭ/	/solliɾn̪t̪ɑ:/	has told (she)
/sollikoɳɖiɾun̪t̪ɑ:ɭ/	/solliʈʈrun̪t̪ɑ:/	was telling (she)
/ɑppɑ: po:jʋiʈʈɑ:ɾ/	/ɑppɑ: po:jʈɑ:ɾ~po:jʈuccɨ/	father had gone
/ɑn̪t̪ɑ pɑkkɑm/	/ɑŋgiʈʈɨ ~ ɑn̪t̪ɑ:ɳʈɑ/	that side
/t̪ɑnijɑ:/	/oɳʈijɑ:~ot̪t̪ɑijɑ:/	alone
/t̪iɾuʋiɻɑ:/	/t̪iɾisɑ:~no:mpi/	festival (at temple)
/po:kɑ ʋe:ɳʈum/	/po:kɑɳum/	want to go (I/we)
/ɑʈit̪t̪u ʋiʈʈɑ:n/	/ɑʈiccuʈʈɑ:n/	had bet (he)
/cejjɑ: ʋiʈʈɑ:l/	/cejjɑ:ʈʈi/	if not done (some one)
/ʋɑn̪t̪ɑ pooʎut̪u/	/ʋɑn̪t̪ɑppə/	when (some one) has come

/-cci ~ -ccɨ/ or /-t̪u/ or /-um/ are the PrNrG markers commonly used in most of the dialects for III person singular masculine and feminine subjects.

Design of Cross-sectional Data Collection

Data were collected from 96 children aged between 1 to 5 years. All the subjects were selected on the basis of the convenience sampling method. Only children with Tamil as a mother tongue were selected. The samples were recorded in the children's home (when playing with parent or peers) or school (when interacting with teacher or peers). Data were also drawn from the TV programme 'Kutty-cutties' – an adult and child interactive programme – for children in the age group 4;6-5;0 of the Urban group (6 children). The samples were sorted according to the age, gender and urban/rural background of the children and tabulated below in Table 10.1.

Table 10.1 Demographic details of typically developing children

Age in years	Rural		Urban		Total no. of Samples
	Boys	Girls	Boys	Girls	
1.0 - 1.6	3	3	3	3	**12**
1.6 - 2.0	3	3	3	3	**12**
2.0 - 2.6	3	3	3	3	**12**
2.6 - 3.0	3	3	3	3	**12**
3.0 - 3.6	3	3	3	3	**12**
3.6 - 4.0	3	3	3	3	**12**
4.0 - 4.6	3	3	3	3	**12**
4.6 - 5.0	3	3	3	3	**12**
Total no. of Samples	**24**	**24**	**24**	**24**	**96**

T-LARSP

Overall design of T-LARSP

Since sections A–D of the LARSP chart are not language-specific, those same sections have been retained in the T-LARSP profile chart. Likewise with the rest of the chart, the Minor /Major Sentence distinction is retained, as are the distinctions between Command, Question and Statement; Connectivity, Clause and Phrase; and the developmental stages I–VII, whereas the category 'word' is labelled as 'morpheme' in T-LARSP due to the morphological complexity of the language. An attempt to analyse Tamil data using LARSP categories shows that there are many constructions and categories found to differ between the two languages. As with the English version, constructions have been assigned to different stages of the T-LARSP chart based mainly on the number of constituent morphemes.

In assigning patterns to Clause, Phrase and Morphological levels, the following criteria were used. As noted earlier, Tamil is a pro-drop language and inflections play both syntactic and morphological roles. They are therefore listed not only in the morphology column, but in the Command and Statement columns as well. Due to the late acquisition of compound verbs in the Tamil children's data, this category without any inflections is placed in the clause column at stage II and analysed as N/ Adj V at stage II phrase level. Also, the sentence pattern in stage II VX and QX has to be XV and XQ for Tamil, i.e. 'come here' is /iŋkɑ ʋɑ:/ – *here come*; 'want water' is /t̪ɑɳɳi ʋe:ɳum/ – *water want* and 'what is this' is /it̪u ennɑ/ *this what*. For the PrN pattern it is NCs, i.e. Noun+case+/(postposition), e.g. /ʋi:ʈʈukku/- 'to house' comprised of /ʋi:ʈu+ku/ (dative case) *house+to*; /ʋi:ʈʈiliɾun̪t̪u/ - 'from the house' is made up of /ʋi:ʈu+il+iɾun̪t̪u/ *house+from* ('from': /il+iɾun̪t̪u/). Also the pattern VO has to be OV; V part has to be part V; and VOA has to be AOV and so on.

Detailed Description

Stage I

For stage I, the data of the children between 1;0 and 1;6 years were recorded, analysed and tabulated. They respond with mm (yes), m..hum (no). They produced nouns that they are exposed to, that are mainly found in their environment. Verbs are very few, like /ṯa:/ 'give', /ʋa:/ 'come', /ko:ṯu/ give', /po:/ 'go', /ukka:r/ 'sit' and /eṯu/ 'take'. Responses and requests like /e:j/ and /ṯe:j/ 'hey' are found. Negatives such as /na:na:/

Table 10.2 The T-LARSP Chart indicating morphological and syntactic structures produced by children of specific groups

A Unanalysed			**Problematic**		
1. Unintelligible	2. Symbolic Noise	3. Deviant	1. Incomplete	2. Ambiguous	3. Stereotypes

B Responses		Normal Response						Abnormal		Problems
		Major					Minor	Structural	φ	
	Repeti-	Elliptical			Reduced	Full				
Totals	tions	1	2	3+						
Stimulus type										
Questions										
Others										
C Spontaneous										

D Reactions		General	Structural	φ	Other	Problems

Stage I 1;0 - 1;6	Noun PN Verb Other (Vocatives Summoners Interjection)				
	Clause			Phrase	Morphology
	Comm.	Ques.	Statement		
Stage II 1;6 - 2;0	XV Pn/NCs	XQ	V^{I} PnCs N_{Neg} OV^{I} NCs CV^{I} Adv.Part.V^{I}	Pn_{ind} Adj N VTsPrNrG DN	Pl. Present Past (all forms) future
Stage III 2;0 - 2;6	XYV V^{Des}	V^{I}s-Q XWhQ	OV^{I} CV^{I} SO SC XV^{I}	D Adj N PnCs NCs $Aux.^{M}$ PrNrG	PrNrG Case
Stage IV 2;6 - 3;0	VV^{Des} PnV^{Neg} PnNCsAV $PnVP_{imp}$	WhQX PnWhQV^{I}	SAV^{I} NCsPp VP SOV^{I} SCV^{I} $S_{t}CO_{1}S_{t}$ 1 SOV^{Neg}	NCsPp Adv. Part.VP Adj. Part.N V_{inf} $Aux.^{M}$ PrNrG	$Aux.^{M}$ (ma:ṯṯu, ve:ṉṯum, illai) $Aux.^{ASP}$ (konṯiru, ʋiṯu) Neg WhQ Q
Stage V 3;0 - 3;6	In(S)V V^{Des} $PnCsV^{Neg}$ $PnCoNV_{imp}$	SWhQV $SV^{I}Q$ $SXV^{I}Q$	S_{t}Neg. S_{t}Emp. S_{t}Verif. SO/CV^{I} $S_{t}Co_{2}$ S_{t} 1 $S_{t}Co_{1}S_{t}$ 1+	Adv.Part.$Aux.^{ASP}$ V_{inf} $Aux.^{VC}$ (caus) Adj. Part.N^{I}	Co Postpositions Negative participle Adjectival participle
Stage VI 3;6 - 4;0	Initiator + Co PnAdj.NPV_{imp} $PnN_{loc}AV_{imp}$	Complex XCoXQ	XCoX 1 1+ Ncl(cl)VP	AVP V_{inf} $Aux.^{VC}$	Adverbial participle

Stage VII 4;0 - 5;0	Discourse		Syntactic Comprehension
	A connectivity others Comment Clause Emphatic Order		Style
	Total no. Sentences	Mean no. Sentences Per turn	Mean Sentence Length

'don't want' and interjections, like /ɑ:h!/, /ɑi!/ are found. Other sounds can be described as babbling. Some of these sequences are able to be identified but others are unintelligible (Table 10.2).

Stage II

There are more differences found between LARSP and T-LARSP at stage II. Under command, XV was the pattern found in Tamil whereas it is VX in LARSP. /pommɑ t̪ɑ:/ *toy give* 'give a toy' and /t̪ɑɳɳi t̪ɑ:/ - *water give* 'give water' /iŋgɑ ʋɑ:/ *here come* 'come here' were the examples for XV. Nouns that name play and food items related to the child were used in this construction.

The structure XQ represents the frequent use of the question pattern /ʋɑn̪t̪ɑ:nɑ:/- *come-past- 3per.m.sg.-Q* 'Did (he) come?', and /pommɑijɑ:/, 'is it a doll?'.

At this stage, it is statements that show the main differences from the English LARSP. The first is the pro-drop feature, i.e. V^I (with ^{I} standing for inflection). Even adults follow this pattern in discourse, like /ʋɑn̪t̪ã:/ *came (he)* 'he came', /po:ccu/ *went (she)* 'she went', /ʋɑɾuʋẽ:/ *will come (I)* 'I will come'. In the above sentences, an overt subject is not found which is grammatically acceptable in Tamil as the verb + inflection specifies the meaning of a complete sentence. Here the PrNrG markers used are /–ccu/, to specify IIIrd person singular (masculine, feminine and neuter) subject and /-ẽ:/ for Ist person singular and /-õ:/ for Ist person plural.

The pattern CV^I was found in utterances like /cu:ʈɑ: iɾukku/ *hot is (it)* 'it is hot'. Even here, the pro-drop feature was followed. Also, negative statements like /pommɑi illə/ *doll (is) not found* 'the doll isn't found', /ɑmmɑ: illə/ *mother (is) not found*, show the verb-less pattern in N_{Neg}.

The NCs pattern found in this stage was the form most often used as a sentence by the children. For questions like 'who is coming?', 'where has grandma gone?', the answer is /sɑʧin/ which means that 'sachin is coming' and /kɑ:ʈukku/ 'to the field'.

Also, N/PnCs was commonly found in this stage, such as /enɑkku/ *me-for* 'it is for me', also /ennut̪u/ 'mine', /unnut̪u/ 'yours' and /ɑkkɑ:kku/ *for-sister* 'this is for sister'.

The OV^I category listed in the Statement column has the pattern / miʈʈɑ:j t̪ɑn̪t̪uccu/ *sweet gave* /kɑ:cu t̪ɑn̪t̪uccu/ *money gave*, /pommɑi ʋɑ:nkunẽ:/ *doll bought*. Recall Tamil is a pro-drop language, and that verbs are inflected for tense and person – number and gender (PrNrG). The pattern Adv.part.V^I was produced in utterances such as /ʋɑ:ŋkɑ po:ccu/ *to buy went* 'she went to buy'.

Turning to the description of categories listed under phrase in this stage, it should be noted that the categories differ from those of English LARSP. For example, the $Pn_{ind.}$ pattern (e.g., /jɑ:roo/ 'somebody') is found.

VTs PrNrG is a verb inflected for tense and person (Pr), Number (Nr) and Gender (G). Example utterances include, /t̪an̪t̪uccu/ 'give-past (he/she/it)', /po:ʋut̪u/ 'go-present (he/she/it)' and /t̪aɾum/ 'give-future'. Here /–ccu/ is the PrNrG marker commonly used for IIIrd person singular subjects for past tense, /-um/ for future, /-t̪u/ for the present tense.

The category Adj.N is found in utterances like /peɾija pommai/ 'big doll', /kuʈʈi pa:ppa:/ 'small child', and DN is found in /an̪t̪a kaɾaʈi/ 'that bear' and /in̪t̪a akka:/ 'this sister'.

Stage III

At stage III, under the command category, XYV and $V^{Des.}$ structures are found. /n̪i: iŋka ʋa:/ *you –here come*; /enakku ca:kle:ʈʈɨ ta:/ *– me-to – chocolates – give* are found under the XYV category. In Tamil, there is no single word equivalent found for 'let', but the suffix – /-la:m/ with the verb provides the notion of 'let'. For example, the form /–la:m/ is added after the infinitive form of the verb, as in /po:ka/ 'to go' /ʋilaja:ʈa/ – 'to play' and /po:la:m/ 'let us go' /ʋilaja:ʈala:m/ 'let us play' etc. This category is termed as $V^{Des.}$ in T-LARSP.

In the question column, the QXY of English LARSP is inappropriate for T-LARSP. /-a:/ is a suffx attached to V^{I} to frame questions as in / po:na:na:/ *did (he) go* 'did he go?'. Children's wh- questions model the adult language pattern of questioning at this stage. The children always put the question word /e:n/ 'why?' to ask for reasons. Also, the pattern XWhQ was seen in /ad̪u ennu/ where the determiner is /ad̪u/- 'that'. Also found were /enna/- 'what' and /eŋka/ 'where', for example, /aɳɳan eŋka/ *brother where?* 'where is the brother?'.

In the statement section of stage III, O/CV^{I} was respresented in the utterances /ʈɾaiʋaɾa: iɾukka:ɾu/ *driver is (he)* and /n̪alla puɭɭa/ *(being) good girl/ boy*. V was missing in SC and SO structures as the copula is not normally used in Tamil.

Category SC was found in utterances like:

/aʋan n̪allaʋan/ 'he is good'
/aʋa˜ a:ji ~ aʋan keʈʈaʋan/ 'he is bad'
/n̪a: n̪alla pullə/ *I good child* 'I am a good child'
and also SO was found in /it̪u pe:na:/ *this (is a) pen* and /at̪u ka:ɾɨ/ *that (is a) car.*

XV^{I} was found in utterances such as /aʋan oʈina:n/ *he run (past)*, /aʋan aʈit̪t̪a:n/ *he beat (past)* and /ɾa:man aʈiccucu/ *raman beat (past)*. PrNrG for kinship terms such as subjects are /–ccu/ for past, /-um/ for future and /-t̪u/ for present in the spoken variety which was used by almost all the children.

Another type of utterance in the category XV^{I} is /pan̪t̪a aʈiccaã/ *hit the ball (he)* 'he hit the ball' where X is NCs, i.e. /pan̪t̪ai/ which is of the form N+Cs. ACs was found in utterances like /aŋka po:ra:n/ 'he goes there'. At the phrase level, the DAdjN structure was found in utterances such as /an̪t̪a periya pommai/ 'that big doll', and the pattern PnCs was seen in /enakku/ 'for me', /avanukku/ 'to him'and /avano:ʈa/ 'with him'.

NCs was seen in /kampa:l/ 'by or with (a) stick', and these forms were commonly found. The pattern Aux.^{M} PrNrG was found in utterances like /ma:ʈʈe:n/ 'won't (I)' and /ve:ɳʈa:m/ 'must not'.

Stage IV

In stage IV, Commands such as VV^{des}, PnV^{Neg}, PnNCsV and PnVP$_{imp}$ (PnAdv.Part.Aux^{M}) were found. Utterances such as /va: po:la:m/ *come go–let-us* and /va: velaja:ʈala:m/ *come play-let-us* illustrate the VV^{des} pattern. Utterances found under the PnV^{Neg} pattern included /n̪i: vara:t̪e:/ *you come-not*, /n̪i: aʈikka:t̪e:/ *you beat-not*, /n̪i: po:va:t̪e:/ *you go-not*, and /n̪i: t̪oʈa:t̪e:/ *you touch-not*.

The category PnNCsV was found in utterances like /n̪i: vi:ʈʈukkɨ va:/ *you home-to come* 'you come home' and /n̪i: kaʈaikku po:/ *you shop-to go*; and PnAdv.Part.Aux^{M} was found in utterances like /n̪i: ca:piʈʈɨpa:ru/ 'you try eating' and /n̪i: ceɲɟɨpa:ru/ 'you try doing'.

In Questions, all wh-words were found used by the children of this age group. The following utterances demonstrate WhQ development: /enna kalar/ 'what colour?'; /enna ve:ɳum/ *what (you) need?*; /ja:ru varra:/ *who comes?*; /enna conna:ŋka/ *what (they) tell-past?*; /eŋka po:riŋka/ *where (you) go-pre.cont.?*; /avan eŋka po:ra:n/ *where he go-pre.?*; /ja:ru caʈʈa/ *whose is (this) shirt?*; and /et̪ukku po:ra:n/ *why (he) go-pre.?*. Also, the PnWhQV[I] pattern emerged at this stage: /avan enna: panra:n/ *he what do-pre.* 'what is he doing?', and /n̪i: eŋka po:kanum/ *you where go-want-to* 'where do you want to go?'.

In the Statement column, SAV[I] was found in utterances such as /avan aŋka van̪t̪a:n/ *he there come-past-PrNrG* 'he came there' and /kannan n̪e:t̪t̪u pa:rt̪t̪a:n/ *kannan yesterday see-past-PrNrG* 'kannan saw yesterday'. SOV[I] was represented in utterances like /n̪a:n avanai pa:rt̪e:n/ *I he-Acc. Cs.-see-past-PrNrG* 'I saw him', /avan enniʈam pe:cina:n/ *he me-to speak-past-PrNrG* 'he spoke to me'. The pattern NCsPpVP was found in utterances like /enkiʈʈe:run̪t̪u piʈiŋkina:n/ *me from grab-past-PrNrG* 'he grabbed from me' and /avanukka:ka van̪t̪a:n/ *he-for come-past-PrNrG* 'he came for him'. SO/CV[I] was found in utterances like /avan aɻaka:ka irukka:n/ *he beautiful is-present-PrNrG* 'he looks beautiful' and /avan kaʈaikku po:ra:n/ *he shop-to go-present-PrNrG* 'he goes to shop'. Category S_t Co_1 S_t was found in utterances like /avanum n̪a:num po:no:m/ *he-*Co_a *me-*Co_a *go-past-PrNrG* 'he and I went' and /kala:vaccum supa:va:ccum va:ŋka/ *kala* Co_a *suba* Co_a *come-future-PrNrG* 'either kala or subha come here'. Also, the category SOV$^{Neg.}$ was found in utterances like /avaɭ sku:lukku po:ka ma:ʈʈa:/ *she-school to-go-future-Neg* 'she won't go to school'.

At the phrase level NCsPp was found in utterances such as /kɑʈɑikku/ *shop-to* 'to the shop', /ɑʋɑnukkɑ:kɑ/ *he-for* 'for him', /u:ɾiliɾun̪t̪u/ *home-town from* 'from the hometown'. Also the category Adv.Participle+ VP was found for example in /cɑ:ppiʈɑ ʋɑccɑ:ŋkɑ/ *eat do-past-PrNrG* 'made to eat' and /uʈkkɑ:ɾɑ ʋɑccucu/ *sit–made-he/she* 'made to sit'. The pattern $V_{inf.}$Aux.^{M}PrNrG was found in the following utterances: /ʋɑɾɑmɑ:ʈʈe:n,/ *come-future-*V_{Neg}. 'won't come', /collɑmɑ:ʈʈe:n/ *say-future-* V_{Neg}. 'won't say', and /cejjɑʋillɑi~cejjɑlɑ/ *do- past-* V_{Neg} 'didn't do'. Adj.part. N was seen in /ɑʈiccɑpɑijɑn/ *beat-past-boy* 'boy who beat' and /killunɑ pɑ:ppɑ:/ *pinch-past-baby* 'child who pinched'.

Stage V

In stage V commands like In[s]VV^{Des} and PnCsV$^{Neg.}$ were found: /e:j (n̪i:) ʋɑ: po:lɑ:m/ hey-come-go-future-PrNrG 'hey come let us go' comes under the In[s]VV^{Des} pattern. Utterances like /ennuʈɑjɑt̪u t̪oʈɑ:t̪e:/ *mine-touch-*V_{Neg}. 'don't touch (it's) mine', come under PnCsV$^{Neg.}$. Pn CoV$_{imp}$ was seen in /n̪i:jum ɑʋɑnum ʋɑ:ŋkɑ/ 'you and he come'.

In Question patterns, example utterances include: /n̪i: eŋkɑ po:ɾɑ/ *you where go-future-Q* 'where are you going?', /ɑʋɑn ennɑ: pɑnɾɑ:n/ *he what do-present-PrNrG-Q* 'what is he doing?' and /ɑn̪t̪ɑ pommɑ jɑ:ɾu t̪ɑn̪t̪ɑ:/ *that doll who give-past(PrNrG)-Q* 'who gave that doll?'. These come under the SWhQV pattern. Also, the children started to ask 'yes' or 'no' type questions at this stage. The SV^{I}Q pattern was found in utterances such as /ɑʋɑn ʋɑn̪t̪ɑ:nɑ:/ *he-come-past-PrNrG-Q* 'did he come?', and SXV^{I}Q in utterances like /ɑʋɑn iŋkɑ ʋɑn̪t̪ɑ:nɑ:/ *he here come-future-PrNrG-Q* 'did he come here?' and /ɑppɑ: n̪ɑ:lɑikku ʋɑɾumɑ:/ *Daddy tomorrow come-future-(PrNrG)-Q* 'will Daddy come tomorrow?'.

In the statement pattern St.Neg. was found in utterances such as /ɑʋɑn ɾɑ:mɑn illɑ/ *he Raman- Neg (no)* 'he is not Raman' and /ɑt̪u kɑ:r illɑ/ *that car- Neg (no)* 'that is not a car'. St.Emph. was represented in /it̪u pommɑt̪ɑ:n/ *this doll-present-Emph.* 'this is a doll only', /it̪u pɑ:ppɑ:t̪ɑ:n/ *this baby-present-(PrNrG)-Emph.* 'this is baby only', /ɑʋɑn po:nɑ:n̪t̪ɑ:n/ *he go-past-Emph.* 'he went only' and /ɑkkɑ colluccut̪ɑ:n/ *sister say-past-(PrNrG)-Emph.* 'sister (really) said it'. The category St.verf. was found in /ɑɳɳɑn colluʋɑ:nlɑ [ɑllɑʋɑ:]/ *brother say-future-PrNrG-Verif* 'brother will say isn't it?' and /ɑkkɑ: tɑɾuʋɑ:llɑ [ɑllɑʋɑ:]/ *sister give-future-PrNrG-Verif* 'sister will give isn't it?'. The pattern Stco$_2$St was found in the utterances /n̪ɑ: conne:n ɑ:nɑ: ke:kkɑ:lɑ/ *I say-past but (he) listen-past-neg* 'I told but he didn't listen', and /ɑppɑ: colluccu ɑt̪ɑnɑ:lɑ ʋɑn̪t̪e:n/ *father say-past so come-past PrNrG* 'father told so I came'. The category $S_tCO_1S_t$ was found in /n̪ɑ:num ɑʋɑnum kɑʈɑikkum pɑ:ɾkkukkum po:no:m/ *I Co$_a$ he Co$_a$ shop Co$_a$ park Co$_a$ go-past PrNrG* 'He and I went to shop and park'.

At the phrase level Adv.part.Aux.^{Asp} was found in utterances like /ʋɑn̪t̪iʈʈɾun̪t̪ɑ:n/ ~ /ʋɑn̪t̪u koɳʈiɾun̪t̪ɑ:n/ *was coming [he]* 'he is coming',

/aʈiccuʈʈa:n/ ~ /aʈittuʋiʈʈa:n/ *had beaten [he]* 'he has beaten', /colliru̪n̪ʈa:(ɭ)/ *Had say-past perfect [she]* 'she has said', and /ʋaccikiʈʈa:n/ 'kept it himself'. $V_{inf.}Aux^{vc}$ was found in /ca:ppiʈa ʋacca:ŋka/ *made [me] eat* 'made me eat' and /t̪o:ŋka po:na:ŋka/ 'went to sleep'. The pattern Adj.part. N^{I} was represented in /ca:pʈa pa:ppa:kku/ *for-eaten baby* 'for the baby to eat'.

Stage VI

Only the (+) section of stage VI of the English LARSP has been included and the (-) part has been left out. Thus, T-LARSP stage VI is structured differently from the original LARSP. The patterns (command, question, statement and phrase) of stage V have been continued into this stage.

In stage VI commands like Ini, PnAdj.NP V_{imp} and $PnN_{loc}AV_{imp}$ are found. Utterances under the category of Ini (initiator) included: /n̪i:ŋka ella:ɾum eŋka ʋi:ʈʈukku n̪a:laikku ʋisɳuʋa ku:ʈʈikkiʈu ʋa:ŋka/ 'all of you come to my home with vishnu'. $PnAdjNPV_{imp}$ was found in /n̪i: periya pommaija t̪a:/ 'you give a big doll' and /n̪i: n̪eraija: sʋi:ʈ t̪a:/ 'you give more sweets', and $PnN_{loc}AV_{imp}$ in utterances like /n̪i:ŋka ʋi:ʈʈukku na:laikku ʋa:ŋka/ 'you come tomorrow to house'. /n̪i: ʋi:ʈʈukku: aparama: ʋa:ŋka/ 'you come (to) home later'.

Under question patterns XCoXQ was found in /amma:ʋum akka:ʋum ʋaɾa:ŋkala:/ 'whether mother and sister are coming?' and /pommaijum ʧa:kle:ʈum ʋa:ŋki ta:ɾiŋkala:/ 'will you buy and give chocolate and (a) doll?'

Among the statement patterns, XCoX represents utterances like / muɾukanum cakt̪ijum enkaʋiʈʈukku n̪e:t̪t̪u ca:jaŋkala:m ʋan̪t̪a:ŋkala: appa na:ŋka ʋeɭaja:ʈuno:m/ 'murugan and sakthi yesterday evening came to my home, then we played'. The utterance /saccinum akilanum enku:ʈa ʋelaya:ʈarappo: canʈa po:ʈʈa:ŋkala: appa amma: ʋan̪t̪uccu, at̪ana:la aʋanuŋka o:ʈipo:jʈa:ŋka/ 'while sachin and akilan were playing with me, they fought themselves (and at) that time mother came after (them so) that they ran (away)' comes under the XCoX 1+ category. Ncl. (cl.) VP was found in /pommaijum t̪a:n ʋaccuɾukre:n/ '(I) also had doll', and /aɳɳanum t̪a:n ʋa:ŋkuna:n/ 'brother also will buy'.

At the Phrase level AVP was seen in utterances like /aʋano:ʈa ʋan̪t̪a:n/ '(he) came with him' and $V_{inf.}$ Aux^{vc} in /ʋaɾa ʋaccan/ 'made him [to] come', and /aʈikka ʋaccan/ 'made him [to] beat'.

Stage VII

In stage VII most of the categories of the English LARSP chart are the same on the T-LARSP chart except existential 'it' and 'there'. Existential 'it' and 'there' do not exist in Tamil. Under comment clause, stereotypical structures are found that do not change the meaning of the overall utterances, for example, /unakku t̪eɾijumla, n̪e:t̪t̪u appa: ʋa:ŋkiʈu ʋan̪t̪a:ŋkala:/ 'as you know, yesterday daddy bought (it) and brought (it)?'. Emphatic involves changing the word order to place a specific emphasis, for example /an̪t̪a pullaiŋka avaŋka t̪a:n enkiʈa vant̪u enkiʈʈa canʈa po:ʈʈa:ŋka/ 'those children, they only came to me and fought with me'. The category 'other' is used for any further constructions which have no category elsewhere on the chart. Syntactic comprehension refers to any cases where syntactic production seems to be in advance of comprehension. Style on the T-LARSP chart may refer to alternative grammatical varieties, styles, or any special forms that may exist in the collected sample, which are still to be explored.

Morphological Level

According to Crystal *et al.* (1989), in English inflections are used systematically from stage III and the list in stage III is based on the inflections of Brown's 14 morphemes (Brown, 1973). The morphology of Tamil is more complex, but the emergence of inflections is seen even at stage II. During stages III and IV most of these inflections are introduced and established.

The markers /-kaɭ/ for plural, and /-a:/ for interrogation emerge initially. By stage III, present, past (all forms), future, and case markers emerge, followed by the wh-words. Regarding PrNrG /–ccu/ is used widely to specify the IIIrd person singular (masculine, feminine and neuter) subject after the past tense suffix, /–um/ after future suffix, and /–t̪u/ after present.

In the example /appa: po:-Ø-ccu/, *father go-past-PrNrG*, the past tense marker /-n-/ is nullified in the spoken form, whereas in the standard form /appa po:na:ɾ/, /–n-/ is past and /-a:ɾ/ is the PrNrG marker and represents the third person masculine singular honorific. /eẽ/ is used for the Ist person singular -- /n̪a: po:neẽ/, /oõ/ is used for Ist person plural -- / n̪a:ma po:noõ/. Here also the marker in the spoken variety differs from that of the standard form. During the final part of stage III, Aux.^{M} patterns /ma:ʈʈu/, /ve:ɳʈu/, /illai/ and Aux.^{ASP} /konʈiru/, /viʈu/ emerged and abundant usage of these was found in stage IV. Some examples: ma:ʈʈeẽ 'won't (I)', /ve:ɳum/ 'need' /ve:ɳa:m/ 'need not', and /illai/ 'no'; and / panniʈʈiɾuka:/ *do-ing (she)*, /panniʈʈa:/ *do-past-Asp.Aux*.

Coordinating and subordinating conjunctions like /–um .... –um/, /-o: ....-o:/, /illana:/, /at̪ana:la/, and /e:na:/ emerged at stage V. Postpositions like /–iɾun̪t̪u/, Adjectival participles like /cejta/, /ceikinʈra/, /ceijum/ and /ceja:t̪a/, Adverbial participles like /po:ka/, /cejt̪a:l/, /cejaʈʈum/, /n̪aʈakkaijil/, /poka:mal/, and Negative participles like /po:ka:t̪u/, /ceja:t̪u/, were seen in their speech by 2;6 years.

Application of T-LARSP to Children with Language Disorders

The T-LARSP was administered to 15 Tamil-acquiring children with language disorders (LD) according to the availability of the participants, and the findings were compared to 15 age-matched typically developing (TD) children. The TD children were chosen from the 75 participants who were previously involved in the study for T-LARSP. Based on chronological age, the participants were divided into five age groups, who fall under the last five stages, i.e. from stage III to stage VII of the T-LARSP. The five age groups each included three children with language disorder (LD) and three typically developing (TD) children. Details of the children with LD are shown in Table 10.3.

The children with LD included children with delayed speech and language (DSL), with cognitive impairment (CD) and with autism (A), who speak Tamil as their native language. They were diagnosed at the Centre for Speech and Language Disability Studies, Annamalai University. They were referred from *Rajah Muthiah Medical College Hospital* (RMMCH), Annamalai University, for speech–language assessment and intervention at the Centre for Speech and Language Disability Studies. The participants were diagnosed using the Madras Developmental Programming System's (MDPS) Behavioural Scale (Jeyachandran & Vimala, 1992). The findings for the Children with LD with regard to each stage of the T-LARSP are tabulated below. TD children are in the numerator and the children with LD in the denominator in the order DSL; CD; A. Thus, in the following tables, the numerator and denominator represent the number of TD children and children with LD in each sub-category who had acquired the grammatical structures specific to that stage.

Table 10.3 Demographic details of children with language disorders

Stages	S.No. of Children	Age	Diagnosis
Stage III (2;0-2;6 years)	1	2;2 years	DSL
	2	2;4 years	CD
	3	2;6 years	A
Stage IV (2;6-3;0 years)	4	2;8 years	A
	5	2;9 years	CD
	6	2;7 years	DSL
Stage V (3;0-3;6years)	7	3;2 years	DSL
	8	3;5 years	CD
	9	3;5 years	A
Stage VI (3;6-4;0 years)	10	3;8 years	A
	11	3;9 years	DSL
	12	4;5 years	CD
Stage VII (4;0-5;0 years)	13	5.8 years	DSL
	14	4;9 years	CD
	15	6.7 years	A

A: Children with Autism; DSL: Children with Delayed Speech and Language; and CD: Children with Cognitive Delay.

Stage III (2;0-2;6 years)

The findings for TD children and children with LD for stage III are tabulated in Table 10.4. According to the data, all the three TD children had acquired syntactic structures of stage I, II and III; conversely, only two children with LD had acquired all the syntactic structures of stage I (1;0-1;6 years) and few syntactic structures of the stage II (1;6-2;0 years). Thus, morphosyntactic and syntactic structures acquired by TD children of 2;0-2;6 years were not found in all the three children with LD of 2;0-2;6 years.

The data have been coded according to the group of children as (TD/DSL;CD; A).

Stage IV (2;6-3;0 years)

The comparative data of TD children and those with LD for stage IV are tabulated in Table 10.5. According to the data, all the three TD children had acquired syntactic structures of stage I, II, III and IV. But the acquisition of the syntactic structures by three children with LD differs in all the four stages. Only two children with LD had acquired all the syntactic structures of stage I (1;0-1;6 years), but the child with autism very rarely produced some of these structures. Also, only one child with LD (DSL) acquired all the structures in stage II; children with CD acquired some structures, and children with A acquired very few in stage II (1;6-2;0 years). So, morphosyntactic and syntactic structures acquired by TD children of stage III (2;0-2;6 years) and stage IV (2;6-3;0 years) were not found in all the three groups of children with LD of 2;0-2;6 years.

Stage V (3;0-3;6 years)

The results of the comparison of language use of TD Children and children with LD at stage V are given in Table 10.6. All the three TD children had acquired syntactic structures up to stage V. On the other hand, children with DSL had acquired all the syntactic structures up to stage IV (2;6-3;0 years) and very few in stage V. Children with CD had acquired all of the stage II (1;6-2;0 years) patterns, and children with A had acquired some features at stage II and all at stage I. However syntactic structures acquired by TD children of 3;0-3;6 years were not found in all the children with LD.

Stage VI (3;6-4;0 years)

As shown in Table 10.7, when TD children are compared with children with LD at stage VI, it was observed that all the three TD children had acquired the patterns of stage VI (3;6-4;0 years); but these patterns were not acquired by the children with LD. Children with DSL had acquired all the syntactic structures up to stage IV (2;6-3;0 years) and very few in stage V, the same as the previous group. Children with CD had acquired all of the stage III (2;0-2;6 years) patterns, and children with A has acquired some features at stage II and all at stage I.

Table 10.4 Comparison of syntactic structures by typically developing children and children with LD at stage III (2;0-2;6 years)

Stage I **1;0 - 1;6**	**Noun** **(3/1;1;0)**	**PN** **(3/1;1;0)**	**Verb** **(3/1;1;0)**	**Other** **(3/1;1;0)**	**(Vocatives**	**Summoners**	**Interjection)**

	Clause				Phrase		Morphology	
	Comm.	Ques.	Statement					
Stage II 1;6 - 2;0	XV (3/1;1;0) Pn/NCs (3/1;1;0)	XQ (3/1;1;0)	V^{I} (3/1;1;0) N_{Neg} (3/1;1;0) NCs (3/1;1;0) Adv.Part.V^{I} (3/1;0;0)	PnCs (3/1;1;0) OV^{I} (3/1;1;0) CV^{I} (3/1;1;0)	Pn_{ind} (3/1;0;0) VTsPrNrG (3/1;0;0)	Adj N (3/1;1;0) DN (3/1;1;0)	Pl. (3/1;0;0) Past (all forms) (3/1;0;0) future (3/1;0;0) Case (3/1;0;0)	Present (3/0;0;0) PrNrG (3/0;0;0) Neg (3/0;0;0)
Stage III 2;0 - 2;6	XYV (3/1;0;0) V^{Des} (3/0;0;0)	V^{I}s-Q (3/1;0;0) XWhQ (3/0;0;0)	OV^{I} (3/0;0;0) SO (3/0;0;0) XV^{I} (3/0;0;0)	CV^{I} (3/1;0;0) SC (3/0;0;0)	D Adj N (3/0;0;0) NCs (3/0;0;0)	PnCs (3/0;0;0) Aux.^{M} PrNrG (3/0;0;0)	Aux.^{M} (mɑ:ṯṯu, ve:ṉṭum, illai) (3/0;0;0) Aux.^{ASP} (koṇṭiru, ʋiṭu) (3/0;0;0) WhQ (3/0;0;0)	Q (3/0;0;0)

The data have been coded according to the group of children as (TD/DSL;CD; A).

Table 10.5 Comparison of syntactic structures by typically developing children and children with language delay at stage IV (2;6-3;0 years)

Stage I **1;0 - 1;6**	**Noun** **(3/1;1;1)**	**PN** **(3/1;1;0)**	**Verb** **(3/1;1;0)**	**Other** **(3/1;1;0)**	**(Vocatives**	**Summoners**	**Interjection)**
	Clause				Phrase		Morphology
	Comm.	Ques.	Statement				
Stage II 1;6 - 2;0	XV (3/1;1;0) Pn/NCs (3/1;1;0)	XQ (3/1;1;0)	V^{I} (3/1;1;0) N_{Neg} (3/1;1;0) NCs (3/1;1;0) Adv.Part.V^{I} (3/1;0;0)	PnCs (3/1;1;0) OV^{I} (3/1;1;0) CV^{I} (3/1;0;0)	Pn_{ind} (3/1;1;0) VTsPrNrG (3/1;0;0)	Adj N (3/1;1;0) DN (3/1;1;0)	Pl. Present (3/1;1;0) (3/1;1;0) Past (all forms) (3/1;1;0) future (3/1;1;0) PrNrG (3/1;0;0)
Stage III 2;0 - 2;6	XYV (3/1;1;0) V^{Des} (3/1;1;0)	V^{I}s-Q (3/1;1;0) XWhQ (3/1;0;0)	OV^{I} (3/1;1;0) SO (3/1;1;0) XV^{I} (3/1;0;0)	CV^{I} (3/1;1;0) SC (3/1;1;0)	D Adj N (3/1;1;0) NCs PrNrG (3/1;1;0)	PnCs (3/1;1;0) $Aux.^{M}$ (3/1;0;0)	Case (3/1;0;0) $Aux.^{M}$ (mɑːʈʈu, veːɳʈum, illai) (3/1;0;0)
Stage IV 2;6 - 3;0	VV^{Des} (3/1;0;0) PnV^{Neg} (3/0;0;0) PnNCsAV (3/0;0;0) $PnVP_{imp}$ (3/0;0;0)	WhQX (3/1;1;0) $PnWhQV^{I}$ (3/1;0;0)	SAV^{I} (3/1;0;0) SOV^{I} (3/1;0;0) $S_{t}CO_{1}S_{t}$ (3/0;0;0) SOV^{Neg} (3/0;0;0)	NCsPp VP (3/1;1;0) SCV^{I} (3/0;0;0) 1	NCsPp Part. VP (3/1;0;0) V_{inf} $Aux.^{M}$ (3/0;0;0) V_{inf} $Aux.^{M}$ PrNrG (3/0;0;0)	Adv. (3/0;0;0) Adj. Part.N (3/0;0;0)	$Aux.^{ASP}$ (koɳʈiru, ʋiʈu) (3/1;0;0) Neg (3/1;1;0) WhQ (3/1;0;0) Q (3/1;1;0)

Table 10.6 Comparison of syntactic structures by TD children and children with LD at stage V (3;0-3;6 years)

Stage I **1;0 - 1;6**	**Noun** **(3/1;1;1)**	**PN** **(3/1;1;1)**	**Verb** **(3/1;1;1)**	**Other** **(3/1;1;1)**	**(Vocatives**	**Summoners**	**Interjection)**
	Clause				Phrase		Morphology
	Comm.	Ques.	Statement				
Stage II 1;6 - 2;0	XV (3/1;1;1) Pn/NCs (3/1;1;0)	XQ (3/1;1;0)	V^{I} (3/1;1;1) N_{Neg} (3/1;1;0) NCs (3/1;1;0) Adv.Part.V^{I} (3/1;1;0)	PnCs (3/1;1;1) OV^{I} (3/1;1;0) CV^{I} (3/1;1;0)	Pn_{ind} (3/1;1;1) VTsPrNrG (3/1;1;0)	Adj N (3/1;1;0) DN (3/1;1;0)	Pl. (3/1;1;0) Present (3/1;1;1) Past (all forms) (3/1;1;0) future (3/1;1;0)
Stage III 2;0 - 2;6	XYV (3/1;1;0) V^{Des} (3/1;0;0)	V^{I}s-Q (3/1;1;0) XWhQ (3/1;0;0)	OV^{I} (3/1;1;0) SO (3/1;1;0) XV^{I} (3/1;0;0)	CV^{I} (3/1;0;0) SC (3/1;0;0)	D Adj N (3/1;1;0) NCs (3/1;1;0)	PnCs (3/1;0;0) $Aux.^{M}$ PrNrG (3/1;0;0)	PrNrG (3/1;1;0) Case (3/1;1;1) $Aux.^{M}$ (mɑːʈʈu, veːɳʈum, illai) (3/1;0;0) $Aux.^{ASP}$ (koɳʈiru, ʋiʈu) (3/1;0;0)
Stage IV 2;6 - 3;0	VV^{Des} (3/1;1;0) PnV^{Neg} (3/1;1;0) PnNCsAV (3/1;0;0) $PnVP_{imp}$ (3/1;0;0)	WhQX (3/1;1;0) $PnWhQV^{I}$ (3/1;0;0)	SAV^{I} (3/1;1;0) SOV^{I} (3/1;1;0) $S_tCO_1S_t$ (3/1;0;0) SOV^{Neg} (3/1;0;0)	NCsPp VP (3/1;1;0) SCV^{I} (3/1;1;0) 1	NCsPp (3/1;1;0) V_{inf} $Aux.^{M}$ (3/1;1;0) V_{inf} $Aux.^{M}$ PrNrG (3/1;1;0)	Adv. Part.VP (3/1;1;0) Adj. Part.N (3/1;1;0)	Neg (3/1;1;0) WhQ (3/1;1;0) Q (3/1;1;0)

(*Continued*)

Table 10.6 (*Continued*)

Stage I 1;0 - 1;6	**Noun (3/1;1;1)**	**PN (3/1;1;1)**	**Verb (3/1;1;1)**	**Other (3/1;1;1)**	**(Vocatives**	**Summoners**	**Interjection)**	
	Clause				Phrase			Morphology
	Comm.	Ques.	Statement					
Stage V 3;0 - 3;6	In(S)V V^{Des} (3/0;0;0)	SWhQV (3/1;0;0)	S_tNeg. (3/0;0;0)	S_tEmɔ. (3/1;0;0)	Adv.Part.Aux.^{ASP} (3/1;0;0)			Co Postpositions (3/1;0;0)
	$PnCsV^{Neg}$ (3/1;0;0)	$SV^{I}Q$ (3/0;0;0)	S_tVerif. (3/0;0;0)		V_{inf} Aux.^{VC} (caus) (3/0;0;0)			(3/1;0;0) Negative participle
	$PnCoNV_{imp}$ (3/1;0;0)	$SXV^{I}Q$ (3/1;0;0)	S_tCo_2 S_t (3/1;0;0)	1	Adj. Part.N^{I} (3/0;0;0)			(3/0;0;0) Adjectival participle
			$S_tCo_1S_t$ (3/0;0;0)	1+				(3/0;0;0) Adverbial participle (3/0;0;0)

Table 10.7 Comparison of syntactic structures by TD children and children with LD at stage VI (3;6-4;0 years)

Stage I 1;0 - 1;6	Noun (3/1;1;0)	PN (3/1;1;0)	Verb (3/1;1;0)	Other (3/1;1;0)	(Vocatives	Summoners	Interjection)

	Clause				Phrase		Morphology
	Comm.	Ques.	Statement				
Stage II 1;6 - 2;0	XV (3/1;1;0) Pn/NCs (3/1;1;0)	XQ (3/1;1;0)	V^{I} (3/1;1;0) N_{Neg} (3/1;1;0) NCs (3/1;1;0) Adv.Part.V^{I} (3/1;1;0)	PnCs (3/1;1;0) OV^{I} (3/1;1;0) CV^{I} (3/1;1;0)	Pn_{ind} (3/1;1;0) VTsPrNrG (3/1;1;0)	Adj N (3/1;1;0) DN (3/1;1;0)	Pl. (3/1;1;1) Present (3/1;1;0) Past (all forms) (3/1;1;0) future (3/1;1;0) PrNrG (3/1;1;1) Case (3/1;1;1) $Aux.^{M}$ (maːt̲t̲u, veːn̲t̲um, illai) (3/1;1;0) $Aux.^{ASP}$ (kon̲t̲iru, ʋit̲u) (3/1;1;0) Neg (3/1;1;1) WhQ (3/1;1;0) Q (3/1;1;1)
Stage III 2;0 - 2;6	XYV (3/1;1;0) V^{Des} (3/1;1;0)	V^{I}s-Q (3/1;1;0) XWhQ (3/1;1;0)	OV^{I} (3/1;1;0) SO (3/1;1;0) XV^{I} (3/1;1;0)	CV^{I} (3/1;1;0) SC (3/1;1;0)	D Adj N (3/1;1;0) NCs PrNrG (3/1;1;0)	PnCs (3/1;1;0) $Aux.^{M}$ (3/1;1;0)	
Stage IV 2;6 - 3;0	VV^{Des} (3/1;1;0) PnV^{Neg} (3/1;1;0) PnNCsAV (3/1;0;0) $PnVP_{imp}$ (3/1;0;0)	WhQX (3/1;1;0) $PnWhQV^{I}$	SAV^{I} (3/1;1;0) SOV^{I} (3/1;0;0) $S_tCO_1S_t$ (3/1;0;0) SOV^{Neg} (3/1;0;0)	NCsPp VP (3/1;1;0) SCV^{I} (3/1;0;0) 1	NCsPp Part.VP (3/1;1;0) V_{inf} $Aux.^{M}$ (3/1;1;0) V_{inf} $Aux.^{M}$ PrNrG (3/1;1;0)	Adv. (3/1;1;0) Adj. Part.N (3/1;1;0)	

(Continued)

Table 10.7 (*Continued*)

Stage I 1;0 - 1;6	Noun (3/1;1;0)	PN (3/1;1;0)	Verb (3/1;1;0)	Other (3/1;1;0)	(Vocatives	Summoners	Interjection)

	Clause				Phrase	Morphology
	Comm.	**Ques.**	**Statement**			
Stage V 3;0 - 3;6	In(S)V V^{Des} (3/1;1;0) $PnCsV^{Neg}$ (3/0;1;0) $PnCoNV_{imp}$ (3/1;1;0)	SWhQV (3/1;1;0) $SV^{I}Q$ (3/0;0;0) $SXV^{I}Q$ (3/0;0;0)	S_tNeg. (3/1;0;0) S_tVerif. (3/0;0;0) $S_tCo_2 S_t$ (3/0;0;0) $S_tCo_1S_t$ (3/0;0;0)	S_tEmp. (3/0;0;0) 1 1+	Adv.Part.$Aux.^{ASP}$ (3/1;1;0) V_{inf} $Aux.^{VC}$ (caus) (3/1;1;0) Adj. $Part.N^{I}$ (3/1;1;0)	Co (3/1;1;0) Postpositions (3/1;1;0) Negative participle (3/1;1;0) Adjectival participle (3/1;1;0) Adverbial participle (3/1;1;0)
Stage VI 3;6 - 4;0	Initiator + Co (3/0;0;0) $PnAdj.NPV_{imp}$ (3/1;1;0) $PnN_{loc}AV_{imp}$ (3/0;0;0)	Complex (3/0;0;0) XCoXQ (3/0;0;0)	XCoX (3/1;1;0) Ncl(cl)VP (3/0;0;0)	 1 1+	AVP (3/0;0;0) $V_{inf.}Aux.^{VC}$ (3/0;0;0)	

Table 10.8 Comparison of syntactic structures by TD children and children with LD at stage VII (4;0-5;0 years)

Stage I 1;0 - 1;6	Noun (3/1;1;1)	PN (3/1;1;1)	Verb (3/1;1;1)	Other (3/1;1;1)	(Vocatives	Summoners	Interjection)

	Clause				Phrase		Morphology
	Comm.	Ques.	Statement				
Stage II 1;6 - 2;0	XV (3/1;1;1) Pn/NCs (3/1;1;0)	XQ (3/1;1;1)	V^{I} (3/1;1;1) N_{Neg} (3/1;1;0) NCs (3/1;1;0) Adv.Part.V^{I} (3/1;1;0)	PnCs (3/1;1;1) OV^{I} (3/1;1;0) CV^{I} (3/1;1;0)	Pn_{ind} (3/1;1;1) VTsPrNrG (3/1;1;0)	Adj N (3/1;1;0) DN (3/1;1;0)	Pl. (3/1;1;1) Present (3/1;1;0) Past (all forms) (3/1;1;0) future (3/1;1;0) PrNrG (3/1;1;1) Case (3/1;1;1) $Aux.^{M}$ (mɑ:ṯṯu, ve:ṇṭum, illai) (3/1;1;0) $Aux.^{ASP}$ (konṯiru, ʋiṯu) (3/1;1;0) Neg (3/1;1;1) WhQ Q (3/1;1;0) (3/1;1;0)
Stage III 2;0 - 2;6	XYV (3/1;1;0) V^{Des} (3/1;1;0)	V^{I}s-Q (3/1;1;0) XWhQ (3/1;1;0)	OV^{I} (3/1;1;0) SO (3/1;1;0) XV^{I} (3/1;1;0)	CV^{I} (3/1;1;0) SC (3/1;1;0)	D Adj N (3/1;1;0) NCs (3/1;1;0)	PnCs (3/1;1;0) $Aux.^{M}$ PrNrG (3/1;1;0)	
Stage IV 2;6 - 3;0	VV^{Des} (3/1;1;0) PnV^{Neg} (3/1;0;0) PnNCsAV (3/1;1;0) $PnVP_{imp}$ (3/1;1;0)	WhQX (3/1;1;0) $PnWhQV^{I}$ (3/1;0;0)	SAV^{I} (3/1;0;0) SOV^{I} (3/1;01;0) $S_{t}CO_{1}S_{t}$ (3/1;0;0) SOV^{Neg} (3/1;0;0)	NCsPp VP (3/1;1;0) SCV^{I} (3/1;0;0) 1	NCsPp (3/1;1;0) V_{inf} $Aux.^{M}$ (3/1;1;0) V_{inf} $Aux.^{M}$ PrNrG (3/1;0;0)	Adv. Part.VP (3/1;1;0) Adj. Part.N (3/1;1;0)	

(*Continued*)

Table 10.8 (*Continued*)

Stage I 1;0 - 1;6	Noun (3/1;1;1)	PN (3/1;1;1)	Verb (3/1;1;1)	Other (3/1;1;1)	(Vocatives	Summoners	Interjection)

	Clause				Phrase	Morphology
	Comm.	**Ques.**	**Statement**			
Stage V 3;0 - 3;6	In(S)V V[Des] (3/1;1;0) PnCsV[Neg] (3/1;0;0) PnCoNV$_{imp}$ (3/0;0;0)	SWhQV (3/1;1;0) SV[I]Q (3/1;0;0) SXV[I]Q (3/0;1;0)	S_tNeg. (3/1;1;0) S_tVerif. (3/1;0;0) $S_t Co_2 S_t$ 1 (3/0;0;0)	S_tEmp. (3/1;1;0) $S_t Co_1 S_t$ 1+ (3/0;0;0)	Adv.Part.Aux.[ASP] (3/1;1;0) V_{inf} Aux.[VC] (caus) (3/1;0;0) Adj. Part.N[I] (3/1;0;0)	Co (3/1;1;0) Postpositions (3/1;1;0) Negative participle (3/1;1;0) Adjectival participle (3/1;0;0) Adverbial participle (3/1;0;0)
Stage VI 3;6 - 4;0	Initiator + Co (3/0;0;0) PnAdj.NPV$_{imp}$ (3/0;0;0) PnN$_{loc}$AV$_{imp}$ (3/0;0;0)	Complex (3/0;0;0) XCoXQ (3/0;0;0)	XCoX 1 (3/0;0;0) Ncl(cl)VP (3/0;0;0)	1–	AVP (3/0;0;0) $V_{inf.}$Aux.[VC] (3/0;0;0)	

Stage VII 4;0 - 5;0	Discourse		Syntactic Comprehension
	A connectivity Comment Clause Emphatic Order	others	Style

Stage VII (4;0-5;0 years)

At the level of stage VII, all three TD children had acquired all the syntactic structures of this stage. On the other hand, acquisition of syntactic structures by children with DSL were limited up to stage IV (2;6-3;0 years), children with CD were limited up to stage III (2;0-2;6 years) and children with A were limited (with very few patterns) up to stage II (1;6-2;0 years) as shown in Table 10.8.

The 15 children classified as LD included five with speech and language delay, five with cognitive delay and five diagnosed as autistic. Comparing these children with TD children throughout stages III to VII, it was the children with autism who seemed to be more disordered or deviant in acquiring the grammatical structures associated with each stage. At stage VII, children with autism do not even have stage III structures. Children with CD seem to be more advanced than children with autism, as they have some structures of stage IV but not the structures of stage V. Children with DSL seem to be one year delayed in acquiring the structures. Thus, when comparing the three groups of children with LD, children with DSL are one to two years delayed, where as children with CD and autism are 3 to 4 years delayed in acquisition.

Notes

(1) See list of abbreviations in the Appendix.
(2) In running text, the English gloss is shown in single quote marks; italics is used for English structural equivalences. An English gloss is not always provided where the meaning of the structural equivalent is clear, and for the later stages of the chart, only an English gloss is provided.

References

Brown, R. (1973) *A First Language: The Early Stages*. London: Allen & Unwin.

Crystal, D. (1979) *Working with LARSP*. London: Edward Arnold.

Crystal, D., Fletcher, P. and Garman, M. (1989) *Grammatical Analysis of Language Disability* (2nd edn). London: Cole & Whurr.

Crystal, D. (1992) *Profiling Linguistic Disability* (2nd edn). San Diego: Singular Publishing Group.

Donaldson, M. (1995) *Children with Language Impairments: An Introduction*. London: Kingsley.

Jeyachandran, P. and Vimala, V. (1992) Madras Developmental Programming System, Vijaya Human Science, 6 Lakhmiperam Street, Chennai–14.

Kothandaraman, P. (1997) *A Grammar of Contemporary Literary Tamil*. Chennai: International Institute of Tamil Studies.

Müller, D.J., Munro, S.M. and Code, C. (1981) *Language Assessment for Remediation*. London: Croom Helm.

Appendix

Abbreviations

Adj.	Adjective
Adv.	Adverb
Aux.^{ASP}	Auxiliary-Aspect
Aux.^{M}	Auxiliary-Modal
Aux.^{VC}	Auxiliary-Voice
C	Complement
Cl.	Clitics
Co	Coordinative
Co_1	Correlative coordination
Co_2	Non- correlative coordination
Cs	Case
D	Determiner
Hon. Pl.	Honorific Plural
Hon. Sg.	Honorific Singular
In./Ini.	Introductory Words
Intg.	Interrogative
Neg.	Negative
N^{I}	Noun Inflection
$N_{loc.}$	Noun + Locative Case
NP	Noun Phrase
N_{st}	Noun Stem
Pl.	Plural marker
Pn	Pronoun
Pp	Post position
PrNrG	Person Number Gender Suffixes
Q	Question
S_t	Sentence
Tns.	Tense marker
V	Verb
V^{I}	Verb with tense and PrNrG inflections
V_{imp}	Verb – Imperative form
VP	Verb phrase
WhQ	‘Wh’ form/ Question words
X	Any Element
Y	Any Element not of X category

11 The Assessment of the Acquisition of Swahili: Towards the S-LARSP

Kamil Ud Deen

Introduction

The Language Assessment, Remediation and Screening Procedure (LARSP, Crystal *et al.*, 1976) was devised as a way to gauge a child's language development relative to their chronological age. The intention was to provide a detailed description of the normal course for the acquisition of syntax. Such a description is potentially of use to a great number of researchers and clinicians, including those interested in the normal acquisition of language, or the acquisition of language amongst disordered populations, or the acquisition of a minority home language, etc.

The LARSP was initially based upon work by Brown (1973) which showed that English-speaking children generally acquire language in a predictable order. That is, children tend to acquire certain structures before others, and that order is relatively invariant from child to child within a language. Two caveats are in order. First, children acquiring the same language may acquire structures in an invariant order, but the age at which they acquire each structure may vary from child to child. Second, the order of structures is generalizable to other languages only to a degree. That is, while there is some uniformity across languages, this tends to be at a broader level.

As its name suggests, the LARSP has emerged as an important tool in the assessment, remediation and screening of language disorders since the assessment of a language disorder can only be done against the backdrop of normative language acquisition. The LARSP, therefore, provides an expectation for normal acquisition which clinicians can use to gauge the speech of children who potentially have a language disorder. Because language disorders occur universally, the LARSP framework is applicable in principle in every language community, and so the developers of the LARSP have (quite rightly) pushed to have the LARSP extended to as many language communities as possible.

In this chapter, we provide an overview of the Swahili adaptation of the LARSP. We begin by discussing the status of Swahili in East Africa, including its various dialects and forms. The next section discusses the linguistic properties of Swahili, followed by a description of the data from which the S-LARSP was developed. We then present a detailed description of the developmental stages that are used in the assessment of the acquisition of Swahili.

Swahili in East Africa

Swahili, also known as KiSwahili, is one of the official languages of Kenya, as well as of Tanzania, and is spoken further west in Uganda and Congo as well as northern Mozambique and in some central areas of the continent. There are great differences in the varieties of Swahili spoken in these areas, and even within a single country, there is a spectrum of varieties of Swahili. The standard variety, referred to as Kiswahili Sanifu, is the variety taught in schools in Kenya and Tanzania, spoken on official mass media, the language of official religion and formal texts. However, spoken Swahili varieties differ greatly from this variety, and are in many cases mutually unintelligible from Kiswahili Sanifu. This makes the development of the S-LARSP particularly difficult, since the standard, formalized variety of the language is not really spoken by very many people.

Nonetheless, there are some characteristics that most varieties of Swahili share, and this is where the S LARSP focuses. These areas of similarity involve the rich verbal and, to a lesser degree, nominal morphology, that is typical of Bantu languages. Other common characteristics include word order and argument structure changing processes (like passivization, causativization, applicati.e. etc.). We discuss these below.

The data (described below) come from children speaking a variety of Swahili spoken in Nairobi, the capital of Kenya. Many in the Swahili-speaking community see Nairobi Swahili (insofar as there is anything like a single dialect within Nairobi) as a less-than-ideal standard bearer for the language. This is because Nairobi is a metropolis with speakers of many languages in close proximity to each other. As such, the language has taken on characteristics of other languages, and has (in the view of some) creolized and changed significantly. But this is true for most varieties of Swahili, bar Kiswahili Sanifu. As such, Nairobi Swahili is as good a variety for this project as any other spoken variety of Swahili.

Importantly, the variety of Swahili used to develop the S-LARSP still retains the crucial characteristics that make Swahili (and Bantu languages in general) so distinctive. For example, while it has lost much of its nominal class morphology, it still retains a rich set of agreement affixes (Deen, 2005) and other verbal inflectional affixation. And so, while at a very detailed level there may be an issue of generalizability of the results from a study on Nairobi Swahili to other varieties, the level at which the S-LARSP operates allows for full generalizability to other varieties.

Linguistic Properties of Swahili

Before presenting the Swahili child data, we first describe the structure of the Swahili verbal complex. Swahili, an eastern African Bantu language, is an SVO language in which the subject and the object are optionally null. This means that many utterances consist of nothing but the verbal complex. The verb occurs in a verbal complex that contains inflectional material as well as grammatical function changing suffixes. This verbal complex is the focus of the S-LARSP, since it is likely the property of Nairobi Swahili most generalizable across various varieties of Swahili. The structure of the verbal complex is given in (1), with an example in (2).

(1) Subject Agr. – Tense – Object Agr. – Verb–Derivational suffixes– Mood

(2) Juma	a -	na -	m –	pend -	a	Mariam
Juma	SA3s-	Pres-	OA3s-	like -	IND	Mariam

'Juma likes Mariam'

The subject agreement marker (SA) is a prefix that occurs on the left edge of most indicative, affirmative verbal clauses, and indexes the person of the subject (1st, 2nd and 3rd person) as well as the number of the subject (singular and plural). Thus, there are six verbal affixes in the subject agreement paradigm (Table 11.1). This is true for nouns that belong to noun classes 1 and 2, which include human referents. Other noun classes take different agreement markers that uniquely index that noun class.

There are several tense/aspect markers (Ashton, 1947; Vitale, 1981), given in Table 11.2. While these are referred to as 'tense' markers, they actually encode other meanings as well, such as aspect, mood, etc. Nonetheless, all these markers occur in the same slot within the verbal complex, and are thus treated as a single class here. These markers occur

Table 11.1 Subject agreement affixes in Swahili

Agreement Marker	Meaning
ni-	1st person singular
m-	2nd person singular
a-	3rd person singular
tu-	1st person plural
mu-	2nd person plural
wa-	3rd person plural

Table 11.2 Tense/aspect morphemes in Swahili

Tense/Aspect Morpheme	Meaning
li	past
na	present on-going/habitual
ta	future
ka	Narrative, resultative
me	present perfect
sha	present perfect completive
ki	conditional
nga	hypothetical
ku	infinitival

in the preverbal position indicated in (1) above, and occur only when the verb is in the indicative mood (see below).

Object agreement (OA), like subject agreement, marks the person and number of the object, though it is slightly more complicated than subject agreement. Object agreement is not obligatory in any varieties of Swahili. On a cursory review of a Swahili corpus, one might think OA is optional in Swahili. But this is not the case: OA is obligatory when the object is specific (as in 3a), while obligatorily absent when the object is non-specific (3b – see Deen, 2005; Ashton, 1947; Vitali, 1981; among others).

(3)	a.	Juma	a –	na –	m –	pend – a	m –	sichana
		Juma	SA3s	pres	OA3s	like IND	1	girl
		'Juma likes the girl.'						
	b.	Juma	a –	na –	pend – a	m –	sichana	
		Juma	SA3s	pres	like IND	1	girl	
		'Juma likes (some) girl.'						

Because of the fact that OA depends on the intended specificity of the direct object, it is not easy to predict when the OA is obligatorily required (though see Deen, 2006 for an effort to do just that). And because of this, it is not possible to measure the rate of supply of this morpheme in obligatory contexts – the gold-standard for measuring when a morpheme has been acquired. And so for the S-LARSP, we rely more heavily on the other inflectional affixes.

The final inflectional affix within the verbal complex is the mood marker, which is the last vowel in the verbal complex. Swahili marks three moods, all with single vowels: the indicative [a], the subjunctive [e] and the negative [i]. The indicative (IND) is the most common mood form and is used in all (true) tensed clauses (2, 3a, 3b). The one major exception to this rule is that the [a] final vowel is used with imperative verbs, which are essentially tenseless, agreementless verbs in the indicative mood, as in (4). This is unusual since the imperative is not strictly an indicative mood.

(4) lal – a sasa hivi!
Sleep IND now
'(Go to) sleep now!'

The negative vowel [i] co-occurs with some other negative morphology in the clause, depending on the intended tense of the clause. The complexity of negation in Swahili has apparently never been investigated in child Swahili, and so this chapter says nothing on this point. Finally, the subjunctive vowel [e] is used when the intended meaning of a clause is either a soft request, or to express obligation or possibility. There are other affixes that occur both before and after the verb root. Prefixes (not covered in detail here) include the various negation prefixes (which typically occur either before the SA marker or in place of the tense marker) and the reflexive prefix (which goes in the place of the OA marker). Suffixes include the passive voice marker, the applicative marker, the causative marker and the reciprocal marker. All of these occur later in development, and are not part of the S-LARSP as described here.

Turning briefly to nouns, in the Bantu languages nouns are organized into a series of classes, each marked with identifying pre-nominal morphology. These prefixes are organized into singular-plural pairs, and Bantu languages typically have 6–12 noun classes. Kiswahili Sanifu is described as having six noun classes, each split into singular-plural (making twelve), plus an additional three classes for nouns that refer to things like locations. However, the variety of Swahili in this study has significantly fewer noun classes (perhaps only four). Because of the large divergence from Kiswahili Sanifu and other varieties of Swahili, noun classes cannot be used as a diagnostic for language competence. Instead, we focus here on verbal morphology, where much more robust comparisons can be made from variety to variety. We turn now to the child data, followed by a description of the S-LARSP.

The Swahili Data

The data collection was conducted over a period of 11 months in Nairobi, Kenya. Biweekly audio recordings were made of naturalistic speech in the homes of four children of differing ages. The children were recruited through personal contacts and referrals. Seven families were considered for inclusion in the study, of which three were deemed unsuitable (on the basis of the linguistic environment of the home, practical issues such as distance and safety of the home, etc.). Table 11.3 provides for each child the age range, the number of recordings, and the starting and ending MLU (calculated as morphemes per utterance).

Table 11.3 Age ranges and number of recordings for each child

Child	Age range	Number of recordings	Start MLU	End MLU
HAW (girl)	2;2.01–2;6.05	07	1.54	2.46
MUS (boy)	2;0.16–2;10.10	23	1.52	3.57
FAU (girl)	1;8.19–2;2.07	10	2.97	3.35
HAS (boy)	2;10.13–2;11.25	04	3.15	4.23

Method

Each session was audio recorded using an external microphone placed in the center of the room. One caregiver (and occasionally a second caregiver) and the investigator were present in the room with the child during all recording sessions (all of which took place at the home of the child). The investigator took contextual notes, while the caregiver engaged the child in speech about a free topic. These contextual notes were later used in transcribing and coding. The data were transcribed using CHAT format (MacWhinney, 2000) and each transcript was then checked by a native speaker assistant and inter-rater reliability was calculated. Any discrepancies were negotiated and addressed.

The children participated in the data collection study at different ages and for different lengths of time. Because of this, one child's data (Mus) spanned a lengthy period of development, and so a method was needed to be able to compare data from the other children to different stages of Mus' data. Each child was assigned to a particular stage or stages according to three measures of grammatical development: MLU, verbs per utterance (Valian, 1991) and proportion of protosyntactic devices (Bottari *et al.*, 1993/1994; Peters, 2001). Each file was examined with respect to the three measures of grammatical development and the stage into which each file fell was determined according to a points system, e.g. an MLU of 2.0 received one point, while an MLU of 2.7 received two points, and an MLU of 3.2 received three points, etc. The stage to which each file was assigned was determined on the basis of the combined points that each file scored across all three grammatical measures. We then pooled the data from each stage (see Deen, 2002 for further details on the children and the establishment of the stages). Because the data from Mus come from such a lengthy time period (almost an entire year), data from this child were divided into three of the four developmental stages (stages 1, 2 and 3) and all analyses were done on the pooled data in each stage. We will refer to these four stages for the initial analyses of Swahili.

We analyse verb forms in child Swahili in terms of what kind of verb stem is produced. Given that the verb must have at least the morphemes SA, T and Mood, and that children often omit inflectional affi.e. we might expect any of the patterns in (5) in child Swahili. Note that here we omit from our analysis OA and the mood final vowel. We omit OA because of the complexity of the specificity condition that is associated with OA (noted earlier), and we omit the mood vowel from our analysis because we found that children never omitted this final vowel. Thus, the following are the remaining possible permutations of the inflectional affixes in child Swahili, along with schematization of each form.

(5)	a.	Full Clause	[SA – T – Verb – Mood]
	b.	[-SA] Clause	[Ø – T – Verb – Mood]
	c.	[-T] clause	[SA – Ø – Verb – Mood]
	d.	Bare Stem	[Ø – Ø – Verb – Mood]

The Full Clause (5a) represents the prescriptive full clause in adult Swahili. An analysis of the adult (child-directed) utterances within the corpus revealed that adults produce full clauses more than 95% of the time. This, therefore, might reasonably be considered the *target* that children are aiming for in their production.

A [-SA] clause (5b) is a full clause minus the SA marker. This results in a clause whose first morpheme is the tense marker. In the child-directed adult tiers of the corpus, this is the second most common clause type, constituting less than 5% of the adult utterances. A [-T] clause (5c), on the other hand, is one in which the SA is produced, but the tense marker is omitted. Such utterances are entirely unattested in adult speech. And finally, Bare Stems (5d) are clauses in which both prefixes are absent (and used in non-imperative contexts). Such utterances are also entirely absent from adult speech in the corpus. Below we report on the rate of these four clause types, and suggest that the relative rates of these four clause types constitute the backbone of the S-LARSP.

Results and assessment

In this section, we present the results of the analysis of the data according to clause type, as well as guidance in using this data as the primary assessment vehicle. The data were analysed initially for all mood types. It was found that for all children, a total of 1342 indicative-marked verbs, 103 subjunctive-marked verbs and 128 negative-marked verbs occurred. Given the preponderance of indicative-marked verbs, further analysis was done on just the indicative verbs. All utterances that denoted indicative, non-imperative force were identified (using contextual clues and notes from the researcher who had been present at the time of recording). These utterances were then coded for morpheme presence or absence, and the results were analysed.

Children produce all four types of verbal clause in (5), though to different degrees. At early stages of acquisition, children with low MLU, V-ratio and rate of protosyntactic devices produce lots of under-inflected forms(5b–d). As children develop, they begin to produce inflectional items to greater degrees, as described in greater detail below. Examples of each clause type are provided in (6–9).

(6) Full Clauses

a.	ni –	na –	zim –	a	tuu	ile	Haw06, line 1160
	SA1s–	pres–	finish–	IND	only	that	(Present tense)
	'I just finish that'						

b.	a –	ta –	lal –	a	Mus10, line 1512
	SA3s–	fut–	sleep–	IND	(Future tense)
	'She will sleep'				

c.	mimi …	ni –	li –	tow –	a	Mus12, line 1546
	I	SA1s–	past–	remove–	IND	(Past tense)
	'I…removed (it)'					

(7) [-SA] Clauses

a.	mimi	Ø –	li –	m –	chap –	a	Fau04, line 116
target :	mimi	ni –	li –	m –	chap –	a	(Past tense)
	I	SA1s–	past–	OA3s–	slap–	IND	
	'I slapped him.'						

b.	ndege	Ø –	me –	end –	a	juu	Mus21, line 172
target:	ndege	i –	me –	end –	a	juu	(Pres.perfect)
	bird	SA–	p.perf.–	go–	IND	up	
	'The bird has gone up.'						

c.	mimi	Ø –	ta –	ingi –	a	apa	ndani	Fau08, line 160
target:	mimi	ni –	ta –	ingi –	a	hapa	ndani	(future tense)
	I	SA1s–	fut–	enter–	IND	here	inside	
	'I will enter here inside.'							

(8) [-T] Clauses

a.	ni –	Ø –	kw –	ambi –	a	Fau04, line 95
target:	ni –	na –	kw –	ambi –	a	
	SA1s–	pres–	OA2s–	tell–	IND	
	'I am telling you.'					

b.	u –	Ø –	kingi –	z –	a ?	Fau07, line 1044
target:	u –	li –	kimbi –	z –	a?	
	SA2s–	past–	run–	causative–	IND	
	'Did you make (him) run?'					

c.	a –	Ø –	sem –	a	nini ?	Fau04, line 464
target:	a –	li –	sem –	a	nini?	
	SA3s–	past–	say–	IND	what	
	'What did he say?'					

(9) Bare Stems

a.	Ø –	Ø –	anguk	–	a	hivi		Haw07, line 210
target:	ni –	li –	anguk	–	a	hivi		
	SA1s–	past–	fall–		IND	like this		
	'I fell like this.'							

b.	Ø –	Ø –	tak –	a	tuwadh –	a	Haw07, line 5
target:	ni –	na –	tak –	a	tuwadh –	a	
	SA1s–	pres–	want–	IND	bathe–	IND	
	'I want to bathe.'						

c.	Ø –	Ø –	ndik –	a	Haw05, line 2946
target:	ni –	me –	andik –	a	
	SA1s–	p.perf.–	write–	IND	
	'I have written.'				

Below we track these four verb forms through the various stages of acquisition and show that the general pattern of development involves the bare stem dominating at earlier stages, followed by a move away from these bare forms towards (initially) tense-marked forms, followed by forms that are agreement- and tense-marked (i.e. full clauses).

Stages of acquisition of Swahili – the backbone of the S-LARSP

Broadly speaking, children go through four discernible stages in acquiring Swahili, and these form the basis for the S-LARSP. The stages are characterized in terms of which verbal morphology was produced and in what patterns. These stages can be summarized as follows:

(10) Stage 1: Variable production of inflectional affixes
Stage 2: Tense production increases; other affixes are variably produced
Stage 3: Subject agreement continues to be omitted; other affixes are reliably produced
Stage 4: Fully inflected verbs are the dominant form (though not the only form)

It should be noted that these stages are defined not by age, but by the nature of the utterances found in the empirical data. That is, while some claims can be made about the age at which children might be expected to traverse one stage or another, that is not the purpose of the scheme presented above (and discussed below). Rather, for the assessment of the acquisition of Swahili, it is recommended that a child be placed into one stage based upon the kinds of utterances that they may be producing, and not on the basis of their age. MLU, or any other commonly used index of language development, *may* be used since the stages were defined on the basis of three such measures (MLU, verbs-per-utterance, and proportion

Table 11.4 Four clause types in child Swahili across the four developmental stages

Stage	1	2	3	4
Full Clause	18%	20%	51%	60%
[-SA] Clause	29%	52%	36%	28%
[-T] Clause	20%	8%	5%	7%
Bare Stem	32%	19%	7%	4%

of protosyntactic devices). The reason that age cannot be used is the children in the corpus were of varying ages, and in some cases, children of very different ages were categorized into the very same stage. So, age is definitely not an indicator of which stage a child is in. Having said that, below, we provide very rough estimates as to the ages at which children might be expected to be in each stage (see also Table 11.4). These are to be taken as general gui.e. and not as the primary source for categorizing a child into a particular stage.

Stage 1

Young children (typically younger than age 2 years) produce verb forms that are predominantly bare of all morphology except for the mood vowel at the end (see column 1 in Table 11.4, row labelled 'Bare Stem').[1] At this stage, however, it is not the case that children omit all inflectional morphology. Rather, they do produce some inflectional morphology, though the largest clause type is clearly the bare stems. Full clauses (fully inflected verb forms, including SA, T and Mood) are produced a paltry 18% of the time. The other two clause types ([-SA] clauses and [-T] clauses) occur to some degree, though none clearly dominate this stage. Overall, the SA marker occurs in only 47% of verbal clauses, and the tense marker occurs in 38% of verbal clauses. Altogether, the under-marked verb forms (bare stems, [-SA] and [-T] clauses) comprise 82% of all verb forms produced at stage 1. Thus stage 1 is best described as a stage in which verbal inflection is variably and unreliably produced.

Stage 2

In the second stage in development, children (likely between ages 2;0 and 2;6) continue to produce bare verb roots/stems, but also begin to produce the tense marker more often. At this stage, children produce the tense marker in approximately 70% of verbal utterances (full clauses and [-SA]clauses), and they produce subject agreement in approximately 30% of utterances (full clauses and[-T] clauses). So the production of subject agreement lags behind that of tense. Bare stems reduce in overall preponderance, and the most dominant form is the [-SA] clause.

Stage 3

This stage (typical of children aged 2;6-3;0) begins to approximate to the adult language, with bare stems observed in less than 10% of all utterances. However, there still remain significant differences between child Swahili and adult Swahili. Specifically, while tense production reaches 87%, subject agreement production lags at 56%. But importantly, for the first time in development, full clauses are the majority of verbal clause types produced in child Swahili. So, stage 3 is characterized by (i) the (almost) adult-like supply of tense morphology, (ii) the remaining noticeable omission of SA, and (iii) the majority of clauses being full clauses.

Stage 4

Children in this stage (typically aged 3 years to 4 years) exhibit improved production rates of subject agreement (67%), but still not to adult-like levels. Moreover, in stage 4, children have essentially mastered the production of tense marking, producing tense markers in 88% of verbal utterances. The two clause types that dominate stage 4 are those that are observed in adult Swahili as well: full clauses (60% in child Swahili, 95% in adult Swahili) and [-SA] clauses (28% in child Swahili, 5% in adult Swahili). This child Swahili begins to resemble adult Swahili in terms of which clause types are most commonly produced, though to be sure, children seem to over-produce [-SA] clauses relative to adults.

The stage that follows this (for which data are not available) would be characterized as a stage in which tense production exceeds 90% and subject agreement approximates that of adults (roughly 90–95%). It is expected that children aged 4 years or more might be in this stage.

Other clause types

In addition to full clauses, [-SA] clauses, [-T] clauses and bare stems, children also produce many other clause types throughout these stages.

Negatives

As mentioned above, there were a total of 128 negative final vowels in the corpus. This suggests that verbal negation is used to some degree, but perhaps not to the degree we might expect. However, negation is complex in Swahili (and Bantu in general) in that there are three locations in which negation can be marked in the verbal complex: as a prefix that precedes the subject agreement marker, as a syncretic morpheme with tense (so in the tense slot), and as a negative final vowel (so in the mood slot – see (1)). Because these other kinds of negation are often omitted, it is not easy to gauge how well children are producing these forms. However, the final vowel is (as mentioned above) always present, and an analysis of the 128 forms reveals that every single one these are indeed used in a negative context. Thus, children use the final negative vowel correctly from the earliest ages. The clause-medial and -initial reflexes of negation, on the other hand, are often omitted. While negation could be a useful area for diagnosis of language disorders, the limited data in this corpus preclude us from including it as a rigorous component of the S-LARSP.

Nonetheless, children in stages 1–2 do use negation, but they generally use it formulaically, in learned phrases. In stages 3–4, children produce negative forms more creatively, and errors do arise (though errors do not occur with the final vowel, but with the prefixes). The typical errors are the omission of the initial negative form, or the use of the affirmative version of the tense marker instead of the negative version (e.g. instead of *sikupiga,* 'I did not hit (it)', children might say *silipiga*, where the affirmative past tense *–li-* is used instead of the negative past tense *–ku-*). Thus, productivity in negation increases in the later stages of acquisition, and omission of negation prefixes becomes less common.

Subjunctives

Subjunctives are a very common form in Swahili, used to mark irrealis, to make requests, to express doubt, etc. This is marked on the verb with the subjunctive [e] final vowel. So, a verb like *pig-a* in the indicative is *pig-e* in the subjunctive. Children in this data set produce subjunctives very frequently, and from early on. In fact, they seem to over-use the subjunctive vowel in contexts where the default indicative is requi.e. such as with imperatives (see Deen & Hyams, 2006 for details). This suggests that the subjunctive is a very early acquisition, and may be something that those assessing children acquiring Swahili would look for. If there is a delay in acquisition, it may turn up in the under-use of subjunctive. This is complicated somewhat by the fact that subjunctives are quite common in the input to children.

Imperatives

Imperatives are very frequent in the input to children and children produce imperatives quite early and quite fluently. There is nothing counter-intuitive about this finding, since it has been found in many languages previously. Moreover, morphologically, the imperative is the simplest form one can get in Swahili, consisting of the verb plus a mood vowel (homophonous with the default indicative vowel, [a]). Thus, in a sense the bare stems observed above are also homophonous with imperati.e. though utterances coded as bare stems were inspected in terms of their context, and there was no imperative force associated with those utterances. Thus, they were clearly intended as indicative utterances, not imperatives. Because there is little morphological learning involved in the imperative, it is not the most useful diagnostic of the acquisition of Swahili for our purposes. We therefore focus the S-LARSP on indicative verb forms since they provide the best construction for diagnostic purposes.

In sum, then, these verb forms constitute the targeted forms for the S-LARSP: the four indicative verb clause types (shown in 5), negative, subjunctive and imperative clauses. The percentages and relative proportions of indicative clauses given in Table 11.4 may be used as a guideline for the assessment of language development.

Other features

As mentioned above, there are numerous other features that Swahili children may or may not exhibit which were not captured in the data used here. Below are some of those features, with some discussion of when they might be expected to be manifested in the speech of a normal child acquiring Swahili.

1. Noun class marking
   Swahili has a rich set of noun class markers, many of which are produced at very young ages. Given the literature on other Bantu languages (e.g. Sesotho, Demuth, 1992; Zulu, Suzman, 1991, among others), we might predict that children acquiring varieties of Swahili in which the noun class system is intact will begin exhibiting knowledge of the noun classes quite young, perhaps even before age 2 years. The issue is whether production of a noun class marker constitutes knowledge of that noun belonging to a particular noun class. In order to conclude such, one would need evidence of that noun in both the respective singular and plural noun classes (e.g. *m-tu* and *wa-tu*, person and people respectively; *ki-ti* and *vi-ti*, chair and chairs, respectively). Such contrasts may not be available in naturalistic data until much later, though they may be elicited in an experimental environment.
2. Argument structure changing suffixes
   Swahili has many suffixes that mark some kind of argument changing function, such as the passive *–w–*, the causative *–ish–*, the applicative *–i–*, the reciprocal *–an–*, etc. Such affixes are observed sporadically in the Swahili corpus here, but not enough to be able to conclude at what age we might expect consistent and reliable use of that suffix. Given what is available in the corpus, coupled with what we know about the acquisition of other Bantu languages, we might predict that the applicative and causative will be acquired by around age 3, with the reciprocal acquired somewhat later, and the passive soon thereafter. The passive is quite controversial, with Demuth (1992) showing that the passive in Sesotho is acquired before age 3. However, the passive in Swahili shows notable differences to its counterpart in Sesotho, and so early acquisition of this kind is not expected in Swahili. Rather, a reasonable target age for the acquisition of the passive might be around age 4 years.

Summary and Conclusion

Children acquiring Swahili go through four discernible stages of acquisition during which they produce different kinds of verbal utterances. Early in development (stage 1, typically younger than age 4), the most dominant clause type is what we refer to as a Bare Stem. These are verbs that are missing all inflectional prefixes (and typically have no argument changing suffixes). The mood vowel is present, although as mentioned above, this may be due to phonotactic reasons.

The second stage is characterized as increased use of tense, but where subject agreement remains unexpressed. In fact, the large majority of utterances are missing subject agreement. The third stage is when the supply of subject agreement begins to approximate adult-use, and for the first time, the most common clause type is the full clause. Stage 4 is when full clauses are by far the most frequent form, well above 50% of all indicative verbs. A stage 5 is assumed to exist (though data for that are not available) in which the child produces more suffixes and some of the more complex prefi.e. such as negation. During most of this development, simple negation strategies are used, though not enough data exist to be able to say any more on this question.

Finally, it is hoped that this chapter will assist those looking to assess children acquiring not only some variety of Swahili, but perhaps of related languages as well. Because this verbal clause structure is relatively common across Bantu languages, the principles observed in the Swahili data are more than likely to transfer to other related languages such as Kikuyu, Luganda, etc. Moreover, the findings here comport well with those reported for languages like Sesotho (e.g. Demuth, 1992), Zulu (Suzman, 1991), Siswati (Kunene, 1979), etc. Given the importance of Swahili in the Kenyan and Tanzanian context, the appropriate and accurate assessment of normal language development is crucial, for social and economic reasons, but for personal and human reasons too. We hope that this chapter will assist in some modest manner in this effort.

Note

(1) It is possible that this mood vowel that children produce at this stage may not be a grammatical morpheme. Swahili requires that all words end in vowels, and so it is possible that this final mood marker is omitted, and then for phonotactic reasons, children insert a vowel to prevent what would otherwise be an ill-formed phonological utterance. For example, for a root like *fuat-* 'follow', a bare verb root ends in a consonant, which is ill-formed in Swahili. Thus children may actually be dropping the mood marker in addition to all the other markers, but it is not detectable because of the insertion of this thematic vowel.

References

Ashton, E.O. (1947) *Swahili Grammar.* London, Longmans, Green and Co.

Bottari, P.P., Cipriani A. and Chilosi, M. (1993) Protosyntactic devices in the acquisition of Italian free morphology. *Language Acquisition* 3 (4), 327–369.

Brown, R. (1973) *First Language: The Early Stages*. London: Allen & Unwin.
Crystal, D., Fletcher, P. and Garman, M. (1976) *The Grammatical Analysis of Language Disability*. London: Edward Arnold.
Deen, K.U. (2002) The acquisition of Nairobi Swahili: The morphosyntax of inflectional prefixes and subjects. Unpublished doctoral dissertation, UCLA.
Deen, K.U. (2005) *The Acquisition of Swahili*. Amsterdam: John Benjamins.
Deen, K.U. (2006) Object agreement and specificity in early Swahili. *Journal of Child Language* 33, 223–246.
Deen, K. and Hyams, N. (2006) The morphosyntax of mood in early grammar with special reference to Swahili. *First Language* 26, 67–102.
Demuth, K. (1992) Accessing functional categories in Sesotho: Interactions at the morpho-syntax interface. In J. Meisel (ed.) *The Acquisition of Verb Placement: Functional Categories and V2 phenomena in Language Acquisition*. Dordrecht: Kluwer Academic Publishers.
Kunene, E. (1979) The acquisition of SiSwati as a first language: A morphological study with special reference to noun prefi.e. noun classes and some agreement markers. Unpublished doctoral dissertation, UCLA.
MacWhinney, B. (2000) *The CHILDES Project: Tools for Analysing Talk* (3rd edn). Mahwah, NJ: Lawrence Erlbaum Associates.
Peters, A. (2001) Filler syllables: What is their status in emerging grammar? *Journal of Child Language* 28, 229–242.
Suzman, S. (1991) Language acquisition in Zulu. Unpublished doctoral dissertation, University of Witwatersrand.
Valian, V. (1991) Syntactic subjects in the early speech of American and Italian children. *Cognition* 40, 21–81.
Vitale, A. (1981) *Swahili Syntax*. Dordrecht: Foris Publications.

12 InuLARSP: An Adaptation of the Language Assessment, Remediation and Screening Procedure for Inuktitut

Shanley E.M. Allen, Catherine B. Dench and Kerry Isakson

Introduction

This chapter presents the first adaptation of the Language Assessment Remediation and Screening Procedure (LARSP) for Inuktitut, an Inuit language spoken in the arctic regions of eastern Canada.

The LARSP is a procedure that profiles children's language ability based on their production of various aspects of grammar such as the structure of noun phrases (e.g. Determiner–Adjective–Noun), the structure of sentences (e.g. Subject–Verb–Object), the structure of questions (e.g. QuestionWord-Auxiliary–Subject–Verb), and the use of words and affixes with grammatical functions (e.g. plural *-s*). The grammatical structures are organized on a LARSP chart, which is divided into stages according to the order in which the structures are acquired by typically-developing children. Each child's individual profile is developed on the basis of a sample of spontaneous speech. The LARSP was initially developed to assess the level of linguistic ability of English-speaking children with language disorders (Crystal *et al.*, 1976). Since then, it has been adapted for numerous other languages as diverse as Hebrew (Berman *et al.*, 1982), Irish (Hickey, 1990) and Chinese (Jin *et al.*, 2012). Reports of many of these adaptations are contained in a set of edited volumes, of which the present volume is the third (Ball *et al.*, 2012; Fletcher *et al.*, 2016; Ball *et al.*, this volume).

Arctic Quebec Inuktitut (hereafter simply Inuktitut), the language discussed in this chapter, is spoken by some 11,000 Inuit throughout the 14 Inuit communities in Nunavik, the northern region of Quebec, Canada

(Dorais, 2010; Statistics Canada, 2011). Virtually all Inuit in this region are native and fluent speakers of the language, using Inuktitut as their main language at home and also usually at work. Inuit children learn Inuktitut at home as their native language, although they later become bilingual in English and/or French through schooling as well as community and media exposure (Allen, 2007). Numerous studies attest to the fluent acquisition of Inuktitut by preschool Inuit children in Nunavik (e.g. Allen, 1996, 2017; Crago & Allen, 1998; Swift, 2004), as well as to the strong Inuktitut abilities of school-aged Inuit children in the early grades (e.g. Allen *et al.*, 2006; Crago *et al.*, 1991; Wilman, 1988; Wright *et al.*, 2000). However, as noted in a 2010 report published by Speech-Language & Audiology Canada (SAC, 2010), there is a critical lack of tools that can be used by speech-language pathologists to assess language ability and language difficulties in children who speak Inuktitut or other indigenous languages. This situation provided the main motivation for adapting the LARSP for use in Inuktitut.

In the present chapter we describe the process and outcome of designing the adaptation of the LARSP for Inuktitut, referred to here as the InuLARSP. The InuLARSP was designed on the basis of already existing Inuktitut child language data collected for previous studies (Allen, 1996; Crago, 1988). Certain aspects of the grammatical structure of Inuktitut, described in the next section, required substantial changes in the items selected for the profile compared to the original English LARSP and to the other adaptations developed to date. In particular, more focus was placed on morphology, and less on syntax, than has been the case for other LARSPs.

Key Grammatical Features of Inuktitut

Inuktitut has three main grammatical features that we took into account in designing the InuLARSP: agglutination, polysynthesis, and argument ellipsis (i.e. subject and object omission). Each of these is described in turn in the following paragraphs.

Agglutination

Agglutination is a process for forming complex words in which several morphemes are affixed to a given root word. In Inuktitut words are made up of two parts: the root, which comes at the beginning of the word, and the derivational and inflectional morphemes, which are suffixed to the root. Words may contain 10 or more morphemes (Dorais, 2010; Fortescue, 1994). Importantly, each morpheme is relatively easily identified within the complex word because there is little to no phonological change at the morpheme boundaries. This easy identification of morphemes differentiates Inuktitut from some other LARSP languages with complex words like

Irish or Hebrew; in the latter languages, the morphemes are often fused together in the process of affixation, and thus not easily distinguishable.

Inuktitut has three classes of roots, as illustrated in the example in (1): noun roots including pronouns and demonstratives (e.g. *tuttu* 'caribou'), verb roots (e.g. *qukiq-* 'shoot') and uninflected particles (e.g. *ilai* 'right'). (A list of the abbreviations used in the glosses of the examples can be found at the end of the chapter.)

(1)	*Tuttualummik*	*qukilaurqutit*	*ilai?*
	tuttu-aluk-mik	qukiq-lauq-vutit	ilai
	caribou-EMPH-MOD.SG	shoot-PAST-IND.2sS	right
	'You shot the big caribou, right?'		

Noun roots and verb roots are often followed by one or more derivational morphemes (e.g. *-aluk* 'EMPH', *-lauq-* 'PAST'). They are not considered complete without an obligatory final inflectional morpheme: case for nouns (e.g. *-mik* 'MOD.SG'), and cross-referencing inflections for verbs (e.g. *-vutit* 'IND.2sS'). Concepts that would be classified as adjectives in English may either be realized as word-internal morphemes like *-aluk* 'EMPH' in (1), or as verbs that take verbal morphology like *piu-* 'be good' in (2).

(2) *Piunngituq.*
piu-nngit-juq
be.good-NEG-PAR.3sS
'It is not good.'

The rich word-internal morphology of Inuktitut includes over 400 derivational morphemes that, as in the morphology of other languages, mark notions such as tense, aspect, emphasis, negation, causation and passive voice. Inuktitut word-internal morphemes also include adjectival and adverbial modifiers (e.g. *-apik* 'little', *-saaq-* 'quickly') as well as nominalizers and verbalizers that serve to change the syntactic class of a word from noun to verb or vice versa (e.g. *-u-* 'be', *-juq* 'that.which').

The word-final inflectional system includes more than 900 verbal inflections that mark modality (i.e. the speaker's expressive intent, including questions and commands) and the person and number of subject and object (e.g. *-jara* 'PAR.1sS.3sO'). The over 300 nominal inflections mark number (singular, dual, plural), case, and information about the person and the number of the possessor, if applicable (e.g. *-ga* 'ABS.1Ssg'). Words may also end with an enclitic – a specific class of morphemes that can be added to either nouns or verbs for various purposes (e.g. *-ai* 'greetings', *-li* 'but', *-ttauq* 'also').

The morphology following the root is typically affixed in order of accumulating semantic scope from the beginning to the end. This does not follow a rigid order as in some other morphologically complex languages, but rather is affixed according to the relative meaning of the morphemes.

Polysynthesis

Polysynthesis is the ability to say in one word what in other languages would require a full sentence (Evans & Sasse, 2002; Fortescue, 1994). This is possible because Inuktitut has a large number of morphemes within the word that serve grammatical functions normally served by individual words and word order in languages like English. For example, as already noted, certain morphemes can turn a noun into a verb (i.e. verbalizers) or a verb into a noun (i.e. nominalizers), and inflectional suffixes on verbs and nouns serve the function of pronouns and possessives. In addition, adjectival and adverbial morphemes within the word express concepts of degree, tense, aspect, negation and the like.

The example in (3) illustrates this characteristic of polysynthesis. The word begins as a noun with a nominal root (*illu* 'house') followed by adjectival affixes (*-juaq* 'big', *-aluk* 'EMPH') and a case affix (*-mut* 'ALL.SG'). It then turns into a verb via a verbalizer (*-uq-* 'go'). Following this are three derivational affixes realizing tense (*-lauq-* 'PAST'), aspect (*-sima-* 'PERF'), and negation (*-nngit-* 'NEG'). The word ends with an obligatory inflectional suffix (*-nama* 'CTG.1sS') and two enclitics (*-li* 'but', *-ttauq* 'also').

(3) *Illujuaraalummuulaursimannginamalittauq.*
illu-juaq-aluk-mut-uq-lauq-sima-nngit-nama-li-ttauq
house-big-EMPH-ALL.SG-go-PAST-PERF-NEG-CTG.1sS-but-also
'But also, because I never went to the really big house.' (Dorais, 1988: 8)

Importantly, none of the morphemes in this word except the initial noun root (*illu* 'house') can stand on its own; all of the other morphemes can only appear within a word.

Subject and object omission

Like in other languages, verbs in Inuktitut require subjects and objects. However, independent subjects and objects are frequently omitted in both speech and writing due to the inflectional morphemes on the verb that mark the person and number of subjects and objects. First and second person subjects and objects are never overtly expressed other than in verbal inflection, while third person subjects and objects are omitted in the majority of instances (Allen, 2000; Allen & Schröder, 2003). This omission is evident in each of the examples earlier. The subject is not realized by an independent word in any of the three examples; rather, it is realized in the inflection at the end of the verbal word. The object in (1) is realized overtly: *tuttumik* 'the caribou'. However, the object in (3) appears as part of the verbal word; it is the root of the word (*illu* 'house') and is followed by a verbalizer (*-uq-* 'go') that turns the noun into a verb.

When subjects and objects are present in the sentence, the predominant word order tends to be subject–object–verb (SOV). However, the word order is fairly flexible since information about the syntactic function of specific elements is encoded in morphology. The actual word order used reflects pragmatic factors.

Taken together, argument omission, polysynthesis, and subject and object omission mean that syntactic relationships in Inuktitut largely play out within the word rather in the relationship between words across word boundaries. This means that Inuktitut is syntactically simpler and morphologically more complex than many other LARSP languages.

Preparatory Analysis for InuLARSP

Given the structure of Inuktitut as discussed in the previous section, we began the process of designing the InuLARSP with the expectation that morphology might play a much larger role than in many of the LARSPs so far, and that syntax might play a much smaller role. There are no large-scale normative data on stages of grammatical development in Inuktitut, and no other assessment tools for morphosyntactic development in Inuktitut. Therefore, we had to start from scratch in our design of the InuLARSP based on information about Inuktitut language development from the literature and from analysis of available Inuktitut child language data.

We first consulted the existing literature on morphosyntactic development of Inuktitut. This has mostly focused on specific phenomena such as passives (Allen & Crago, 1996), causatives (Allen, 1998), noun incorporation (Allen, 1996; Parkinson, 1999), argument realization (Allen, 2000; Allen & Schröder, 2003), verbal inflection (Allen, 2013; Crago & Allen, 2001; Wilman, 1988) and temporal reference (Swift, 2004). Two overview articles provide more general information about the overall developmental trajectory of Inuktitut in preschool children (Allen, 2017; Crago & Allen, 1998). However, none of this literature offered enough detail about which morphemes and syntactic structures are learned at which age and stage to serve as a basis for designing the InuLARSP. We thus decided to perform further analyses on the original data on which this literature was based.

Data analysed

The data we analysed come from two studies of Inuktitut child language development (Allen, 1996; Crago, 1988). Spontaneous speech samples were recorded from eight monolingual Inuktitut-speaking children living in small communities in northern Quebec. The children were videotaped in naturalistic situations at home, interacting with friends and family members and engaging in their normal daily activities. Four children (Jini, Lucasi, Sarah, Tumasi) were aged between 1;0 and 1;9 at the onset of taping and were taped on four occasions at four-month intervals

(Crago, 1988; ages are given as years; months). The other four children (Elijah, Lizzie, Louisa, Paul) were between 2;0 and 2;10 at the onset of taping and were taped on three occasions at four-month intervals (Allen, 1996). All of the speech spoken by and to the eight children during the taping sessions had previously been transcribed by native speakers of Inuktitut using conventions of the CHILDES Project (MacWhinney, 2000), and had been coded for morphology and syntax by trained research assistants and the first author.

Stages

Stages of development are a central part of the LARSP. Therefore, the first step in our analysis was deciding how to determine the relevant stages for our data set, and thus for the InuLARSP.

Two methods for determining stages have been described by the authors of other LARSP adaptations. For languages for which data samples are available for many children, stages are typically assigned by age (e.g. 1;6-2;0, 2;0-2;6, 2;6-3;0), and then morphemes and syntactic structures are assigned to ages using statistical criteria (e.g. structure used by 50% of children in a given age range). For languages for which data samples are available from only a limited number of children, authors have typically (and understandably) been cautious about assigning stages by age, and have rather used the number of elements (i.e. words) as the determining factor for stages. Typically this method assigns one-element sentences to stage I, two-element sentences to stage II and so on.

Both of these approaches were problematic for the InuLARSP adaptation. First, data were available for only eight children, including one linguistically precocious child whose samples would skew any organization by age. Thus, assigning stages by age was not likely to be useful. Second, the number of elements in a sentence is far less relevant as a developmental measure for Inuktitut than for languages such as English, Dutch and Icelandic. Rather, the number of morphemes in a sentence, as well as the morphological complexity of the sentence, are more relevant indicators of development in Inuktitut (Allen, 2017; Allen & Dench, 2015). As a result, a slightly different approach was used for assigning developmental stages in the InuLARSP.

In their first two taping sessions, the children in the Crago study used only one-morpheme utterances; the data from these sessions was used as the basis for stage I of the profile. The data from the remaining 20 taping sessions (two each for the four younger children, three each for the four older children) were analysed to develop stages II to V. We extracted the first 200 child utterances from each session to create samples of equal size for each child at each age. A mean length of utterance in morphemes (MLUm) was calculated for each sample on the basis of the first 100 utterances in the sample (see details in Allen & Dench, 2015). The data samples are listed in Table 12.1.

Table 12.1 Data used for analysis, including age in months and mean length of utterance in morphemes

Child	Age in Years;Months	Mean Length of Utterance in Morphemes
Jini	1;8	1.71
Tumasi	1;9	1.27
Sarah	1;11	1.55
Jini	2;0	1.73
Elijah	2;0	1.73
Tumasi	2;1	1.85
Lucasi	2;3	1.36
Sarah	2;4	1.53
Elijah	2;5	3.74
Lizzie	2;6	3.00
Paul	2;6	2.07
Lucasi	2;8	1.54
Elijah	2;9	2.95
Louisa	2;10	1.88
Lizzie	2;10	2.62
Paul	2;11	2.57
Louisa	3;2	2.12
Lizzie	3;3	3.02
Paul	3;3	3.26
Louisa	3;6	2.77

We preliminarily grouped the 20 language samples from Table 12.1 into four stages (stages II to V) with three to six samples per stage, using a combination of mean length of utterance in morphemes (MLU(m)) and age as determining factors. We then used the distribution of morphemes and syntactic structures across samples to reassess the assignment of samples to stages. This last step is described in the next section.

Determining Morphemes and Syntactic Structures to Include

The most important component of the LARSP is the morphemes and syntactic structures that are included in the chart. We selected the morphemes and syntactic structures for the InuLARSP according to three main guidelines. First, we aimed to include enough morphemes and syntactic structures in the chart to adequately represent the diversity present in the language of preschool children, but not so many that it would make the assessment unmanageable. Second, we focused on elements that appeared frequently enough to be representative of typical child speech.

Third, we put high priority on morphemes and syntactic structures that would distinguish children's development across the five stages. In the process of selecting elements to include, we treated morphology and syntax separately.

As noted earlier, morphology in Inuktitut is highly complex with over 1500 derivational and inflectional morphemes available. It would be impossible to list all of the morphemes in the developmental profile. Therefore, we began construction of the morpheme section of the chart by listing all the morphemes that appeared in the child data, and then determining the frequency of occurrence of each morpheme at each stage. A total of 99 morphemes appeared in the data on at least one occasion.

We then analysed the twenty 200-utterance language samples for the presence of these 99 morphemes. In order to be a useful item on a profile, an item must be produced frequently and consistently by a variety of children. As a result, we first eliminated any morpheme produced fewer than 10 times in total across the 20 samples. Second, we eliminated any morpheme produced fewer than 15 times unless it was strongly and stably represented across the various samples (e.g. used in at least three of the five samples at a particular stage), and/or if it appeared only at stages IV and V. Third, we divided each of the 200-utterance samples into two 100-utterance samples (the size of sample typically used for the LARSP), creating two sets of twenty 100-utterance samples. We then eliminated any morpheme that appeared fewer than 10 times in either of these sets of samples. After applying these three criteria, 59 candidate morphemes remained.

For the syntax sections, the twenty 200-utterance samples were analysed for the presence of multiword utterances with syntactic structures. As expected, there were relatively few of these: the majority of utterances were one word in length, with the longest utterance being only three words in length. A total of 25 syntactic structures were identified. Certain of these structures were observed only once or twice in the data, and these were either removed from the analysis or combined with other similar structures (e.g. all the three-word utterances were collapsed as XYZ), leaving 10 candidate structures.

The selected morphemes and syntactic structures were provisionally placed at the profile stage at which they first appeared consistently. Following inspection of the resulting morphological and syntactic profiles, the language samples were then reclassified into the four stages, with five samples at each stage. Each morphological and syntactic item was then given a final classification into a stage, based on its use by at least three of the five children at that stage.

Description of InuLARSP

As shown in Figure 12.1, the InuLARSP is divided into three main sections. The first section records demographic information about the

	Name:			**Date of birth:**			**Date of recording:**		
	Therapist:			**Age:**			**Remarks:**		
A.	**Unanalyzed** Unintelligible: Symbolic Noise: Deviant:			**Problematic** Incomplete: Ambiguous: Stereotypes:			**B.** Total number of utterances: Analyzed utterances: MLU(m):		
Minor	***Responses***			***Vocatives***		***Other***		***Problems***	
Stage I	'N'			'V'		Other		Baby Words	
	Questions			***Commands/Statements***					***Word + Morph***
	Syntax	***Word***	***Inflections***	***Clause/Phrase***	***Nominal Elements***	***Nominal Inflections***	***Verbal Elements***	***Verbal Inflections***	
Stage II	Q	*suna* *nauk*	Q+inf		LOC *maani* EMPH *-aluk* Greeting *-ai* NZ *-juq*	ABS (1Ssg) *-ga*	Polite *-lauq-*	IMP (2sS/3sO) *-guk* IMP (2sS) *-git* PAR (3sS) *-juq*	X+1 X+2 X+3
Stage III		*kina*	ENCL *-li*	SV/VS OV/VO CS/SC AX/XA	CONJ *-li* CONJ *-lu*	LOC (SG) *-mi* ALL (SG) *-mut* POSS (SG) *-up* ABS (PL) *-it*	PASS *-jau-* COP *-it-* AV *-guma-* NEG *-nngit-*	IMP (1dS) *-luk* CTG (1sS) *-gama*	X+4
Stage IV					DEM *uminga* DEM *ukua* PRO *uvanga* DIM *-apik* ADJ *-nnguaq*		FUT *-langa-* FUT *-laaq-* AV *-nnguaq-* COP *-u-* CAUS *-tit-*	IMP (3sS) *-li* IND (1sS) *-vunga* PAR (1sS) *-junga* PAR (1sS/3sO) *-jara* CTG (3sS) *-mmat*	X+5 X+6
Stage V	QX	*nani*	INT (2sS) *-vit*	XYZ V Vsub NPoss N Det N	DEM *kanna* NZ *-jaq*	ABS (2Ssg) *–it* ABS (3Ssg) *-nga*	PAST *-kainnaq-* PAST *-lauq-* FUT *-niaq-* AV *-gunnaq-* VZ *-qaq-*	IND (3sS) *-vuq*	X+7
Errors	missing inflection:			missing tense morpheme:		overuse of pronoun:	filler morpheme:	other:	

Figure 12.1 InuLARSP Chart

participant as well as numbers of utterances of various types in the sample. The second section records numbers of each type of morpheme and syntactic structure, organized into five stages of development. The final section notes any errors appearing in the data. Each of these sections is described in turn.

Demographic and utterance information

The first section of the InuLARSP is very similar to that of most other LARSPs. The top section records the name, date of birth and age of the child, as well as the name of the therapist, the date of recording, and any remarks that are relevant to the interpretation of the chart. Next, Section A records the number of utterances that were not analysed due to being unintelligible, deviant, or only containing symbolic noise. It also records the number of utterances that are problematic for analysis due to being incomplete, ambiguous and stereotypical, all using identical definitions to those described in the 1981 LARSP revision (Crystal, 1982: 16). Section B records the total number of utterances spoken and the total number of utterances analysed in the next section, as well as the mean length of utterance in morphemes (MLU(m)).

Morphological and syntactic development

The second part of the InuLARSP profile begins with a section recording *Minor* utterances – utterances, or portions of utterances, that are not relevant to grammatical analysis. These include responses to interlocutor questions (e.g. *auka* 'no', *aaa* 'yes'), vocatives (e.g. *Anaana, ...*; 'Mom, ...'), interjections (e.g. *haa* 'huh?', *ilai* 'right'), greetings (e.g. *ai* 'hi'), and the like, as well as any problem utterances.

The following section – stages I through V – is the heart of the chart. Here the relevant morphemes and syntactic structures of Inuktitut are listed according to the stage at which they consistently appear in the data samples. As already noted, the InuLARSP focuses more on morphology than most LARSP adaptations. Statements and commands are differentiated in Inuktitut by morphology rather than different syntactic constructions, and as a result are placed together on the InuLARSP chart.

In the following sections, we describe the elements listed at each stage. We first describe stage I on its own, since the elements present at this stage are stand-alone roots and thus different from all the other stages. We then describe each of the elements contained in the remainder of the chart (e.g. Questions, Nominal Elements), and present the stages of development separately for each element.

Stage I

Stage I in Inuktitut, as in other languages, is very simple. Language at this stage is typified by one word /one morpheme utterances that consist of a noun root (4a), a verb root (4b), and utterances classified as *Other*, such as an interactional term (4c) or the early-developing demonstrative pronoun *una* (4d).

(4) a. *Piipi.*
'Baby.' (Sarah, 1;3)
b. *Amaaq.*
'Carry on back.' (Sarah, 1;3)
c. *Atiilu?*
'Again?' (Sarah, 1;3)
d. *Una.*
'This one.' (Lucasi, 1;8)

Also common at stage I are baby words, a nursery vocabulary used by and to children up to about 3 years of age (Crago *et al.*, 1998). A baby word typically bears no similarity to the adult equivalent and is often phonologically simpler, as in the example in (5).

(5)	*Apaapa.*	[adult:	*Niqi* OR	*Niri-guma-junga.*]	
	food/eat	[	food	eat-want-PAR.1sS]	
	'Food/eat.'	[	'Food'	'I want to eat.']	(Jini, 1;0)

Questions

The first section in stages II to V of the InuLARSP chart focuses on questions. Three columns appear under the *Questions* heading: the

Syntax column records whether a question word appears alone in the utterance or with another word, the *Word* column records the presence of particular question words, and the *Inflection* column records the use of inflections used to mark questions. Each of these are treated in turn in the following paragraphs. Inuktitut, like other languages, also allows utterances with no question word or interrogative inflection to be used as questions, typically signalled with intonation. As in the English LARSP, this form is not recorded in the *Questions* section of the InuLARSP because it is not relevant to morphosyntactic ability.

Syntax

Single-word questions are already evident at stage II, as represented by Q on the chart. These may appear as just a question word alone as in (6a), or a question word with additional verbal (6b) or nominal (6c) morphology. More complex two-word question utterances appear at stage V – most frequently a question word with a subject as illustrated in (6c). Given the overall low frequency of these structures, however, a question word and any other element is represented as QX.

(6) a. *Nauk?*
nauk
where
'Where?' (Lizzie, 2;6)
b. *Naniilirqa?*
nani-it-liq-va
at.where-be-INCP-INT.3sS
'Where is it now?' (Lizzie, 3;3)
c. *Una kinaup?*
u-na kina-up
this.one-ABS.SG who-ERG.SG
'Whose is this?' (Paul, 3;3)

Word

Question words are typically used to form content questions. Two question words appear consistently at stage II: *suna* 'what' and *nauk* 'where'. The latter is illustrated in (6a). A further question word appears at stage III: *kina* 'who', as shown in (6c). The question word *nani* 'at where' appears at stage V, as illustrated in (6b).

Inflections

The first nominal and verbal inflections attached to question words begin to appear at stage II. These may be either interrogative inflections as in (6b), or inflections of other types as in (6c). Since no particular inflection appears consistently enough to merit specific mention on the chart, this is listed as Q+inf on the chart. At stage III we see the first consistent use of the question-marking enclitic *-li* 'where'. This morpheme can be affixed on nominal stems to form a *where*-question, as shown in (7a). Finally, verbal inflections in the interrogative mood can be used on any verb root to form a yes-no question. At stage V, the interrogative inflection *-vit* 'INT.2sS', shown in (7b), begins appearing consistently.

(7) a. *Jaikuli?*
Jaiku-li
Jacob-where
'Where is Jacob?' (Elijah, 2;0)
b. *Aanii atjiliurtaulangaviit?*
Aani atjiliuq-jau-langa-vit
Annie film-PASS-FUT-INT.2sS
'Annie, are you going to get your picture taken?' (Tumasi, 2;1)

Commands and statements: Clause / phrase

As noted earlier, commands and statements are recorded together on the InuLARSP chart because they both have the same syntactic structure, unlike in other languages where commands and statements have different syntactic structures. Five aspects of commands and statements are differentiated within the InuLARSP, each recorded in a separate column: *Clause/Phrase*, *Nominal Elements*, *Nominal Inflections*, *Verbal Elements* and *Verbal Inflections*. We treat each of these in turn, beginning here with *Clause/Phrase*.

Although Inuktitut syntax is primarily encoded in word-internal morphology, some syntax is signalled through the relationships between words – either within verbal clauses (e.g. subject and verb within a sentence) or within noun phrases (e.g. possessive noun and a second noun representing the thing that is possessed). These syntactic relationships are listed in the *Clause/Phrase* column of the InuLARSP chart. Because word order is flexible in Inuktitut, both possible orderings between words are indicated on the chart (e.g. SV and VS for ordering of subject and verb).

Verb clause constructions

Verb clause constructions that contain two words begin appearing at stage III. Four such constructions are common enough to be included on the chart: subject–verb constructions (SV/VS) as in (8a), object–verb constructions (OV/VO) as in (8b), subject–complement constructions (SC/CS) as in (8c) and adverbial constructions where an adverb is used with another element (AX/XA) as in (8d).

(8) a. *Maaki langavuq.*
Maaki langa-vuq
Maggie FUT-PAR.3sS
'Maggie will be (coming)'. (Jini, 1;8)

b. *Imiq pijariirtitara.*
imiq pi-jariiq-tit-jara
drink PLEON-already-CAUS-PAR.1sS.3sO
'I finished the drink.' (Paul, 2;6)
c. *Ukuait iirqait.*
u-kua-it iirqak-it
this.one-ABS.PL-ABS.PL pill-ABS.PL
'These are pills'. (Tumasi, 2;1)
d. *Aamutu maani.*
aamu-juq ma-ani
sleep(BW)-PAR.3sS here-LOC
'You are sleeping here'. (Jini, 1;8)

Three-word verb clause constructions appear consistently for the first time at stage V. The most frequent structures are subject–verb–adverb (SVA) and verb–adverb–adverb (VAA), but subject–object–verb (SOV) and subject–complement–adverb (SCA) are also seen. Such structures are very rare; we found only 12 in the 4000 utterances coded. Therefore, they have been collapsed together as XYZ. An example of the VAA structure is in (9a). The first subordinate clause structures also appear at stage V, indicated as V Vsub in the chart, as shown in (9b).

(9) a. *Qaupasaaq kisiani siqinnilaartu.*
qaupasaaq kisiani siqinniq-laaq-juq
day.after.tomorrow only be.sunny-FUT-PAR.3sS
'It's going to be sunny only in two days.' (Elijah, 2;5)
b. *Piirunnailugu anilangammat.*
piiq-gunnaq-it-lugu ani-langa-mmat
remove-can-NEG-ICM.XxS.3sO go.out-FUT-CTG.3sS
'It can't be taken off because she's going out.' (Lizzie, 2;10)

Noun phrase constructions

Noun phrase constructions first appear consistently at stage V, and typically contain only two words. The two constructions represented are possessive noun–noun structures (Nposs N) as in (10a), and determiner–noun phrases (Det N), as in (10b).

(10) a. *Mirquluup pialuanik.*
Mirquluk-up pi-aluk-nganik
Mirquluk-ERG.SG thing-EMPH-MOD.3Ssg
'Mirquluk's thing.' (Elijah, 2;0)
b. *Una siqurngujaq surqajanngituq?*
u-na siqurngujaq suq-qajaq-nngit-juq
this.one-ABS.SG clock do-can-NEG-PAR.3sS
'This clock doesn't work?' (Elijah, 2;9)

Commands and statements: Nominal elements

The second column under the *Commands and Statements* heading on the InuLARSP records information about nominal elements. This comprises a range of grammatical words and morphemes related to nouns. We discuss each type of element in turn, including how that element is represented across the developmental stages.

Personal pronouns (PRO)

Inuktitut has only first and second person personal pronouns; all third person pronoun reference is indicated through demonstrative pronouns. First and second person pronouns are not permitted as subjects or objects of sentences; reference to first and second person subjects and objects is achieved through inflections on verbs. Thus, first and second person pronouns are relatively rare in Inuktitut compared with other languages. They typically appear alone (11a) and in equational constructions (11b), often in response to questions about who will do something or who owns a particular object. Note that the subject, object, and possessive forms of personal pronouns are identical in Inuktitut.

(11) a. *Uvangali.*
uvanga-li
I/me/my/mine-and
'It's my turn.' (Paul, 3;3)
b. *Una ivvit.*
u-na ivvit
this.one-ABS.SG you/your/yours
'This is yours.' (Lizzie, 3;3)

Only the first person pronoun *uvanga* appears with sufficient frequency to appear on the InuLARSP chart, and then only at stage IV.

Demonstrative pronouns (DEM)

Inuktitut has a complex demonstrative system. There are two sets of roots, singular and plural, with ten members each that denote different meanings of proximity, movement, and spatial position (e.g. *ma-* 'this moving one here', *pikku-* 'those stationary ones up there'). The roots are also inflected for eight cases (see information on nominal inflections). In our data, the children did not produce all of these forms, but rather used a few forms very frequently. The most commonly used demonstrative, *una* 'this stationary one here (ABS)', was already present at stage I as illustrated in (4d); it is placed in the *Other* category on the chart. Two other demonstratives – *uminga* 'this stationary one here (MOD)', shown in (12a), and *ukua* 'these stationary ones here (ERG/ABS)', shown in (12b) – appear at stage IV. The only other demonstrative used frequently and consistently enough across children to be useful on the InuLARSP is *kanna* 'that stationary one down there (ABS)', shown in (12c), which appears at stage V.

(12) a. *Aarqisulaurluk uminga Saalati.*
aarqisuk-lauq-luk u-minga Saalati
repair-POL-IMP.1dS this.one-MOD.SG Charlotte
'Let's repair this one, Charlotte.' (Louisa, 3;2)
b. *Ukua sinigumajut.*
u-kua sinik-guma-jut
this.one-ABS.PL sleep-want-PAR.3pS
'These ones want to sleep.' (Lizzie, 2;10)
c. *Kanna paajaulangamijuq.*
katsu-na paa-jau-langa-mi-juq
that.one.down.there-ABS.SG beat-PASS-FUT-also-PAR.3sS
'That one down there will also get beaten up.' (Elijah, 2;9)

Localizers (LOC)

Inuktitut has eleven localizer root forms denoting various locations with respect to the speaker. These forms can be inflected with one of four inflections denoting 'in/at', 'to', 'from', or 'through' (e.g. *kanani* 'at down here', *avunga* 'to there further away'). As with demonstratives, Inuit children use a few forms frequently and the others rarely. Only one localizer is used consistently – *maani* 'here' – which appears at stage II and is shown in (13).

(13) *Maani itsivalaurli.*
ma-ani itsiva-lauq-li
here-LOC sit-POL-IMP.3sS
'Let her sit right here.' (Lizzie, 2;10)

Nominalizers (NZ)

Nominalizers are used in Inuktitut, as in other languages, to turn words that begin as verbs into nouns. Although several nominalizers are available in Inuktitut, only two are used consistently by the children in our data. The form *-juq* is the simplest and most frequent, and is also the earliest to develop, appearing at stage II. The form *-jaq* carries a passive meaning, and appears at stage V. These are exemplified in (14).

(14) a. *Qangattajuurtualuk.*
qangattajuuq-juq-aluk
fly.airplane-that.which-EMPH
'The one who is flying the plane.' (Elijah, 2;0)
b. *Qimaniartaaluvu?*
qimaq-niaq-jaq-aluk-vut
leave.behind-FUT-that.which.PASS-EMPH-ABS.1Psp
'(Is it) our one that will be left behind?' (Paul, 2;11)

Enclitics (ENCL)

Inuktitut has a number of enclitics – morphemes that can be suffixed to either nouns or verbs for various purposes. Four are used consistently and frequently enough to appear on the InuLARSP, and are salient in samples of child language. The greeting enclitic *-ai*, which is suffixed to names as in (15a), appears at stage II. The emphatic (EMPH) enclitic *-aluk*, used both for emphasis ('big/very') and as a pejorative ('bad'), also appears at stage II, as illustrated in (14a). Two conjunctions (CONJ) are placed at stage III: *-li* 'and' and *-lu* 'and'. The latter is shown in (15b).

(15) a. *Ataataai.*
ataata-ai
father-hi
'Hi, Dad.' (Jini, 2;0)
b. *Pamiuqatsunilu, panik.*
pamiuq-qaq-tsuni-lu panik
tail-have-CTM.4sS-and daughter
'He also has a tail, daughter.' (Paul, 3;3)

Adjectival morphemes (ADJ)

As noted earlier, words that are adjectives in English can be realized either as verbs as shown in (2), or as morphemes suffixed to noun stems. Three of the latter are used consistently enough in child language to appear on the InuLARSP. The morpheme *-aluk* 'EMPH', the same form as the enclitic *-aluk* mentioned in the previous section, appears at stage II as illustrated in (14b). The diminutive (DIM) *-apik* occurs at stage IV, as shown in (16a). The adjectival morpheme *-nnguaq-* 'pretend' also appears at stage IV, as shown in (16b).

(16) a. *Nukaapiga.*
nuka-apik-ga
sibling-little-ABS.1Ssg
'My little sibling.' (Elijah, 2;9)
b. *Annuraannguanga.*
annuraaq-nnguaq-nga
clothes-pretend-ABS.3Ssg
'Her toy clothes.' (Lizzie, 2;10)

Commands and statements: Nominal inflections

The third column on the InuLARSP chart under *Commands and Statements* is reserved for nominal inflections. The nominal inflection system in Inuktitut is complex. It includes three numbers – single, dual and plural – as well as eight cases – ergative (subject of transitive verb), absolutive (subject of intransitive verb or object of transitive verb), modalis (second or indirect object), locative ('at, in'), allative ('to'), ablative ('from'), vialis ('through') and equalis ('like'). An additional set of inflections for possession marks case as well as person and number of the possessor(s) and number of the possessed item(s). In general, Inuit children begin using singular inflections before plural inflections, while dual inflections are relatively infrequent. Simple inflections also typically appear before inflections marking possession, with one exception: the absolutive first person singular possessive *-ga* 'ABS.1Ssg' (= 'my'). Note that the most basic inflection, the absolutive singular form, is null and thus is not included in the InuLARSP.

At stage II, only one nominal inflection is used consistently enough to appear on the chart: the absolutive first person singular possessive *-ga* 'ABS.1Ssg' (= 'my') as illustrated in (16a) and (17). At stage III, three unpossessed singular endings appear: the ergative/possessive singular *-up* 'ERG.SG' (see (6c) and (10a)), the locative singular *-mi* 'LOC.SG' (= 'in/at'; see (20c)), and the allative singular *-mut* 'ALL.SG' (= 'to'; see (21c)). One unpossessed plural ending also appears at stage III: the absolutive plural *-it* 'ABS.PL' (see (8c)). At stage IV, no new nominal inflections appear. At stage V, two nominal inflections appear: the second person possessed ending *-it* 'ABS.2Ssg' (= 'your'; see (21d)) and the third person possessed ending *-nga* 'ABS.3Ssg' (= 'his/her/its'; see (16b)).

Commands and statements: Verbal elements

The fourth column of the *Commands and Statements* section of the InuLARSP records information about verbal elements. This comprises a range of grammatical morphemes related to verbs. We discuss each type of element in turn, including how that element is represented across the developmental stages.

Politeness marker (POL)

Inuktitut indicates politeness not by words such as the English *please* but by a politeness marker *-lauq-*, used preceding imperative inflections, that functions to soften commands. An example is shown in (17). Inuit children use this marker quite early, at stage II.

(17) *Piipiga qailauruk.*
piipi-ga qai-lauq-guk
baby-ABS.1Ssg come-POL-IMP.2sS.3sO
'Please bring me my baby.' (Lizzie, 2;10)

Negation (NEG)

Negation in Inuktitut is indicated most frequently by the morpheme *-nngit-*, as shown in (18). This morpheme appears by stage III in the data.

(18) *Nirilanganngina ma.*
niri-langa-nngit-gama
eat-FUT-NEG-CTG.1sS
'I will not eat.' (Paul, 2;11)

Verbalizers (VZ)

Verbalizers are a key characteristic of the polysynthetic structure of Inuktitut. They are a set of morphemes that typically appear as independent verbs in other languages, but are suffixes in Inuktitut. They suffix onto noun stems, turning the noun stems into verbs. One verbalizer appears at stage III: the copula *-it-* which is affixed to locative stems, as shown in (19a). Another form of the copula appears at stage IV, *-u-*, which is affixed to all other types of noun stems, as shown in (19b). At stage V, the verbalizer *-qaq-* 'have' appears consistently, as shown in (19c). Although several other verbalizers are used by the children, none are consistent or frequent enough to be useful in distinguishing stages in the InuLARSP.

(19) a. *Maaniilaurit!*
ma-ani-it-lauq-git
here-LOC-be-POL-IMP.2sS
'Be here!' (Louisa, 3;6)
b. *Mikijuunnginama.*
miki-juq-u-nngit-gama
be.small-that.which-be-NEG-CTG.1sS
'I'm not small'. (Paul, 2;6)
c. *Nukaapiqarqunga.*
nukak-apik-qaq-vunga
younger.sibling-cute-have-IND.1sS
'I have a cute little brother.' (Elijah, 2;9)

Affixal verbs (AV)

Affixal verbs are a second set of morphemes that typically appear as independent verbs in other languages but are suffixes in Inuktitut. They suffix onto verb stems, adding further meaning to the verb. The first affixal verbs appear at stage III: the desiderative *guma-* 'want to' and the passive *-jau-* 'PASS', both illustrated in (20a). Two more appear at stage IV: the causative *-tit-* 'CAUS' illustrated in (20b), and the verb *-nnguaq-* 'pretend' illustrated in (20c). The modal *-gunnaq-* 'can' is used at stage V, as shown in (20d).

(20) a. *Kalijaugumajunga.*
kalik-jau-guma-junga
pull-PASS-want-PAR.1sS
'I want to be pulled.' (Elijah, 2;9)

b. Niarquatitara?
niarquaq-tit-jara
bump.head-CAUS-PAR.1sS.3sS
'Did I bump its head?' (Louisa, 3;6)

c. *Pirsialummi qamulitinngualaujunga.*
pirsiq-aluk-mi qamulitik-nnguaq-lauq-junga
storm-EMPH-LOC.SG ride.sled-pretend-PAST-PAR.1sS
'I played riding a sled in the big storm.' (Elijah, 2;9)

d. *Makitagunnatuq.*
makit-taq-gunnaq-juq
stand-repeatedly-can-PAR.3sS
'It can stand up.' (Lizzie, 3;3)

Tense (TNS)

Inuktitut has multiple morphemes to denote the past and future tense, encoding distinctions in how close to the present the event took place. In general, the children in our data indicated the future more frequently and earlier than the past (Swift, 2004). Two future morphemes appear at stage IV: *-langa-* (near future; see (17d) and (18)) and *-laaq-* (tomorrow or later; see (9a)). An additional future morpheme appears at stage V: *-niaq-* (later today; see (14b)). Two past morphemes also appear at stage V: *-kainnaq-* (very recent past; see 21b)) and *-lauq-* (yesterday or earlier; see (20c)).

Commands and statements: Verbal inflections

The fifth and final column on the InuLARSP chart under *Commands and Statements* is reserved for verbal inflections. The verbal inflection system in Inuktitut consists of some 900 portmanteau morphemes that mark subject and object agreement for four persons – first, second, third, and fourth (= a third person different from the third person referent in the main clause) – and three numbers – singular, dual, and plural. In addition, they mark one of ten moods: indicative, participial (used as an indicative in this dialect of Inuktitut), imperative (command), interrogative (question), contingent (reason or cause), conditional (condition), dubitative (signalling doubt), contemporative (two events occurring at same time), incontemporative (two events occurring at different times), and contemporative negative. As a general rule, the children use inflections marking only subject agreement earlier and more frequently than inflections marking both subject and object agreement. Not surprisingly, they use more forms for first person subjects than for the other persons. They also use imperative and indicative (including participial) inflections earlier than they use inflections for the other moods.

Imperative verbal inflections (IMP)

There are 72 possible imperative inflections in Inuktitut, but the children only produced a few of them. However, these are some of the first verbal inflections to be used with frequency and variety. Two imperative endings appear at stage II: *-git* 'IMP.2sS' (see (19a)) and *-guk* 'IMP.2sS.3sO' (see (17)). Other forms *-luk* 'IMP.1dS' (see (12a)) and *-li* 'IMP.3sS' (see (13)) appear at stage III and stage IV respectively.

Participial verbal inflections (PAR)

The participial inflection is known by this term since it forms participles in some Inuit languages such as West Greenlandic. However, in the language we are dealing with here (Inuktitut as spoken in northern Quebec), the so-called participial inflection is used as an indicative form and appears much more frequently in both child and adult speech than the indicative form itself. The first participial ending appears at stage II: *-juq* 'PAR.3sS' (see (12c) and (20d)). Two more endings are added at stage IV: *-junga* 'PAR.1sS' (see (20a) and (20c)) and *-jara* 'PAR.1sS.3sO' (see (8b) and (20b)).

Indicative verbal inflections (IND)

Indicative inflections do not appear in the chart until relatively late. The inflection *-vunga* 'IND.1sS' (see (19c)) appears at stage IV, while *-vuq* 'IND.3sS' (see (8a)) appears at stage V.

Contingent verbal inflections (CTG)

Contingent inflections first appear consistently at stage III with the form *-gama* 'CTG.1sS' (see (18) and (19b)). This is followed at stage IV by *-mmat* 'CTG.3sS' (see (9b)).

Interrogative verbal inflections (INT)

As noted earlier, only one interrogative inflection appears consistently enough to be noted on the InuLARSP. This is the inflection *–vit* 'INT.2sS', which appears at stage V and is exemplified in (7b).

Highest number of morphemes per word

As previously stated, the bulk of grammatical development in Inuktitut occurs in the use of increasingly complex morphology. Up to this point in the chart, we have focused on the particular morphemes that appear at different stages. Another indicator of development is the number of morphemes children produce on each root, regardless of what the morphemes are. This number increases as children develop – both the average number of morphemes produced per root, and the maximum number of morphemes produced per root. The maximum number of morphemes produced with a root is included in the chart since it is the easiest of these two figures to record.

At stage II, children typically produce utterances consisting of a root word plus a maximum of three morphemes, as illustrated in (21a). At stage

III, the maximum number of morphemes added increases to four, as shown in (21b). At stage IV, the number slightly increases to six morphemes, as exemplified in (21c). Words with 7 or more added morphemes start appearing at stage V, as illustrated in (21d).

(21) a. *Angijualumii?*
angi-juq-aluk-mik
be.big-that.which-EMPH-MOD.SG
'Is it a big one?' (Jini, 2;0)

b. *Qiniriakainnanginakku.*
qiniq-giaq-kainnaq-nngit-gakku
look.for-begin.to-PAST-NEG-CTG.1sS.3sO
'I didn't begin to look for it.' (Lizzie, 3;3)

c. *Imamuutupalliajuq.*
imaq-mut-uq-juq-u-vallia-juq
water-ALL.SG-arrive.at-that.which-be-gradually-PAR.3sS
'It's gradually going into the water.' (Paul, 2;11)

d. *Kililangannngitaaluinuna?*
kiliq-langa-nngit-jaq-aluk-it-u-na
cut-FUT-NEG-that.which.PASS-EMPH-ABS.2Ssg-this.one-ABS.SG
'You're not gonna get cut?' [lit. 'this will not be your cut one']
(Elijah, 2;5)

Errors

The final section on the InuLARSP is the *Errors* section. The original LARSP contains an error line that reflects mistakes made by typically developing English-speaking children. Typically developing children learning Inuktitut generally do not make errors of this sort, because of differences in the language typologies of English and Inuktitut (Crago & Allen, 1998). However, numerous errors were recorded in one study of an Inuktitut-speaking girl aged 5;4 with specific language impairment (Crago & Allen, 2001). This child, named Lina, had normal hearing, no history of chronic middle ear disease, and no signs of social and emotional disabilities or neurological deficit. She was considered comparable to her peers in cognitive and motoric domains by her teachers and family. She was not tested on any standardized tests since none existed for language development in Inuktitut. However, she was considered significantly language impaired by her family and community members (Inuit nursing assistant, special education teacher, and pedagogical counsellor). As compared to an age-matched peer and an MLU-matched peer, she had a restricted lexicon with word-finding difficulties, frequent use of an all-purpose word meaning 'thing', missing verbal inflections on both verbs and locatives, missing tense morphemes, overuse of pronouns, use of filler morphemes, and a lack of passive constructions. Representative examples of her utterances are provided in (22) through (25), where (a) is the child's utterance and (b) is the target utterance.

(22) a. *Maani ivvit.*
ma-ani ivvit
here-LOC you/your/yours
'Here you.' (Lina, 5;4)
b. *Maaniigit.*
ma-ani-it-git
here-LOC-be-IMP.2sS
'Be here.' (target utterance; Crago & Allen, 2001: 95)
(23) a. *Sininngua.*
sinik-nnguaq-
sleep-pretend-
'Pretend to sleep.' (Lina, 5;4)
b. *Sininngualuk.*
sinik-nnguaq-luk
sleep-pretend-IMP.1dS
'Let's pretend to sleep.' (target utterance; Crago & Allen, 2001: 92)
(24) a. *Aaa, qaisi.*
aaa qai-si-
yes come-PRSP-
'Yes, is coming.' (Lina, 5;4)
b. *Aaa, qaisijuq.*
aaa qai-si-juq
yes come-PRSP-PAR.3sS
'Yes, he/she/it is coming.' (target utterance; Crago & Allen, 2001: 93)
(25) a. *Puatjukumi anaanaganut maunga.*
puitjuk-ku-MI anaana-ganut ma-unnga
swim-?-FILLER mother-ALL.1Ssg here-ALL
'Swim to my mother to right here.' (Lina, 5;4)
b. *Puitjutuq anaanaganut.*
puitjuq-juq anaana-ganut
swim-PAR.3sS mother-ALL.1Ssg
'He/she/it swims to my mother.' (target utterance; Crago & Allen, 2001: 94)

Although based on a single case study, these possible errors have been listed in the *Errors* section of the InuLARSP in the expectation that they might also reflect errors found in atypical language development of other Inuit children.

Application

In order to illustrate how the InuLARSP is implemented with actual data, we have provided two examples of completed profiles in Figures 12.2 and 12.3. The first profile (Figure 12.2) shows data from

Name: Louisa	**Date of birth:**	**Date of recording:**
Therapist:	**Age:** 3;1 years	**Remarks:**
A. Unanalyzed Unintelligible: 6 Symbolic Noise: 0 Deviant: 0	**Problematic** Incomplete: 1 Ambiguous: 0 Stereotypes: 0	**B.** Total number of utterances: 100 Analyzed utterances: 93 MLU(m): 2.87

Minor	***Responses*** 12	***Vocatives*** 7	***Other*** 8	***Problems*** 0
Stage I	'N' 0	'V' 4	Other 0	Baby Words 0

	Questions			***Commands/Statements***					***Word + Morph***
	Syntax	***Word***	***Inflections***	***Clause/Phrase***	***Nominal Elements***	***Nominal Inflections***	***Verbal Elements***	***Verbal Inflections***	
Stage II	Q 0	*suna* 0 *nauk* 1	Q+inf 1		LOC *maani* 1 EMPH *-aluk* 13 Greeting *-ai* 2 NZ *-juq* 7	ABS (1Ssg) *-ga* 16	Polite *-lauq-* 1	IMP (2sS/3sO) *-guk* 1 IMP (2sS) *-git* 2 PAR (3sS) *-juq* 7	X+1 38 X+2 25 X+3 11
Stage III		*kina* 0	ENCL *-li* 0	SV/VS 2 OV/VO 3 CS/SC 5 AX/XA 3	CONJ *-li* 2 CONJ *-lu* 3	LOC (SG) *-mi* 0 ALL (SG) *-mut* 0 POSS (SG) *-up* 0 ABS (PL) *-it* 0	PASS *-jau-* 0 COP *-it-* 1 AV *-guma-* 3 NEG *-nngit-* 9	IMP (1dS) *-luk* 0 CTG (1sS) *-gama* 3	X+4 5
Stage IV					DEM *uminga* 5 DEM *ukua* 0 PRO *uvanga* 1 DIM *-apik* 4 ADJ *-nnguaq* 1		FUT *-langa-* 3 FUT *-laaq-* 0 AV *-nnguaq-* 0 COP *-u-* 2 CAUS *-tit-* 0	IMP (3sS) *-li* 0 IND (1sS) *-vunga* 0 PAR (1sS) *-junga* 0 PAR (1sS/3sO) *-jara* 3 CTG (3sS) *-mmat* 0	X+5 4 X+6 0
Stage V	QX 0	*nani* 0	INT (2sS) *-vit* 2	XYZ 1 V Vsub 0 NPoss N 0 Det N 1	DEM *kanna* 0 NZ *-jaq* 2	ABS (2Ssg) *–it* 0 ABS (3Ssg) *-nga* 2	PAST *-kainnaq-* 0 PAST *-lauq-* 0 FUT *-niaq-* 1 AV *-gunnaq-* 0 VZ *-qaq-* 0	IND (3sS) *-vuq* 0	X+7 0

Errors	missing inflection: 5	missing tense morpheme: 0	overuse of pronoun: 0	filler morpheme: 0	other: 0

Figure 12.2 Completed InuLARSP Chart for Louisa, typically developing, age 3;1

Louisa, a typically-developing child aged 3;1 years. A 100-utterance language sample, from a different session than the one used to develop the InuLARSP profile, was analysed according to the principles described above. The profile shows strong representation of grammatical features at stage III with the exception of questions (which depend on context)

Name: Lina	**Date of birth:**	**Date of recording:**
Therapist:	**Age:** 5;4 years	**Remarks:**
A. Unanalyzed Unintelligible: 2 Symbolic Noise: 0 Deviant: 0	**Problematic** Incomplete: 0 Ambiguous: 2 Stereotypes: 0	**B.** Total number of utterances: 100 Analyzed utterances: 96 MLU(m): 2.5

Minor	***Responses*** 26	***Vocatives*** 1	***Other*** 13	***Problems*** 0
Stage I	'N' 0	'V' 4	Other 0	Baby Words 0

	Questions			***Commands/Statements***					***Word + Morph***
	Syntax	***Word***	***Inflections***	***Clause/Phrase***	***Nominal Elements***	***Nominal Inflections***	***Verbal Elements***	***Verbal Inflections***	
Stage II	Q 1	*suna* 0 *nauk* 2	Q+inf 1		LOC *maani* 5 EMPH *-aluk* 3 Greeting *-ai* 0 NZ *-juq* 0	ABS (1Ssg) *-ga* 4	Polite *-lauq-* 0	IMP (2sS/3sO) *-guk* 0 IMP (2sS) *-git* 4 PAR (3sS) *-juq* 3	X+1 45 X+2 17 X+3 6
Stage III		*kina* 0	ENCL *-li* 1	SV/VS 3 OV/VO 1 CS/SC 5 AX/XA 2	CONJ *–li* 6 CONJ *-lu* 3	LOC (SG) *-mi* 1 ALL (SG) *-mut* 1 POSS (SG) *-up* 0 ABS (PL) *-it* 0	PASS *-jau-* 0 COP *-it-* 1 AV *-guma-* 0 NEG *-nngit-* 2	IMP (1dS) *-luk* 0 CTG (1sS) *-gama* 0	X+4 1
Stage IV					DEM *uminga* 0 DEM *ukua* 2 PRO *uvanga* 4 DIM *-apik* 0 ADJ *-nnguaq* 3		FUT *-langa-* 0 FUT *-laaq-* 0 AV *-nnguaq-* 5 COP *-u-* 0 CAUS *-tit-* 0	IMP (3sS) *-li* 0 IND (1sS) *-vunga* 2 PAR (1sS) *-junga* 1 PAR (1sS/3sO) *-jara* 0 CTG (3sS) *-mmat* 0	X+5 1 X+6 0
Stage V	QX 0	*nani* 0	INT (2sS) *-vit* 2	XYZ 5 V Vsub 0 NPoss N 0 Det N 1	DEM *kanna* 0 NZ *-jaq* 0	ABS (2Ssg) *-it* 0 ABS (3Ssg) *-nga* 2	PAST *-kainnaq-* 0 PAST *-lauq-* 0 FUT *-niaq-* 1 AV *-gunnaq-* 0 VZ *–qaq-* 0	IND (3sS) *-vuq* 1	X+7 0

Errors	missing inflection: 10	missing tense morpheme: 2	overuse of pronoun: 4	filler morpheme: 3	other: 4

Figure 12.3 Completed InuLARSP Chart for Lina, specific language impairment, age 5;4

and nominal inflections. There is also fairly strong development at stage IV, particularly in the area of nominal elements, and even evidence of development at stage V.

The second profile (Figure 12.3) is that of Lina, the child aged 5;4 with specific language impairment mentioned earlier. Although Lina is more than two years older than Louisa, the two children have similar mean lengths of utterance, and thus Louisa can be considered a language match for Lina.

Given the similarity in mean length of utterance, one might expect the InuLARSP profiles of the two children to also be similar. Indeed, they do have fairly similar patterns in the profile's Sections A and B as well as for the *Minor* utterances, although Lina has twice as many responses (yes, no, alright) as Louisa. The two children also share similar patterns in the *Questions* section, both in terms of syntax and in terms of words and inflections used. However, clear differences in the profile are evident in the remaining sections of the InuLARSP. In the *Commands/Statements* section, the child with language impairment seems to be more advanced in terms of syntax, producing more three-word utterances. In terms of morphology, however, the profile of the language match, Louisa, shows greater variety and overall use of nominal and verbal elements than that of Lina. Their use of nominal and verbal inflections is similar in terms of the range of inflections used, but once again the typically developing Louisa uses the inflections more frequently. Louisa also uses more morphemes per word: she regularly produces words with four and five morphemes in addition to the root while Lina, the child with language impairment, rarely uses words with more than three morphemes in addition to the root. Another major difference relates to errors. Louisa makes few errors, generally restricted to occasional missing inflections. In contrast, Lina, the child with language impairment, makes multiple errors including missing inflections on both verbs and locatives, omission of other required morphemes, inappropriate overuse of pronouns, and the use of filler morphemes.

In general, we conclude that the InuLARSP profile can be used to document the stages of language development of both typically developing and language-impaired children. We also see that the InuLARSP profile brings to light a variety of differences in the language competence of the two children that might not be expected from examining a measure like the mean length of utterance alone.

Conclusion

In order to serve language impaired children who speak Inuktitut as their first language, assessment tools for Inuktitut are of great value. Creating a LARSP for Inuktitut is an important step in that direction. In the present chapter, we reported the steps in creating the InuLARSP and the resulting chart. Although we had a limited data sample on which to base this first version of the InuLARSP, we nonetheless expect that the tool will serve as a solid basis for assessing the language development of Inuit children and developing further relevant assessment instruments. Future research should verify the stages and entries in the InuLARSP with more children in the relevant age ranges, both typically and atypically developing.

Acknowledgements

The research on Inuktitut reported here was funded by grants to Shanley Allen and to Martha Crago from the Kativik Ilisarniliriniq, the school board of Northern Quebec and from the Social Sciences and Humanities Research Council of Canada. We are very grateful to all the children and their families who participated in the studies discussed here. We also thank Lindsay Coffin and Mary Elliot for assistance in data analysis, and the Kaiserslautern Scientific Writing Group for comments on earlier versions of this chapter.

References

Allen, S.E.M. (1996) *Aspects of Argument Structure Acquisition in Inuktitut*. Amsterdam: John Benjamins.

Allen, S.E.M. (1998) Categories within the verb category: Learning the causative in Inuktitut. *Linguistics* 36 (4), 633–677.

Allen, S.E.M. (2000) A discourse-pragmatic explanation for argument representation in child Inuktitut. *Linguistics* 38 (3), 483–521.

Allen, S.E.M. (2007) The future of Inuktitut in the face of majority languages: Bilingualism or language shift? *Applied Psycholinguistics* 28 (3), 515–536.

Allen, S.E.M. (2013) The acquisition of ergativity in Inuktitut. In E.L. Bavin and S. Stoll (eds) *The Acquisition of Ergative Structures* (pp. 71–105). Amsterdam: Benjamins.

Allen, S.E.M. (2017) Polysynthesis in the acquisition of Inuit languages. In M. Fortescue, M. Mithun and N. Evans (eds) *Handbook of Polysynthesis* (pp. 449-472). Oxford: Oxford University Press.

Allen, S.E.M. and Crago, M.B. (1996) Early passive acquisition in Inuktitut. *Journal of Child Language* 23 (1), 129–155.

Allen, S.E.M, Crago, M.B. and Pesco, D. (2006) The effect of majority language exposure on minority language skills: The case of Inuktitut. *International Journal of Bilingual Education and Bilingualism* 9 (5), 578–596.

Allen, S.E.M. and Dench, C. (2015) Calculating mean length of utterance for Eastern Canadian Inuktitut. *First Language* 35, 377–406.

Allen, S.E.M. and Schröder, H. (2003) Preferred argument structure in early Inuktitut spontaneous speech data. In J.W. Du Bois, L.E. Kumpf and W.J. Ashby (eds) *Preferred Argument Structure: Grammar as Architecture for Function* (pp. 301–338). Amsterdam: John Benjamins.

Ball, M.J., Crystal, D. and Fletcher, P. (2012) *Assessing Grammar: The Languages of LARSP*. Bristol: Multilingual Matters.

Berman, R.A., Rom, A. and Hirsch, M. (1982) *Working with HARSP: Hebrew Adaptation of the LARSP Language Assessment Remediation and Screening Procedure*. Tel Aviv University.

Crago, M. (1988) Cultural context in communicative interaction of Inuit children. Unpublished doctoral dissertation, McGill University, Montreal, QC.

Crago, M.B, and Allen, S.E.M. (1998) Acquiring Inuktitut. In O. Taylor and L. Leonard (eds) *Language Acquisition across North America: Cross-cultural and Cross-linguistic Perspectives* (pp. 245–279). San Diego, CA: Singular Publishing Group.

Crago, M.B. and Allen, S.E.M. (2001) Early finiteness in Inuktitut: The role of language structure and input. *Language Acquisition* 9 (1), 59–111.

Crago, M.B., Allen, S.E.M. and Pesco, D. (1998) Issues of complexity in Inuktitut and English child directed speech. In E.V. Clark (ed.) *Proceedings of the 29th Annual Stanford Child Language Research Forum* (pp. 37–46). Stanford: CSLI.

Crago, M.B., Annahatak, B., Doehring, D. and Allen, S.E.M. (1991) Evaluation of Inuit children's first language by native speakers. *Journal of Speech-Language Pathology and Audiology* 15 (2), 43–48.

Crystal, D. (1982) *Profiling Linguistic Disability*. London: Edward Arnold.

Crystal, D., Fletcher, P. and Garman, M. (1976) *The Grammatical Analysis of Language Disability*. London: Edward Arnold.

Dorais, L.-J. (1988) *Tukilik: An Inuktitut Grammar for all*. Laval, QC: Association Inuksiutiit Katimajiit.

Dorais, L.-J. (2010) *Language of the Inuit: Syntax, Semantics, and Society in the Arctic*. Montreal, QC: McGill-Queen's Press.

Evans, N. and Sasse H.J. (2002) Introduction: Problems of polysynthesis. In N. Evans and H.J. Sasse (eds) *Problems of Polysynthesis* (pp. 1–13). Berlin: Akademie Verlag.

Fletcher, P., Ball, M.J. and Crystal, D. (2016) *Profiling Grammar: More Languages of LARSP*. Bristol: Multilingual Matters.

Fortescue, M. (1994) Polysynthetic morphology. *The Encyclopedia of Language and Linguistics* 5, 2600–2602.

Hickey, T. (1990) ILARSP: A grammatical profile of Irish. *Clinical Linguistics and Phonetics* 4, 363–376.

Jin, L., Oh, B.L. and Razak, R.A. (2012) C-LARSP: Developing a Chinese grammatical profile. In M.J. Ball, D. Crystal and P. Fletcher (eds) *Assessing Grammar: The Languages of LARSP*. Bristol: Multilingual Matters.

MacWhinney, B. (2000) *The CHILDES Project: Tools for Analyzing Talk* (3rd edn). Mahwah, NJ: Erlbaum.

Parkinson, D.P. (1999) The interaction of syntax and morphology in the acquisition of noun incorporation in Inuktitut. Unpublished doctoral dissertation, Cornell University, Ithaca, NY.

SAC (2010) *Speech, Language and Hearing Services to First Nations, Inuit and Métis Children in Canada, with a Focus on Children 0 to 6 Years of Age*. Ottawa: Speech-Language and Audiology Canada.

Statistics Canada (2011) Aboriginal languages in Canada. Language, 2011 Census of Population. Retrieved September 20, 2014 from http://www12.statcan.gc.ca/census-recensement/2011/as-sa/98-314-x/98-314-x2011003_3-eng.pdf

Swift, M.D. (2004) *Time in Child Inuktitut: A Developmental Study of an Eskimo-Aleut Language*. Berlin: Mouton de Gruyter.

Wilman, D. (1988) The natural language of Inuit children: A key to Inuktitut literacy. Unpublished doctoral dissertation, University of New Mexico, Albuquerque, NM.

Wright, S.C., Taylor, D.M. and Macarthur, J. (2000) Subtractive bilingualism and the survival of the Inuit language: Heritage- versus second-language education. *Journal of Educational Psychology* 92, 63–84.

Appendix

Abbreviations

The following abbreviations are used in glosses throughout this chapter:

Nominal Case: ABS = absolutive; ALL = allative; ERG = ergative; LOC = locative; MOD = modalis.

Verbal Modality: CTG = contingent; CTM = contemporative; ICM = incontemporative; IMP = imperative; IND = indicative; INT = interrogative; PAR = participial (functionally equivalent to indicative in Inuktitut).

Word-Internal Morphology: BW = baby word; CAUS = causative; EMPH = emphatic; FUT = future; INCP = incipient aspect; NEG = negative; PASS = passive; PAST = past; PERF = perfective aspect; POL = politeness softener; PLEON = pleonastic; PRSP = prospective aspect.

Verbal Inflection (e.g. PAR.3sS): 1 = first person; 2 = second person; 3 = third person; 4 = fourth person; X = any person; s = singular; d = dual; p = plural; x = any number; S = subject; O = object

Nominal Inflection (e.g. ABS.SG): SG = singular; DU = dual; PL = plural.

Possessed Nominal Inflection (e.g. ERG.3Ssg): 1 = first person possessor; 2 = second person possessor; 3 = third person possessor; 4 = fourth person possessor; S = singular possessor; D = dual possessor; P = plural possessor; sg = singular possessum; du = dual possessum; pl = plural possessum.

Author Index

Subject Index

The alphabetical arrangement of the index is letter-by-letter. Grammatical terms and abbreviations in LARSP charts are not indexed